BETWEEN HEAVEN AND EARTH

A GUIDE TO CHINESE MEDICINE

天地之間

BETWEEN HEAVEN AND EARTH

A GUIDE TO CHINESE MEDICINE

HARRIET BEINFIELD
L. A c.
AND EFREM KORNGOLD
L. A c., O. M. D.

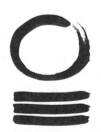

BALLANTINE BOOKS
NEW YORK

This book is not intended to replace the services of a licensed health care provider in the diagnosis or treatment of illness or disease. Any application of the material set forth in the following pages is at the reader's discretion and sole responsibility.

Grateful acknowledgment is made to the following for
permission to reprint previously published material:

FRIENDS OF THE EARTH: Four poems from *Of All Things Most Yielding* selected by Marc Lappé, edited by David R. Brower. Copyright by Friends of the Earth, Washington, D.C.

SIMON & SCHUSTER, INC.: Fourteen lines from *The Sonnets to Orpheus* by Rainer Maria Rilke, translated by Stephen Mitchell. Copyright © 1985 by Stephen Mitchell. Reprinted by permission of Simon & Schuster, Inc.

Library of Congress Cataloging-in-Publication Data

Beinfield, Harriet.
Between heaven and earth : a guide to Chinese medicine /
Harriet Beinfield & Efrem Korngold.—1st ed.
p.   cm.
Includes bibliographical references and index.

ISBN 0-345-35943-7

1. Medicine, Chinese. 2. Herbs—Therapeutic use.
3. Materia medica, Vegetable—China. 4. Acupuncture.
I. Korngold, Efrem. II. Title.
R601.B45 1991
615'.321'0951—dc20   90-93214   CIP

Manufactured in the United States of America

Book design by Alex Jay/Studio J

First Edition: June 1991

10 9 8 7 6 5 4 3 2 1

Heaven, Earth, and I are living together, and all things and I form an inseparable unity.

Chuang Tzu

The organic pattern in Nature was for the medieval Chinese the Li, and it was mirrored in every subordinate whole. . . . Li signified the pattern in things, the markings in jade or the fibres in muscle, like the strands in a piece of thread, or the bamboo in a basket . . . it is dynamic pattern as embodied in all living things, in human relationships and in the highest human values. . . . Li, in its most ancient meaning, is the principle of organization and pattern in all its forms.

Joseph Needham

What pattern connects the crab to the lobster and the orchid to the primrose and all four of them to me? And me to you?

Gregory Bateson

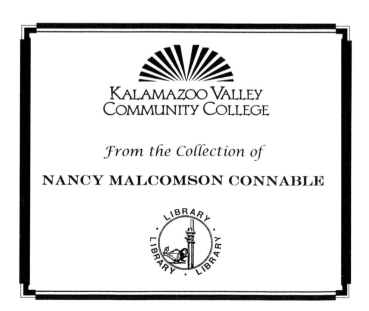

CONTENTS

FOREWORD

FOR OVER TWENTY-THREE CENTURIES ACUPUNCTURE NEEDLES AND GIN-
seng have mended what is now one-quarter of the world's population, yet it
is only in the last two decades that most Americans have even heard of
them. In 1971, the year before the "Bamboo Curtain" lifted, *New York Times*
journalist James Reston became ill while on assignment in China. After having his appendix removed, he was treated with acupuncture for postsurgical
pain. The front-page stories he sent home reported, "I've seen the past, and
it works!" At that moment Chinese medicine entered mainstream American
consciousness.

Efrem and I began to practice acupuncture shortly after that in 1973.
Since then we've treated thousands of Americans. One was Sam, a thirty-six-
year-old biochemist, who had an excruciating pain in his abdomen diagnosed by his doctor as gallstones. Although he felt skeptical about Chinese
medicine, he was more frightened by the prospect of surgery. After two
months of acupuncture, herbs, and dietary modification, Sam expelled scores
of stones, and a sonogram confirmed that surgery was no longer necessary.
Esther, a retired seventy-five-year-old nurse, had severe arthritis. After a year
she was free of pain and had recovered the use of her joints and limbs.
Fifteen years later she'd had no recurrence. Yet another person was Suzanne,
who at age twenty-eight, after three miscarriages and two gynecological sur-
geries, was unable to conceive. In the eighth month of treatment, she became
pregnant and later delivered a healthy daughter, now a teenager.

These people and many like them had their intellect aroused by their
success with acupuncture and herbs. Having been impressed, they wanted
to be informed. We began writing this book in response to their request,
"Where can I read more about it?" Although other books exist on the subject,
none give the uninitiated a comprehensive yet comprehensible overview. So
we set out to explain our sense of what Chinese medicine is—how it thinks,
how it works, what it can do.

Numerous schools of thought and various methods are found within the
vast historical tradition of Chinese medicine. It has never been a monolithic
institution. After all, millions of doctors over the millennia have practiced
its techniques and developed its theories. It sustained itself in part by adjusting to changing conditions and will continue to develop differently in
each country and era in relation to the social demands and belief systems
that prevail there. In *Medicine in China: A History of Ideas*, Paul Unschuld
comments:

The travel of ideas is different from the travel of merchandise. The latter can be handed on, from one region to the next, by different means of transportation, without itself undergoing any change. Ideas must be transmitted by the head, and, of necessity, will undergo change. Where could a foreign idea be accepted, assimilated, or transmitted without being influenced by the particular situation it meets, by the changing languages that serve as its means of transportation, and by the preconditioned patterns of thought cherished by the final receiver?

As Chinese medicine takes root in our terrain, it evolves to adapt to our environment. Does a botanist hiking along steep slopes move through the same forest as the native tribesman who once dwelled among the evergreens? Is a mountain that endures the ages the same even though climbers see variable landscapes from epoch to epoch? What the mountain means to people and how they use it changes with each traveler or caravan. Ideas, more mutable and malleable than landmasses, are even more liable to change form. The ancient Chinese had their own mythos, language, circumstances, preoccupations, and we have ours. This book represents a nexus, a point of convergence, a meeting of worlds.

As we traveled the curved footpaths around mountains of Chinese medical thought, we made choices about what to include, what to leave out, and how best to express our version of these ideas. *Between Heaven and Earth* is a product of continuous dialogue between dual authors—an unfinished conversation, the most coherent statement we can express at this time. It's not the definitive summary of Chinese medicine, the last word, but a starting point for new discourse that invites the next utterance. The "we" refers to our collaborative voice, whereas the "I" belongs to Harriet, who sometimes chooses to convey ideas through her personal narrative.

Between Heaven and Earth is a cross-cultural transmission and transplantation. In transposing Chinese ideas into our own idiom, our challenge has been to bridge gaps—between mind and body, theory and practice, therapy and self-care, practitioner and patient, ancient and modern, convention and invention, East and West. We have dug into and mined the rich ore of Chinese medicine for the purpose of creating new metal, a refined alloy. Through cultural blending, we are transmuting wisdom from early China into what has relevance for us today. Welcome to an ongoing process.

We have divided our discussion of Chinese medicine into three overlapping parts:

- Theory: the ideas—about nature, the human body, and the self—upon which the medicine is based

- Types: the psychology in Chinese medicine—how five archetypes symbolize human character, illuminating our personal tao, the way we are
- Therapy: the treatment methods of acupuncture, herbs, diet—what they are and how to use them

The first section, "Theory," introduces you to the essential principles of traditional Chinese medicine and explains the beliefs upon which this foreign medicine rests. We also examine how these beliefs differ from the assumptions we take for granted in Western medicine—the conceptual baggage we carry with us from home. After establishing the philosophical grammar, the logic and vocabulary through which Chinese medicine speaks, you can begin to acquire the fluency to converse in its language.

As we worked on the second section of the book, "Types," we played with Chinese theory, elaborating upon it to suit American conditions and needs. Our intellectual chemistry commingled with Eastern thinking, propagating reactions of its own. What came out of this was an articulation of the psychology implicit in Chinese medicine yet not explicitly developed by the Chinese.

For Americans, psychology—the study of how people think, feel, and behave—captures immense interest. In contrast, the gaze of Chinese culture is averted away from the individual and instead directed toward social groups (the family, collective, and state), so psychology in China is quite underdeveloped, and its medicine has focused primarily upon physical symptoms. But because Chinese medical theory assumes human process unfolds as a consequence of the tension and unity between interacting systems, mental phenomena are not considered to be altogether separate or distinct from physical events.

We have fused Chinese theory with outlooks from Western psychology for the purpose of transcending our cultural practice of isolating physiology from psychology so that we can begin to knit together the fracture that splits body from mind. Toward that end, we have generated a schema of types: five metaphors for the emotional, physical, and spiritual dynamics that organize us. Each of these types has idiosyncratic traits, motivations, and struggles—five styles of being in the world. You are invited to discover how your style of interpreting reality fits within these categories and discern who you are:

- The *Pioneer*, determined to make things happen
- The *Wizard*, seeking magic and excitement
- The *Peacemaker*, constantly arranging and harmonizing the world
- The *Alchemist*, who masters form and function
- The *Philosopher*, relentlessly in pursuit of truth

By identifying people's archetypes, the sources of their virtues, strengths, dilemmas, and limitations become apparent. These depictions help to counteract the discomfiting image many of us have of ourselves as a haphazard collection of disjointed events and shifting identities. Instead there is a pattern in our tapestry—woven through us and by us—we embody and manifest its design. Examining its fabric informs us about how we are predisposed to suffer and derive satisfaction in particular ways. An outcome of self-recognition can be self-acceptance, often a precursor to self-mastery. This system is a lens, a model, a paradigm through which we can understand, explain, and help ourselves and others.

Although this book is not a manual or textbook, we want to encourage you to experience as well as comprehend the potential this medicine offers. So the third section of the book, "Therapy," explains methods of treatment and the thought process used by each one. Acupuncture need not be intimidating; herbal medicine need not be mystified; and the promise of Chinese food therapy has not yet begun to dazzle our palates.

In addition to explanation, we provide practical counsel by guiding you toward the herbal remedies and foods appropriate for you. To do this, we devised a system that simplifies yet preserves the art of prescribing. Since Chinese herbs can be purchased over-the-counter, we outline a set of herbal formulas and herbal food recipes so that those of you so motivated can put your understanding into action.

As you read this book you may want to selectively navigate your passage, reading the text out of sequence, skipping to sections that most engage you. Some will be intrigued by the ideas, others by traditional Chinese diagnosis and physiology, others will search for the right herb formula, and still others will be immediately drawn to the middle of the book to identify themselves and their family within the schema of the five archetypes, returning later to the other chapters.

Many people in our culture have been nurturing a shift in consciousness as they search for alternatives to the threatening political and environmental dilemmas our civilization has created. Our overarching concern, the meta-purpose of this book, is to demonstrate that to think through the mind of Chinese medicine, to see through its eyes, is in itself a healing process.

What makes Chinese medicine distinct, even more than its needles and herbs, is its metaphysics (assumptions about reality), epistemology (ways of acquiring knowledge), and ideology (system of beliefs and values), all of which find their expression in the Taoist imperatives of preserving life and living in accord with nature. To the extent that we learn to live with nature—with our own nature, each other, and the earth—we have freedom, power, and purpose and can enjoy life. To the extent that we do not, we suffer. For us, the ethic of Chinese medicine is to assist us in this striving.

I
THEORY

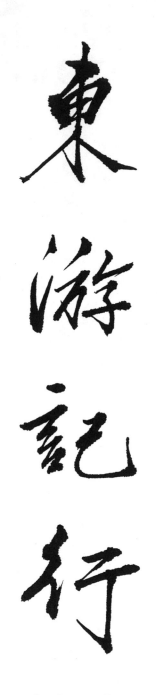

Our Journey East:
Exploring Foreign Territory

CHAPTER ONE

OUR JOURNEY EAST: EXPLORING FOREIGN TERRITORY

Lying motionless, gazing at a chart on the wall showing streams of force connecting the little toe with the corner of the eye in a web of continuous loops, I feel my breath soften and my vision sharpen.

Delicate pins protrude from my elbow, ankle, and knee. My arms and legs are flooded by tiny rivulets of current. It's not like a hypodermic needle that injects a foreign substance—what I'm feeling is simply more of myself. It's strange, in the sense of odd and unfamiliar, but as a sensation not unpleasant. In fact, the edges of my mouth are cradling a silly smile.

The skin is stretched less tightly over my bony frame as my pores relax. I sense movement as I lie quiet, aware of impulse within my mind at rest. Thoughts tumble into consciousness, roll over, and shuffle off.

With my eyes closed, and perception directed inward, simultaneous layers of activity play like instruments in concert with each other. I am the composer and the composed, the musician and the listener, the instrument and its player.

SUBTLE YET PALPABLE, MY INITIAL ENCOUNTER WITH ACUPUNCTURE LEFT me tantalized by mystery and promise. Mystery, in that tiny needles could extend my field of awareness and completely alter the state of my being. Promise, in that by burrowing into the conceptual soil of this system, I could deepen my self-understanding.

As the daughter of a surgeon and the granddaughter of two surgeons, my early life was steeped in the cauldron of medicine brewed over several generations. Enthusiasm for healing was contagious, and I became infected. As a child I was impressed by my father's devotion and satisfaction. He rushed to the hospital day or night to operate on a man lacerated in a motorcycle accident or a child threatened by a ruptured appendix. Lives would have been lost without his heroic intervention.

The role of doctor and the appeal of medicine came naturally—but why Chinese medicine? The ideology of Chinese medicine immediately captivated me by its stark contrast to the perspective of Western medical science. I had never been comfortable thinking of myself in my father's language of electrolytes and blood-gas ratios, a collection of quantities and statistics. The Chinese medical vocabulary contained metaphors from nature like *Wood*, *Fire*, *Earth*, *Metal*, and *Water*, *Heat*, *Wind*, and *Cold*.* This cosmological description of human process confirmed what I knew intuitively to be so—that what moves the world outside moves within me—that subject and object are two aspects of one phenomenal world. As peculiarly outside my cultural context as it was, Chinese medicine felt familiar. What enticed me even more than my sense of continuity with family tradition was the affinity I felt with its concepts, and I wondered if the ancient wisdom embedded within its construction of reality could untangle some of our modern predicaments.

When Efrem and I were first introduced to acupuncture at a seminar at Esalen in the spring of 1972, there was tremendous upheaval in the world. The Chinese were in the midst of a cultural revolution, and so were we. During the sixties the concerns I wrestled with were more social than medical. Many of us were seeking to antidote the toxicity of racism in the American social body and heal the wounds inflicted by a decade of violence in Vietnam. I struggled to understand and reconcile how Western civilization, having achieved some outstanding accomplishments, could so often contribute to rather than alleviate human suffering. How could it perpetuate vast environmental insult and the threat of nuclear disaster and yet be building a better future?

To remake the world it seemed we needed to rethink it. After all, solutions depend on how problems are framed, the context within which they exist. At issue for me was in part how we defined reality—and the reality assumed by Chinese medicine made sense.

Chinese medicine echoes the logic of quantum physics, which suggests that we exist in a relative, process-oriented universe in which there is no "objective" world separable from living subjects. The essential questions cannot be resolved by measuring static "things"; rather, answers become stories about interactions and relationships. Within this paradigm contradictions are not only sanctioned but prevail, and truth is purely contextual. In contrast with our conventional Western tendency to draw sharp lines of distinction, Chinese thought does not strictly determine the boundaries between rest and motion, time and space, mind and matter, sickness and health.

---

*Specially defined Chinese medical terms are italicized and capitalized throughout the text to differentiate them from their common meaning, such as heart as an anatomically located organ in the chest versus *Heart* as an *Organ Network*, or wind that dances through the trees versus *Wind* that represents an adverse pathological phenomenon. The glossary will assist in clarification.

Chinese medicine transcends the illusion of separation by inhabiting the reality of a unified field, an interwoven pattern of inseparable links in a circular chain.

THE ANCIENT CHINESE WORLDVIEW

The ancient Chinese perceived human beings as a microcosm of the universe that surrounded them, suffused with the same primeval forces that motivated the macrocosm. They imagined themselves as part of one unbroken wholeness, called Tao, a singular relational continuum within and without. This thinking predates the dissection of mind from body and man from nature that Western culture performed in the seventeenth century.

From when I first encountered it, this fusing of the mind with the body and people with their world had a magic, seductive lure. I was eager to imagine myself as integrated and interrelated, an active participant in a system in the continuous process of transforming itself. I learned that Chinese philosophers and physicians have studied nature over thousands of years, divining how to interact with it to cultivate and guide *Qi* (pronounced "chee"), life's animating force and substance. The Chinese concept of *Qi* symbolizes life in all its forms: thoughts and emotions, tissue and blood, inner life and outer expression. I wanted to reap and share the benefits of their knowledge.

I was startled to find that my father considered Chinese medicine quackery. Even though I could appreciate that surgery and antibiotics were often necessary, my father could not entertain the value of acupuncture and herbs. Though I could appreciate the worth of a microscope to identify tissue alterations and bacteria, my father could not fathom the notion of *Qi*. It probably should not have surprised me, since Chinese medicine does not rest solely upon the tangible, measurable phenomena upon which his medicine relies. That I was drawn to a system outside his Western conceptual framework unsettled and offended him. Yet I recognized the Chinese view as inclusive, not exclusive. Within that view the subtle, ephemeral, and invisible were as significant as what could be seen, touched, and counted, and caring for the human spirit was no less essential or real than caring for the human structure, nor separate from it.

THE MODERN PREDICAMENT

Western philosophy was more akin to Eastern until the Renaissance of the seventeenth century, when our civilization revolutionized its thinking. It was then that the scientific philosophy of the 1600s began to consider people as   5 independent of the living systems that surround them and assumed that we could dominate and exploit nature without being affected by it. We escaped from dependency on and attachment to the natural world, pursuing invulnerability, invincibility, and immortality. Four hundred years later many of us regret this stance, aware, as anthropologist Gregory Bateson puts it, that "an organism that destroys its environment destroys itself."

The long-term survival of our species has been placed at risk by an unbridled lust for short-term gains coupled with a false postulation of civilization's autonomy from nature. Human beings have befouled their own nest, a sure sign of either madness or disease when observed in the rest of the animal kingdom. Contamination of rivers and seas puts fish in peril and threatens our potable water supply, the ozone layer is nibbled by fluorocarbons, rain forests perish so that cattle can graze, soil depletion and pesticides diminish the quality of our food, urban horizons shimmer with heavy ocher air . . . The litany seems endless. The disruption of our global respiration seems the consequence of burning fossil fuels (which fill the air with carbon dioxide and other gases, trapping heat) and of denuding forests (whose trees release oxygen, consume carbon dioxide, and attract water vapor to cool the earth's surface). Known as the "greenhouse effect," this upset in the relationship between the primal elements of heat and cold, fire and water, produces a fever of land, sea, and air with disastrous repercussions—upon weather conditions and marine, animal, and human life as we know it.

The gravity of issues like this has motivated burgeoning numbers of us to re-form our consciousness about who we are and how to live with each other upon the earth. We are being obliged to see how that which appears to be separate affects and fits within a pattern, and we are seeing, as Bateson points out, that "the patterns connect." Reluctantly we are entertaining the idea that it may be necessary to transcend thinking of ourselves solely as entities with private interests (nation-states, corporate bodies, individual persons) and instead view ourselves and our world as one organic system.

Today many of us seek to reclaim the sense of connectedness that existed universally in ancient culture, when human fate was wholly entwined with nature. The ecological assumption within these cosmologies held that all things were inextricably bound together. The world was seen as a symbiotic entity in which each living system interacted with and mutually supported every other. The growing popularity of Chinese medicine, which embodies these values, is itself part of a pattern. Chinese medicine instructs us to perceive the way the world functions and re-create harmony within the context of the whole.

TAOIST PHILOSOPHY IN ACTION

Protecting human life by preserving the conditions within which it thrives is the purpose of Chinese medicine. Each of us is pictured as an ecosystem as well as living within one. The balance of forces within us (*Yin-Yang, Heat-Cold, Blood-Qi*) determines our internal climate, our health or disease.

Chinese medicine embraces the logic that the best remedy for calamity is to avert it—the best cure for sickness is prevention. The *Nei Jing*, a medical classic written in the second century B.C., states:

> Maintaining order rather than correcting disorder is the ultimate principle of wisdom. To cure disease after it has appeared is like digging a well when one already feels thirsty, or forging weapons after the war has already begun.

The true physician teaches the Tao—how to live. Traditional Chinese doctors are trained to cultivate wellness as well as to correct ill health. Planning ahead, Chinese medicine knows that storms interrupt clear weather, that illness stalks and gains a foothold when we are vulnerable. Its strategy is to enable us to withstand the storm without becoming disabled by it and to accumulate resources in times of good weather, peace, and plenty.

The technology of Chinese medicine—simple, inexpensive, and highly portable—was what first ignited Efrem's imagination. A traditional doctor in China need carry only a few needles and gather local herbs from the countryside to minister to his patients. Because this medicine was so accessible, after the revolution in 1949 many thousands of "barefoot doctors" were trained to serve the unmet needs of the Chinese people for medical care. This equipped ordinary people with the tools to gain control of their own lives.

In contrast with this model, American medical doctors are assigned the active (powerful) roles while patients are resigned to passive (powerless) ones. Efrem felt a kinship with the Taoist physician who performed skillfully to mitigate distress but also acted as teacher, sharing knowledge and power. Doctor and patient then engaged in the mutual endeavor of grasping the problem and accomplishing the healing.

Sages describe a state without suffering and a way to get there. That way is not to search for a single remedy, a panacea, a "magic bullet," but to engage in the ongoing process of learning to become more animated, more connected: more charged with life. Both Efrem and I were struck by the notion that Chinese medicine was about just that—striving toward greater integration through the cultivation of *Qi*. The excitement was and remains that Chinese medicine offers an approach that includes, yet moves beyond, issues of physical health.

By the summer of 1972, at a time when few Americans had heard of acupuncture, and at the risk of being considered cultural renegades, we struggled to cross over ethnic, social, and intellectual barriers, riveted by the idea that with Chinese medicine we could both understand the world and change it. Just as my younger sister was finishing medical school, we were exploring foreign territory, making our journey east.

THE NATURE OF REALITY SHIFTS

After the acupuncture seminar at Esalen, the intrigue escalated. Efrem and I read what we could, but it wasn't enough. Like hounds on the scent of a fox, we were pulled irresistibly by the magnet of Chinese philosophy and driven to discover whether these ancient healing techniques really worked. At that time no schools offered study programs in the United States, and China had not yet been opened to American students. So we traveled to England in the fall of 1972 to enroll in the College of Traditional Chinese Acupuncture.

We were part of the first class of Americans to study at this college. Half of our group were Western medical doctors. We all went through major readjustments during our course of study as our presumptions about the nature of reality, ourselves, health, and healing were pulled apart, stretched, and rewoven into new cloth.

I began to experience myself as a little tao, a galaxy of internal planets spinning through time and space. These planets became named as five transformative phases: *Wood, Fire, Earth, Metal,* and *Water.* Each one functioned as an energetic field linked with the visceral organs of *Liver, Heart, Spleen, Lung,* and *Kidney,* whose lines of force coursed through channels in my body like a lattice of waterways crosses the earth. Physiological functions, personality characteristics, even single impulses could be classified within this new language.

We came to recognize that each class member could be characterized by the attributes of one *Organ* and *Phase.* For example, an enthusiastic cardiologist became easily excited, had a nervous laugh, and liked to give running commentary about his experience as he lived it. We identified him as expressing the influence of *Fire.* A methodical and serious graduate student who dressed fastidiously and set high standards for herself and others reflected the influence of *Metal.* A dynamic, impatient psychologist who took the initiative to set up the school's first training clinic exhibited typical *Wood* characteristics. A socially reticent, intense nonconformist who plunged into the learning, absorbing all he could in his fertile mind, manifested a strong *Water* aspect. And an internist able to heal with his compassionate touch and smile, who assumed care of us when the stress of our studies took its toll, had the phase of *Earth* speaking through his personality.

Just as I could see myself as a little tao, our class too became a projection of a single body. We each performed our own function, a distinct role appropriate to our individual nature. Our physical shape, the quality of our movement and manner, our symptoms, the tastes and flavors we preferred, the odor of our flesh, the color of our tongue, the sound of our voice, the feeling of our pulse, revealed ways our persona organized and expressed itself within the context of these new categories.

THE REALITY OF MEDICINE SHIFTS

We experienced a radical shift of focus from what we'd known. We learned to feel the pulse in six positions on the radial artery of both wrists, each position corresponding to a channel associated with an *Organ Network*. This was particularly dramatic for the doctors. Since medical school they had accepted as an article of faith and an assumption of science the existence of only one pulse, which reflected the function of the heart alone. The notion that the shape, force, and rhythm of the blood pulsing through the radial artery was not merely determined by the activity of the heart, but was the outcome of the interaction of all forces coalescing in the human body at any given time, diverged sharply from their medical education.

Alongside our training, we were experiencing acupuncture for our own maladies. In the midst of a particularly intense week of uninterrupted study, Efrem felt flushed, agitated, and had the unpleasant sensation of his pulse pounding throughout his body. His blood pressure was abnormally high, 140/90. Our teacher inserted one needle along the outer edge of his hand and another along the front border of his neck muscle. The change was striking—within minutes his blood pressure normalized, the pounding ceased, and he felt an expansive calm. What had been a pervasive mood of anxiety and melancholy became one of exhilaration and repose. He experienced acupuncture as simultaneously alleviating the distress in his body and restoring his good humor. This imprinted upon him that within this medical system, mental discomforts need not be ignored nor invalidated as being "only in your mind."

CHANGING DEFINITIONS

Although I had always considered myself to be in perfect health, my self-image was chipped away by the chisel of this new perspective. As a child, whenever I had a sniffle my father gave me a powerful pill to squelch it, and as a result, I never got sick. Later, even though my stamina was capricious and I had low blood pressure, my father considered this a blessing—no need

9

to worry about high blood pressure. In my family, as long as you weren't sick, you were healthy. But bothersome aspects of my physical and emotional life that I'd previously dismissed as idiosyncratic began to appear as lifelong signs of a pattern that betrayed less than optimal function. It dawned on me that although I was not sick, I could feel better.

For years my hands and feet were ice blocks under the covers at night and my lower back ached periodically. Cuts became easily infected, and frequent canker sores burned in my mouth, aggravated by the sweets that I craved. Sometimes a lingering hunger persisted after meals, and in the evenings when I was tired, my hearing diminished to the hum of a dim tuner. Restful sleep eluded me if I remained awake past eleven P.M., and rising the next morning could seem an Olympian feat. Yet more limiting than any of these minor body afflictions was a nagging sense of fatigue. There was constantly more on my agenda than I had energy to accomplish. In the early afternoon I could be easily overcome by a muddled feeling that left me sluggish, unable to focus, and unproductive for several hours of prime time during the work day. I felt hopeful and optimistic but lacked the steady strength to fulfill my ambitions.

I had never assembled these vague complaints. My father would have dismissed them since they didn't make particular sense within his framework, and besides, there was nothing in his repertoire to "fix" any of them. From his point of view I was normal. But within the context of Chinese medicine, each sign and symptom assumed new meaning.

Although Western lab tests would have indicated normal kidney function, the coldness, tiredness, and hearing loss represented a weakness of *Water*, the *Kidney Network*. The sores in my mouth and surge of energy late at night were characteristic of an imbalance of *Wood*, the *Liver Network*. Sleeping problems were associated with a deficiency of *Fire*, the *Heart Network*. Overall, my character was most dominated by *Earth*, the *Spleen Network*. A sunny disposition, an eagerness to help other people, and constant reflection upon how to generally improve the human condition are traits of *Earth*. A fixation with details, a sometimes obsessive need to get things done, and that sudden soggy, muddled feeling are associated with disharmonies of *Earth*.

As I received acupuncture treatment, and later herbal medicine, my resources increased and steadied; in addition, I could relieve my monthly irritability, water retention, and insomnia. As my complaints receded, I experienced myself as a more effective captain of my vessel, guiding fate by altering the givens, assuming control over tendencies and reactions that I had presumed came with my territory.

All of us established relationships between physical and emotional patterns, connecting what had otherwise seemed unrelated. In Western medicine, cold extremities, back pain, hearing loss, and fatigue are not associated with each other or with the kidney. Troubled sleep, excitability, and laughter are not associated with the heart. Menstrual problems are unrelated to the liver. But in Chinese medicine, a weak *Kidney* may mean not only having a backache, poor hearing, and fatigue, but also being fearful, stingy, withdrawn, and apathetic. The *Organ Networks* of Chinese medicine were not equivalent to the anatomical organs of Western medicine. *Organ Networks* were defined functionally, not structurally. As such, they included emotional and mental function as well as physiological performance, and even their physiology was defined differently.

Furthermore, within this logic, problems are not isolated from the context in which they occur, so a single symptom is understood in relation to the entire body environment. The strategy is to adjust the field, reorganizing the process out of which symptoms grow, coercing them into retreat by eliminating the milieu in which they thrive.

Stimulated and unsettled, many of us underwent personal as well as professional transformation. The sun still rose each morning and traded places with the moon at night, but our perception of ourselves and the world around us altered.

After reading these chapters, you will also learn how to interpret yourself within the context of these concepts so that you can say, "I am an *Earth* type who has conflict with *Wood* and weakness in *Water*. My primary therapeutic focus will be in these areas." That is a purpose of this book.

THE CROSS-FERTILIZATION OF MEDICINE:
EAST GOES WEST AND WEST GOES EAST

From the late Middle Ages on, traditional Chinese medicine trickled into foreign lands. A comprehensive Chinese herbal text written in 1587 found its way into the hands of German physicians around 1605. In 1810 a French physician named Louis Berlioz reported successfully treating neurogenic diseases with acupuncture. In 1929, after serving as French consul in China, Dr. Soulie de Mourant translated a Chinese text, furthering the practice of acupuncture in France.

During the mid-1800s Chinese immigrants building railroads and mining gold in the United States brought their medicine with them. For the most part it remained within the Chinese community. However, a few exceptions occurred in the Northwest, where local settlers benefited from the care of Chinese doctors. Historical records from the towns of John Day, Oregon, and Boise, Idaho, indicate that Chinese doctors successfully treated respiratory, digestive, and reproductive infections, as well as arthritis and symptoms of cardiovascular disease. Pioneer women who were unable to conceive were helped to bear healthy children.

Meanwhile, European and American missionaries had been exporting Western medicine to China. The Chinese were very impressed with surgical technique, vaccinations, and the means of hygiene and sanitation that helped reduce the spread of infectious diseases, wound sepsis, and the mortality of women following childbirth. Western industrial and medical technology came to be associated with progress. By the time penicillin was developed in the 1940s, traditional medical institutions in China had been significantly replaced by the more highly prized Western medical schools.

In 1949, the year of the Chinese revolution, there were 10,000 Western-trained doctors for 400 million people. At this time the 550,000 traditional doctors recovered their stature within the medical establishment because of the dire need for more doctors and a fervent desire to reassert faith in China's own cultural legacy. Since 1949 traditional medicine has been revived and incorporated as a mandatory part of the training in many modern medical schools. Researchers there now investigate the biochemistry of herbal constituents and the electrophysiology of acupuncture points to trace their impact on the healing mechanisms of the body.

Still, in many life-threatening situations, only Western medical and surgical techniques are appropriate. Functional disorders constitute a middle ground where either system may be elected. In chronic degenerative illnesses for which Western medicine has little to offer, traditional medicine is a welcome option. Some Chinese hospitals accommodate alternate floors for Western and traditional care, with doctors selecting what best suits their patients' needs. In some circumstances both systems work in concert. For instance, Western surgery, radiation, or chemotherapy is used to control cancer, while traditional Chinese medicine is used to strengthen the body and enhance immunity, enabling the person to better tolerate treatment.

During the 1950s and 1960s when traditional medicine was being re-integrated in its homeland, travel, commerce, and exchange between the United States and China was highly restricted. In 1972, the year when then-President Nixon unstrapped the political restraints upon our relationship with the People's Republic, acupuncture needles passed from East to West. At this time our class of Americans at the College of Acupuncture was preparing to use these needles on American bodies.

While in China, *New York Times* journalist James Reston had an emergency appendectomy, and his postoperative abdominal pain was relieved by an acupuncture needle in his leg. It appeared particularly spectacular because it was so little understood. Realizing that *Qi* traverses the body through channels, it becomes less enigmatic that toothaches can be relieved by the stimulation of a point along a pathway that connects the mouth to the hand or foot. Learning that white fungus reduces blood cholesterol levels, it no longer seems a miracle that people who live in regions in China where it is part of the diet have lower incidences of heart attacks. It is common knowledge among Chinese that pseudoginseng powder stops hemorrhage, chrysanthemum flower tea will relieve a bilious headache, and black mushrooms increase immunity.

Since the dawn of this century the West has been exporting medical technology and pharmaceuticals to the East. In the last quarter of this century the medicinal treasures of the Orient have been imported to the West. In 1976 Efrem and I were among the first two hundred and ten practitioners to receive an acupuncture license from the California State Board of Medical Quality Assurance. Nationally there are now between six and ten thousand practitioners of Chinese medicine, and two dozen other states have instituted licensure programs. Two decades ago there were no colleges of Chinese medicine in this country; now there are more than twenty. What began as a handful of books on the subject has grown to a library of more than four hundred titles, many of which are translations of Chinese texts.

MIRACLES EAST AND WEST

The advantages of integrating Western and Chinese medicine were dramatized for Efrem and me following the birth of our son in 1975. Born with two gaping holes in a swollen heart, Bear's life would have been eclipsed without surgical intervention. After diagnosing his problem by injecting a dye into his heart that projected an image on a video screen, our cardiologist determined it was possible for the holes to be closed with Dacron patches. If he had been born twenty years earlier when open-heart surgery for infants had not yet been developed, his heart could not have been repaired. We were grateful that miracles existed in the West.

Following surgery, because of his fragile constitution, he was subject to countless bouts of bronchitis and upper-respiratory infection. In San Francisco we studied herbs with local Chinese doctors. When Bear was able to swallow herbal pills, they became incorporated into his routine along with breakfast and lunch. We used certain formulas for overcoming acute illness and others as a tonic for strengthening him, improving his resistance. Eventually he rebuffed the onslaught of winter colds even when his schoolmates succumbed. Now as a teenager Bear radiates the health we had hoped for from his birth. We were grateful for miracles of the East as well.

In 1980, after eight years of practicing acupuncture, Efrem went to China to further study the use of herbs and experience Chinese medicine in its native habitat. A Western-style dispensary stood alongside the herbal pharmacy at the Kunming Railway Workers Hospital. A special kitchen brewed individual herb teas, delivering fresh medicine to both inpatients and outpatients.

Efrem's teacher, Dr. Zheng Wen Tao, was first trained as a Western physician. Later he was asked to return to school to study traditional medicine. He combined classical knowledge with the findings of modern research, producing herbal formulas particularly effective for treating cardiovascular and immune disorders. Dr. Zheng Wen Tao was particularly renowned for his treatment of intractable diseases. Efrem witnessed the gradual remission of scleroderma in a young woman after one year of herbal treatment. Scleroderma, an autoimmune disease, is marked by the progressive hardening of connective tissue, considered both fatal and untreatable by Western medicine. This young woman had been told that she had one year to live. Instead, during that year she reversed the course of her illness and regained health. Zheng Wen Tao is the epitome of the modern Chinese medical hero, able to unite modern science with classical tradition. When Efrem returned home, we expanded our use of herbal medicine in the treatment of our acupuncture patients, setting up an herbal pharmacy in our acupuncture clinic.

A FOREIGN CULTURE PLANTED ON HOME SOIL

Some people tend to dismiss Chinese medicine for not conforming to the modern medical model, while others tend to romanticize and mystify it. Some discount it because it is not modern, others revere it because it is old. The former group considers it eccentric quackery, and the latter considers it a panacea. It is clear to us that it is a system unto itself, altogether distinct from a trendy health fad or other therapies considered to be holistic or alternative. It has endured for centuries not only because its techniques produce tangible results, but because it embodies a coherent philosophy that integrates many aspects of human life.

Western medicine has had a monopoly not only on our medicine cabinets, but also on our minds. Now other possibilities exist. More and more people are receiving acupuncture, so far several million Americans, and Chinese herbs are finding the way onto their shelves. Within the next decade medicinal foods will be simmering in stainless-steel pots, making the exotic aromas and flavors of China as familiar to us as chicken soup. Americans, like the Chinese, are quite pragmatic—Chinese medicine meets their need, so people try it; it helps, so they come back for more.

By familiarizing yourself with its concepts, you will be able to judge if and when it is a fitting option for you. Spotting yourself within its categories will help you better understand your behavior and feelings, the ways you express your health, and the ways you fall ill. By the end, we hope you will be able to interpret yourself amply enough to acquire the rudimentary know-how to initiate personal change.

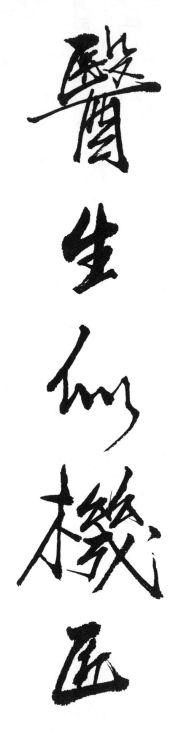

Philosophy in the West:
The Doctor as Mechanic

CHAPTER TWO

PHILOSOPHY IN THE WEST: THE DOCTOR AS MECHANIC

> Cartesianism is the unspoken philosophical substratum of contemporary medicine—the source of many of its great strengths and equally of its deficiencies.
>
> Pellegrino and Thomasma
> *A Philosophical Basis*
> *of Medical Practice*

BECAUSE OUR PERCEPTION OF THE WORLD INFLUENCES HOW WE LIVE IN it, our consciousness sculpts reality. Conversely, our experience shapes our thinking, so our reality molds consciousness. Our minds create what is real, and our lived experiences generate our thoughts. There is a reciprocity between beliefs and observations—what we look for affects what we see, so describing "just the way things are" from the Chinese and Western vantage point is not necessarily the same. Each makes sense of the body according to a different set of beliefs.

It became clear to us that to penetrate Chinese medicine we needed to examine how reality itself was defined, East and West. Because taken-for-granted assumptions are buried just beneath the skin of our conscious awareness, in this chapter we peel that skin back to expose our Western philosophic presumptions about how things are. Upon understanding ourselves, we can approach the unfamiliar and proceed to probe the East on its own terms.

SCIENCE: THE NEW RELIGION OF THE WEST

During the Middle Ages, people in Western Europe had a unified view of their universe: seeing themselves as an integral part of everything that was both seen and unseen. They were connected with Heaven through God and with Earth through Nature. The break with this organic sensibility came with the decline of feudal society as cities grew where there were once feudal kingdoms. As the pervasive authority of the Roman Catholic church was undermined by the Protestant Reformation, the people of Europe believed they could attain mastery in the world through their own willful efforts. No longer were they solely dependent on the spiritual community of the Church.

In the Christianity of this new era, the realm of Heaven existed outside of Nature, apart from it, barely within human reach. Earth and Heaven were divided into separate realms. The dark, sinister, mysterious forces of Earth were juxtaposed with the enlightened, righteous, and supernatural forces of Heaven. Instead of being an ally, Nature became an adversary to be overcome and conquered. Man stood outside of it, apart from and above it. The Earth was no longer intimately connected to the life of our own body, instead it became an object that could be manipulated and exploited. Human beings were the battleground in which Man and Nature, good and evil, spirit and body, wrestled with each other. A unified reality was sacrificed for dominion over Nature, for technology, for "progress."

A schism occurred between the sacred and the secular, Heaven and Earth, life and death. Before this, with God for protection and guidance, it was unnecessary to question and understand Nature. But without divine providence, the unpredictable chaos of Nature was perceived as forbidding and dangerous. Death, associated with the dark forces, became irreconcilable with life, rather than an inevitable transition in the cycle of existence. The best protection against Nature was through domination and control: to gain power over Nature was to conquer death.[1] A new set of values and beliefs was created to explain and organize the world. This new "religion" was that of science, and its priests were the mathematicians, physicists, and mechanical engineers.[2]

DESCARTES: NATURE AND THE BODY AS MACHINE

In the West the philosophy of science is based on the premise that humans are separate from nature, and that the world, like a machine, can be dismantled and reduced into constituent parts. Reality is located in the tangible structure of matter: that which can be measured, quantified, and analyzed. Events occur according to unchanging laws. The foundation for this scientific thinking was buried in the soil of Aristotle's "empirical materialism," excavated during the Renaissance. With Aristotle, reality came to mean that which could be substantiated materially. Matter was understood to be fixed and unchanging, therefore real.

In the seventeenth century, the French mathematician Descartes ushered in the Western scientific revolution. His introduction of analytic, reductive reasoning formed the basis of a new philosophy of science, which became the philosophy of modern medicine as well. His thinking had such profound influence that the principles underpinning modern science came to be referred to as Cartesian.

Descartes believed there could be absolute, certain truth, commenting, "All science is certain, evident knowledge. We reject all knowledge which is merely probable and judge that only those things should be believed which are perfectly known and about which there can be no doubts."[3] Through the use of reductive, deductive logic, Descartes felt on the verge of comprehending the fundamental workings of the universe. He conceptualized the world and everything in it as a machine, stating, "I do not recognize any difference between the machines made by craftsmen and various bodies that nature alone composes."[4] Mechanical laws were said to universally govern all phenomena. The exact sciences formulated to dominate and control nature were applied to human beings as well. Descartes considered the human body a machine, likening a healthy man to a well-made clock. He also erected a firm division between mind and matter, asserting, "There is nothing in the concept of body that belongs to the mind; and nothing in that of mind that belongs to the body."[5]

This mechanistic view of nature led to the fixed and absolute physical laws devised by astronomer and mathemetician Isaac Newton, which outlined the cause-and-effect method of explaining the material universe. This logic formed the basis of the scientific method, which even today remains essentially unchanged. Perhaps unaware that many logical systems of knowledge exist, most Westerners consider this to be the only valid way of understanding the world.

Within this worldview, nature and humans are machines governed by mechanical laws: systems that do work, tools of production. Western medicine, correspondingly, is the study of how the human machine works. When people are like machines, doctors become like mechanics. The mechanic occasionally performs routine maintenance but mostly intervenes to execute emergency repairs. He plunges into the working parts, replacing the nonfunctioning elements, and puts the machine back into working order. It follows that the doctor as mechanic fixes the broken body-machine.

In this schema, the body is reduced to structural parts, proceeding from organs to tissues, tissues to cells, cells to molecules. The doctor as mechanic separates the whole into parts in order to discern the nature, proportion, and function of each constituent. Sorting out the parts enabled early Western doctors to conceptualize a diseased entity as the faulty component and sever it from the organism as a whole. They could thereby remove it or treat it in isolation from other organ and tissue parts.

THE RISE OF WESTERN MEDICINE

The findings of the early anatomists validated the mechanistic view that the body is made out of distinct and separate parts, connected and yet autonomous. They divided the body into systems analogous to mechanical processes that corresponded precisely with structural descriptions of organs and tissues. The circulatory system comprises the heart as a mechanical pump that pushes the blood through the pipes of the veins and arteries. The lungs are like a bellows, the nervous system like an elaborate electrical telephone network.

For the mechanic, it is best if the parts of the machine are standardized and uniform. That way the parts are interchangeable, easily replaced, and the ways in which they break down become predictable from one body to the next. Standardized diseases develop from established causes, and protocols of treatment are fixed. Uniform parts sit on the shelf. This view focuses entirely on the ways in which all people are alike and tends to overlook the ways in which people are unique and dissimilar. When a group of people receives the same diagnosis, they receive the same treatment. Science and industry have enabled medicine to be practiced on a mass basis. The same mechanistic philosophy that inspired mass production in industry also inspired mass medicine and health care.

The marriage of science, industry, and medicine spawned an age of innovation and specialization. As a result the human body and mind were divided and reduced into ever more diverse and refined areas of investigation.

For example, chemists began to perceive the body as a chemical factory controlled and regulated through the balance of molecular compounds. The practice of pharmaceutical therapy was the by-product of the tremendous discoveries made in chemistry. Penicillin, aspirin, digitalis, cortisone, and smallpox vaccine were just a fraction of the wonder drugs discovered to treat specific diseases and remove specific pathogens or causative factors. The physicists, on the other hand, perceived the body as an atomic structure and developed radiation technology for diagnosis and treatment. The X-ray machine furthered diagnostic precision and inhibited the spread of many cancers.

For their part, the engineers perceived the body as a mechanical structure composed of discrete parts. They invented surgical tools and methods for removing and replacing faulty parts. The body as a machine could be stopped, taken apart, repaired, and put back together. Remarkable developments in surgical technology enabled doctors to do open-heart repair, skin grafts, appendectomy, cesarean section, attachment of severed limbs, and bone setting. These innovations contributed to the resolution of potentially devastating health-care crises and constituted the wonders of modern medicine.

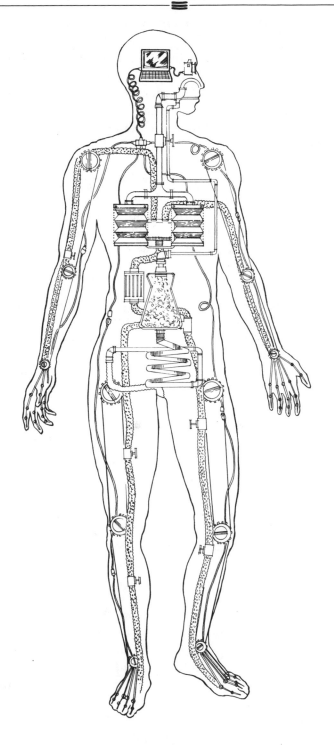

The Body As Machine

THE NARROWING DEFINITION OF DISEASE

Another fundamental shift occurred in the mid-1800s, when Louis Pasteur located the origin of disease outside the body, in the form of germs. His analytic research isolated a particular prior cause, triggering a given effect. The germ theory of disease postulated that a single microorganism could produce specific symptoms of disease in healthy organisms. This theory helped to explain epidemics and plagues and to develop effective remedies against them.

However, this "doctrine of specific cause" became generally invoked to explain all diseases. And because only the single cause was sought, the multitude of contributing factors occurring simultaneously in any given sick person were ignored. That the total condition of the person profoundly affected his or her susceptibility to a disease was excluded by this conceptual model.

For example, insulin was discovered when experimenters were able to produce the high blood sugar symptoms of diabetes in healthy animals by damaging the pancreas. According to the doctrine of specific cause, it was then concluded that the cause of diabetes was a deficiency in the production of insulin by the pancreas. This was a major lifesaving discovery of modern medicine. As remarkable as it was, however, the belief that insulin was a cure prevented people from searching for the real basis of the disease, the degenerative course of which remained unaltered.

The narrow view of specific cause has limited the scope and effectiveness of modern medicine, which often equated the control of symptoms with the cure of the disease. This belief in single cause diverted medicine from an appreciation of the context and complexity of human process from which degenerative diseases emerged. Although many involved in health care are increasingly aware that disease is not separable from the human life that cradles it, the ideology of Western medicine does not accommodate this insight. Referring to the "crisis in health care," H. R. Holman, M.D., of Stanford University cites shortcomings and suggests the need for philosophical and social remedies:

> Longevity has changed little, and the major illnesses such as malignancy and cardiovascular disease remain unimpeded. . . . Illnesses disproportionately affect the poor, major environmental and occupational causes of illnesses receive little attention and less action . . . clearly, there is a crisis in health care, both in its effect upon health and in its cost. . . . Some medical outcomes are inadequate not because appropriate technical interventions are lacking, but because our conceptual thinking is inadequate.[6]

Modern medicine directs its gaze through a microscope so that detail is gained at the expense of a restricted visual field. Specialists look at smaller and smaller fragments, gaining more and more positive information in the form of descriptive data but losing a sense of the integrity of the system as a whole. How did this medical model gain exclusive ascendance in America?

NARROWING THE INSTITUTION OF MEDICINE

In the beginning of the century a survey of medical schools was subsidized by the Carnegie and Rockefeller foundations. Its purpose was to find out which schools would be most interested in promoting "scientific medicine," therefore promoting the newly developing drug- and hospital-based technology industries. The Flexner Report, issued in 1910 by the American Medical Association following this survey, recommended that financial support from the foundations be awarded only to medical schools committed to scientific research based on models developed in the nineteenth century. All therapies not based on the Cartesian model were considered unscientific and would therefore be disenfranchised. Only 20 percent of the existing medical schools survived. The other 80 percent adhered to the "vitalist doctrine," which asserted that "man assists, but nature heals." Naturopathy, homeopathy, and herbology were forced out of the mainstream and relegated to the status of folk medicine. They were ultimately driven under by lack of funds and political harassment.

Formerly the majority of physicians were helpers, allies, and comforters to people struggling with maladies in their daily life. The new doctor became the exclusive source of specialized knowledge and the heroic slayer of disease. Increasingly a delegation of authority and power went to the doctor. Patients were educated to believe that doctors alone knew what made them sick and that only their technology or drugs could make them well.

As the depth and breadth of scientific information about the body grew, both doctors and people lost faith in the capacity of the human organism to heal itself. How could anyone but an enlightened and sophisticated engineer run such an awesomely complex and vulnerable machine? This faith was withdrawn from the body's self-healing abilities and put into the hands of the "experts"—the physicians.

OUTCOMES OF THIS MEDICAL MODEL

Medicine was not set up to advise people on how to stay or become well. The doctor could only fix what had broken down. He could miraculously remove evil (tumors, infections, stones) with drugs and surgery. He could manipulate function (thyroid hormones, diuretics, steroids) and replace worn parts (plastic hips and hearts). As a heroic soldier he could wage a valiant short-term battle. He could remove the "evil," but there was no mechanism built into the system to discern or promote the "good." Medicine's strengths were the source of its weakness. The research and clinical institutions of medicine are still defined by the existing conceptual model and more oriented toward intervention than prevention.

Furthermore, as doctors became the experts, they acquired a type of power over their patients. Mastery of medicine became a technically sophisticated and exclusive high priesthood. The common person could not possibly gain access to and interpret the data necessary to administer medical care. Even the medical profession itself diversified into more highly specialized fields: the general practitioner who cared for a whole person was replaced by the cardiologist, who cared for the heart; the orthopedist, who ministered to the bones; the neurologist for the nerves; the oncologist for the cancer; the psychiatrist for the mind; and so on.

When power was taken from the person by the general practitioner, and from the general practitioner by the specialist, there was no longer one doctor who cared for the whole person and knew her in the context of her total environment. The once intimate relationship between helper and helped shifted to an impersonal one between strangers. Doctors lost knowledge of their patients as real people.

This shift in the organization of medicine taught people to feel that science knew more about them than they could ever know or understand about themselves. People as patients began giving away the responsibility to care for their own health. The phrase *health-care delivery system* suggests the doctor is like a mail carrier who can deliver health at the doorstep. This situation is reminiscent of Plato's image of a "household" in which the "master," the mind, knows but does not act and the "slave," the body, acts but does not know. Doctors function as the master (mind) and patients as the slave (body). Now divided, the body loses its intelligence and the mind loses its power to actualize: not only is self-understanding undermined, but possibilities for action are limited as well. People mistakenly feel that the power to cure comes from outside themselves, administered by an alien intelligence.

This distortion of power often instigates an antagonistic relationship between doctors and patients. When doctors cannot perform the heroic role and fix the broken machine, they sometimes blame the victim, judging patients guilty of not getting better. Isolated, abandoned, undermined, and invalidated, patients then feel condemned to a circle of pain with no escape. Along with their physical pain, they are frustrated and angered by their feelings of powerlessness. They then become quick to blame the doctor for their problems, jumping into malpractice litigation. Suing for malpractice becomes an act of revenge, an attempt on the part of the patient to gain power over the doctor, not a reclamation of true self-power. The doctor is either a hero or villain—heralded for recovery or blamed for poor outcomes.

OTHER PARADOXES

Power, no matter who has it, does not confer wisdom. Doctors sometimes equate their authority with sagacity. Some interventions produce disastrous long-term effects on health. Iatrogenesis, or doctor-induced illness, can result from drugs, surgery, radiation, and chemotherapy. Iatrogenesis is one of the leading causes of fatal disease. Approximately one out of every five people admitted to a research hospital acquires an iatrogenic illness.[7]

Nobel prize–winning microbiologist René Dubos describes the new threats to health arising out of technological innovation. He says it is a painful and richly documented paradox that every drug of proven worth can itself become a cause of disease.

> Some of the toxic effects are extremely indirect and delayed. They result from disturbances in the physiological and ecological equilibrium of the organism. Their mechanism does not reside in chemical or physiological reactions involving direct cause-effect relationships, but rather in complex interrelated responses made by the whole integrated organism, including its indigenous microbiota.[8]

Another consequence of focusing more attention on the disease than the patient is that the doctor can eradicate the tumor but has no means of promoting the health of the patient. This enables one to say, "The treatment was a success, but the patient died." For example, chemotherapy claims success at treating the disease and yet cannot necessarily improve the longevity of the patient. John Cairns of the Harvard School of Public Health states:

> Each year about 3,000 patients under age 30 are being cured by chemotherapy who would otherwise have died. Only two percent of the patients who die of cancer are under 30, however. For the vast majority of cancers, which arise in older patients, the results of chemotherapy are much more controversial. . . . Apart from the success with Hodgkin's disease, childhood leukemia and a few other cancers, it is not possible to detect any sudden change in death rates for any of the major cancers that could be credited to chemotherapy.[9]

25

The other major paradox of the Western medical model is that it separates the indivisible. Western medicine has so successfully dissected the human body that it suffers from "overseparation," where the whole is no longer perceived as a meaningful entity. What was one indivisible circle, an unbroken continuum, became a straight line of successive causality in which events became random, losing their intrinsic relationship to each other. The mind has been separated from the body; the disease from the person who has it; the specific pathogen from the disease process as a whole; the parts from each other; the symptoms from the source of the ailment; and the patients from their self-responsibility and self-power.

This overseparation occurred at the dawn of modern Western civilization when matter was severed from the immaterial, human from nature, and process was frozen in fixed and absolute laws. Dualism shattered unity. This division has made us susceptible to an inversion of process whereby the means (technological, industrial, and scientific innovation) governs our ends (human values) and people become the "objects" rather than the "subjects" of their own activity. This has distorted our image of what the world is and who we are within it. The world man has made is impressive but lacks integrity—it no longer fits together, and neither do we know our place within it. When people are like machines, modern medicine becomes obliged to keep the machine running. Its purpose is defined as avoiding death rather than enriching life. Bodies must be kept alive at all costs because to die is considered intrinsically evil—death is the enemy to be conquered. Life and death are no longer part of a continuous cycle.

In ancient culture nothing was intrinsically good or evil, it was simply a matter of how one stood in relation to it. For an old person, it could be a gift to die with grace and ceremony just as it had been a gift to live—to preserve the tissue without the spirit would have been an offense, an insult worse than death.

The center of Western civilization has been commerce, industry, and information—the proliferation of economic transactions, manufactured products, and data. As Westerners we have been able to produce the world we live in, to control it by achieving power over nature. But the Western model is exclusive. It excludes the mysterious and intangible from its reality because the immaterial cannot be tamed, contained, and controlled. In an effort to achieve mastery over the world, connectedness with nature and humanity often perish.

Physicist Roger Jones comments upon the legacy of Descartes: "His genius, which has cleanly cut through the dense web of primitive mystery, has also severed our felt connection to the universe." This is where the Chinese model, still based on ancient principles, can help the Cartesian separation become whole again. Science historian Joseph Needham tells us that "the mechanical view of the world simply did not develop in Chinese thought, and the organicist view in which every phenomenon was connected with every other . . . was universal among Chinese thinkers." Rather, he continues, "The harmonious co-operation of all beings arose, not from the orders of a superior authority external to themselves, but from the fact that they were all parts in a hierarchy of wholes forming a cosmic and organic pattern and what they obeyed were the internal dictates of their own natures."

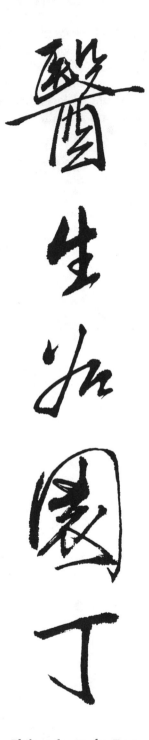

Philosophy in the East:
The Doctor As Gardener

CHAPTER THREE

PHILOSOPHY IN THE EAST:
THE DOCTOR AS GARDENER

Everything observable by the senses is subject to change and therefore in motion . . . there are interlocking cycles of change . . . one
cannot bid the winds and waves to cease, but one can learn to
navigate treacherous currents by conducting ourselves in harmony
with the prevailing processes of transformation—and thus weather
the storms of life.

> John Blofeld
> *I Ching*

EASTERN PHILOSOPHY IS BASED ON THE PREMISE THAT ALL LIFE OCCURS
within the circle of nature.[1] Things within this matrix are connected and
mutually dependent upon each other. Nature is one unified system, the Tao,
with polar and complementary aspects: *Yin* and *Yang*. Nature is in constant
motion, following cyclic patterns that describe the process of transformation.
When the elements of nature are in balance, life is harmonic and flourishes.
When the balance of polar forces is upset, disaster looms.

Within the Eastern worldview, the human being is a microcosm of Nature, a smaller universe. Human beings represent the juncture between
Heaven and Earth, the offspring of their union, a fusion of cosmic and ter-
restrial forces. The Chinese ideogram for human being pictures a figure rooted
like a tree in the Earth with hands outstretched like branches toward the
heavens, receiving power from above and below. Sustained by the power of
Earth and transformed by the power of Heaven, humanity cannot be separated from Nature—we *are* Nature, manifest as people. As a cosmos in miniature, we are propelled by the same forces. Good and bad are relative, not
absolute. Life and death balance each other. Seen and unseen, soma and
psyche,* are aspects of one continuous process, by definition everchanging
and in flux.[2]

---

*Psyche and soma comes nearest to conveying the meaning of the Chinese concepts *Shen* and *Jing*.
Shen refers to the organizing force of the self, reflected in the mental, emotional, and expressive
life of an individual. *Jing* refers to the material substance, physical structure, and sensate life of a
person. When referring to the totality of a person, the expression *Shen-Jing* is used, encompassing
both the intangible and tangible realms of experience.

Since everything is connected by the circle, health is understood broadly, defining the whole being within the social and natural order. What is good for nature is good for humanity, what is good for one is good for all, what is good for the mind is good for the body, and so on. To harm a part is to harm the whole. What is bad for the heart is bad for the body, what damages one person damages all people, what injures the earth injures me. Conversely, to restore and preserve the good health of one body and mind is to foster the well-being of the whole, the earth and all life upon it.

The center of most ancient cultures, from China in the second century B.C. to twentieth-century native America, was the earth. Human welfare was attached to the rains upon the soil, the wind of the heavens, and pliable trees embedded in an abundant forest. Chief Seattle, in 1854, summed up this ancient view of how humanity stands in relation to the world: "This we know—the earth does not belong to man, man belongs to the earth. All things are connected like the blood that unites one family. Whatever befalls the earth befalls the sons of the earth. Man did not weave the web of life; he is merely a strand of it. Whatever he does to the web, he does to himself."

Most ancient cultures, engaged in tilling, sowing, cultivating, and harvesting the soil, depended on the fruits of the land for survival. Agrarian cultures experienced power through nature and aspired to be in harmony with the seasons, rhythms, and patterns that connected all things with each other. Within this reality, the world was like a garden. The garden was nature—the living earth, the human person, the biosphere, the circle of all life.

When people are like gardens, then doctors are like gardeners. The role of the Chinese doctor is to cultivate life.

THE MOTIVE FORCE: QI

That which animates life is called *Qi* ("chee"). The concept of *Qi* is absolutely at the heart of Chinese medicine. Life is defined by *Qi* even though it is impossible to grasp, measure, quantify, see, or isolate. Immaterial yet essential, the material world is formed by it. An invisible force known only by its effects, *Qi* is recognized indirectly by what it fosters, generates, and protects.

Matter is *Qi* taking shape. Mountains forming, forests growing, rivers streaming, and creatures proliferating are all manifestations of *Qi*. In the human being, all functions of the body and mind are manifestations of *Qi*: sensing, cogitating, feeling, digesting, stirring, and propagating. *Qi* begets movement and heat. It is the fundamental mystery and miracle.

Life cannot be separated from the way it manifests. When the heart beats and the breath is warm, it is understood that life exists within the body. When the heart stops beating and the body becomes cold, the life force, or *Qi*, is no longer present. Life force and *Qi* are one. Like fresh air, healthy *Qi* moves freely; like stale air, stagnant *Qi* is heavy, oppressive, constrictive, and congestive.

Like air, *Qi* has its own movement and also activates the movement of things other than itself. Just as the wind moves the trees, grasses, and water, so *Qi* moves the chest, causing inhalation and exhalation. People do not inhale *Qi*. Rather, *Qi* is the motive force that establishes respiration. In this way, *Qi* is the cause and also the effect.

The essence of food is also a form of *Qi*. This highly refined essence is the source from which the material form of the body is constructed. When the *Qi* of food and the *Qi* of air enter the body, they become one entity known as "pure" or "righteous" *Qi*. *Air Qi* represents the immaterial motivating aspect of *Qi* and *Food Qi* the material or constructing aspect. *Qi* is both the foundation of structure and the catalyst of transformation and movement.

Scholar Nathan Sivin relates that by the year 350 in Chinese writings about nature, the word *Qi* meant "basic stuff." He comments that in Chinese thought there was a tendency

> to think of stuff and its transformations in a unitary way. . . . [Qi is] simultaneously "what makes things happen in stuff" and (depending on context) "stuff that makes things happen" or "stuff in which things happen." . . . Qi is often the material basis of activity, but the activity itself is often also described as Qi. . . . This is not an easy idea for moderns, with their clear distinction between substance and function, to grasp. The ambiguity is impossible to overlook, but discourse was adapted to it, and the readers for whom it was intended did not complain that it is confusing. By the time a medical literature developed, its authors tended to use Qi predominantly in the functional sense.[3]

Medical understanding was generated from ideas about nature. According to the ancient Chinese art of practical ecology, known as *Feng Shui* ("Wind Water"), the earth has veins of energy that course through it, hold it together, and act as a grid from which all life derives its power. The movement of wind and water reflects the activity of *Qi*.

The forces of *Qi* can work to our advantage or disadvantage. By closely observing the formation of mountains, growth of trees, flow of water, movement of wind, and patterns of light and shadow, the practitioner of *Feng*

Shui places us in a favorable relationship to these forces, to derive maximum benefit from the environment. The object is to align human dwellings, objects, and activities with the current of *Qi*. The point of focus is the relationship between the person and the patterns of *Qi*. This protects and enhances our power and good fortune. The doctor as gardener practices *Feng Shui* in that he seeks to place human beings in a beneficial relationship to *Qi*.

THE MOTIVE FORCE: QI

Qi (pronounced "chee") can be understood as the creative or formative principle associated with life and all processes that characterize living entities. All animate forms in nature are manifestations of *Qi*. *Qi* is an invisible substance, as well as an immaterial force that has palpable and observable manifestations.

Qi has its own movement and also activates the movement of things other than itself. *Qi* begets motion and heat. Within the context of the human person, *Qi* is that which enlivens the body and is differentiated according to specific functional systems. All physical and mental activities are manifestations of *Qi*: sensing, cogitating, feeling, digesting, stirring, propagating.

One Chinese ideogram for *Qi* is composed of an upper radical representing "rising vapor" and a lower radical denoting "grain." The steam that spirals from a pot of cooking rice symbolizes distilled essence, hence *Qi* can be translated as the vapor of the finest matter. The highly refined essence of food (*Food Qi*) and air (*Air Qi*) in the body become one entity known as "pure" or "righteous" *Qi*. *Defensive Qi* (*wei*) is the activity of adapting to influences such as weather or mobilizing resistance to pathogenic microorganisms and noxious substances in the environment. *Qi* refers to resources the human organism consumes, transforms, and transmits.

HEALTH IN THE GARDEN

A garden is a dynamic self-regulating system that transforms sunlight (*Yang*) and water (*Yin*) into the living tissue of vegetation. Within the cycle of seasons, there is a time for sprouting, maturing, ripening, harvesting, and composting. Through this process of transformation the garden continuously sustains and re-creates itself. This interplay of *Yin* and *Yang* is what enables life to mushroom.

Maximum growth in the garden derives from the proper balance between the heat and light of the sun with the cool moisture of water. The garden is healthy when rich growing conditions prevail and when plants are resilient enough to tolerate adversity. An occasional period of drought, a spring storm, an infestation of insects, or the moldy fungus that grows during periods of extended humidity can be overcome by a vigorous ecosystem, adaptable enough to recover once the hardship has passed.

The gardener does not make the garden grow. Nature does. The gardener is an ally who prepares the soil, sows the seeds, waters, and removes the weeds, placing plants in the proper relation to each other and the sun. If the gardener did not tend the garden, it would lose its unique identity and grow wild, merging completely with its surroundings to blend with the larger environment. The gardener protects the integrity of the garden by promoting growth in some areas, restricting it in others, adding compost to keep the soil fertile. He observes and nurtures the interaction between the garden and environment.

HEALTH IN THE MICROCOSM OF A HUMAN BEING

Both the garden and the human body are microcosms of nature. The processes, cycles, and conditions that exist in a garden can also be observed in the life of a human being.

Like the earth, the human body is enveloped and permeated by streams of *Qi* that link and enliven all its activities. The human body is subject to similar rhythms and cycles as the garden. A person both embodies and interacts with cycles—daily, monthly, seasonal, and lifelong. Over millennia doctors observed cycles in nature and conceptualized the body in these terms. They saw a human being as a complete system unto itself with constellations of subsystems within it. The body is not conceived of as cells, tissues, and other structural components. Rather it is understood in terms of the relationships among the constituents of form and process that generate, regulate, and accumulate *Blood, Moisture,* and *Qi.*

Just as earth is comprised of land, ocean, and atmosphere, so the body is organized as *Blood, Moisture,* and *Qi.* The *Blood* governs tissue, the material form of the body. The *Moisture* governs the internal environment, the body's inner ocean. The *Qi* governs the shape and activity of the body and its process of forming and organizing itself. *Qi* also means the totality of *Blood,*

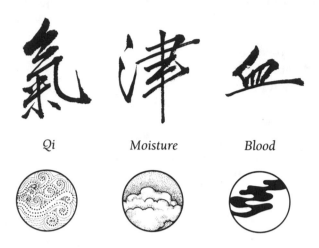

Qi   Moisture   Blood

QI, MOISTURE, BLOOD

Just as earth is comprised of land, ocean, and atmosphere, so the body is organized as *Blood*, *Moisture*, and *Qi*. *Blood* governs tissue, the material form of the body. *Moisture* governs the internal environment, the body's inner ocean. *Qi* governs the shape and activity of the body and its process of forming and organizing itself. *Qi* also implies the totality of *Blood*, *Moisture*, and *Qi*, the total summation of the life of the organism.

Blood is a material substance as well as the process of generating, distributing, and storing nutrients. *Moisture* is an amorphous substance as well as the process of generating, distributing, and storing fluid. *Qi* is an invisible substance, as well as an immaterial force that manifests as movement and activity through which it is palpable and observable. *Moisture* cannot be separated from the function of moisturizing, *Blood* from nourishing, nor *Qi* from moving. They are part of a continuum of tangible forms and immanent functions.

Within the body, every phenomenon is a product of the interaction of *Blood*, *Moisture*, and *Qi*. Without proper *Moisture*, the *Qi* becomes hot and agitated and the *Blood* dries up and congeals. Without *Blood*, *Moisture* is dispersed and *Qi* is scattered. Without *Qi*, *Moisture* and *Blood* stagnate, coagulate, and cease circulating. Each constituent exists as an individual entity and yet depends completely upon the larger system, the body. All functions and processes are interdependent, cogenerating, and mutually regulating.

Moisture, and *Qi*, earth, sea, and air, the total summation of the life of the organism, body, or world.

Within the body, every phenomenon is a product of the interaction of *Blood*, *Moisture*, and *Qi*. Without proper *Moisture*, the *Qi* becomes hot and agitated and the *Blood* dries up and congeals. Without *Blood*, *Moisture* is dispersed and *Qi* is scattered. Without *Qi*, *Moisture* and *Blood* stagnate, coagulate, and cease circulating. Each constituent exists as an individual entity and yet depends completely upon the larger system, the body. All functions and processes are interdependent, cogenerating, and mutually regulating.

Together, *Blood*, *Moisture*, and *Qi* represent the visible and invisible, gross and refined, substance and process of the soma and psyche. *Blood* is a material substance as well as the process of generating, distributing, and storing nutrients. *Moisture* is an amorphous substance as well as the process of generating, distributing, and storing fluid. *Qi* is an invisible substance, as well as an immaterial force that manifests as movement and activity through which it is palpable and observable. *Moisture* cannot be separated from the function of moisturizing, *Blood* from nourishing, nor *Qi* from moving. They are part of a continuum of tangible forms and immanent functions. Just as ice, water, and steam are three manifestations of the same molecular entity, *Blood*, *Moisture*, and *Qi* are three manifestations of the same "life force." In death, a disorganization of the continuum occurs: tissue and spirit become separated from form and process.

PATTERNS OF HARMONY IN THE HUMAN GARDEN

Nature, like a symphony, is composed of complex interweaving patterns of form and movement. These patterns are recapitulated in every smaller system. The body is to nature as a violin is to an orchestra. The strings are to a violin as the organs are to the body. The musical vibrations of each string are like the functions of each organ. For the orchestra to play a symphony in harmony, all the instruments must be tuned to each other—all the strings of each instrument and all the notes of each string must be played in tune. If a single instrument is out of tune, the whole sound is dissonant rather than harmonious.

This illustrates an aspect of Chinese philosophy known as the theory of correspondence. Simply, this theory states that in order for a larger system to be in balance as a whole, each smaller system within it must itself be balanced. This principle of harmony is the same at each level of complexity. Patterns of harmony in one system both reflect and generate patterns of harmony in other systems, as well as at greater and lesser orders of complexity.

Correspondence thinking postulates that events occur in association with each other, linked by a mutual force regardless of their location in time and space. Qi is the medium that links all events with each other, transcending time and space because patterns are formed that persist beyond their moment of origin. Causal thinking, which dominates Western philosophy, postulates that events occur in a series, like a line of falling dominoes, one act triggering another in spatio-temporal sequence. As we have seen, Western medicine emphasizes the single cause that triggers a particular pathologic or physiologic process. The linear continuum of time and space links events, and an occurrence in the past only influences a current condition indirectly through the causal chain. Chinese medicine, on the other hand, presumes that if you reorganize the existing pattern of disharmony into a harmonic pattern of relationships, the original cause will disappear because the conditions in which it was rooted cease to exist. Chinese medicine treats conditions, whereas Western medicine treats causes. For the doctor of Chinese medicine the issue is the same as for the conductor of a symphony: it is not how the instrument makes sound, but rather the pattern of sound that the instrument emits.

LOSS OF ADAPTIVE ABILITY: DISEASE

In Chinese medicine, health is the ability of an organism to respond appropriately to a wide variety of challenges in a way that insures maintaining equilibrium and integrity. Disease represents a failure to adapt to challenge, a disruption of the overall equilibrium, and a rent in the fabric of the organism.

The source of disease is any challenge to the body with which it is unable to cope, whether it is a harmful substance or a bad feeling. Disease is a manifestation of an unstable process, a pattern of disharmonious relationships. When defenses are weakened and resources exhausted, a multiplicity of factors conspire to permit illness. The adage "The man is not sick because he has an illness, but has an illness because he is sick" aptly expresses this view.

Lack of sunlight, depletion of the soil, overgrowth of weeds, all restrict the bounty of the garden. Similarly, deficiency or excess of Qi, inadequate nutrition, or poor circulation of Blood and Moisture weaken health. Too much sun burns the plants, too much wind dries them out, too much water rots their roots. Yet in the absence of light, water, and air, the plants cannot germinate or grow. The climates, emotions, and activities of life are not

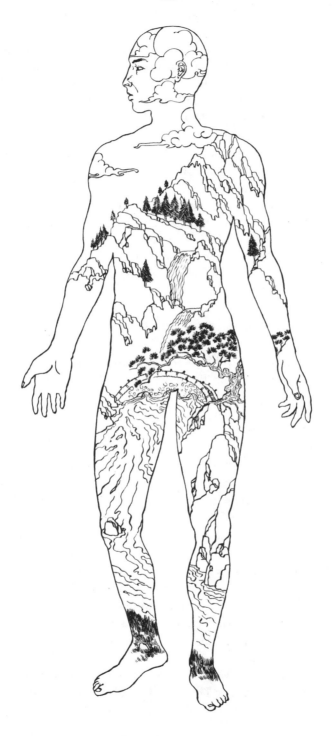

The Body As Garden

intrinsically good or bad. It is their excess or deficiency that distorts the pattern of flow.

The gardener may occasionally need to apply strong measures like poison or fire to control marauding insects or weeds. But he has to be careful not to damage the garden irreparably while he is attacking the pest. Doctors as gardeners protect the Qi at the same time as they attack the disease. Simultaneous with the struggle to fight the disease, the doctor of Chinese medicine strives to restore the resilience and strength of the body. This adaptability and fortitude constitutes the condition of health. If in the process of attacking the disease the Qi is dissipated, this undermines a person's capacity to recover health.

The gardener is like the herbalist when he nourishes with compost or adds minerals to the soil, using material substances to promote growth. And he is like the acupuncturist when he builds fences, digs ditches, ponds, and channels for irrigation, adjusting the flow of water and wind.

OBSERVING THE SIGNS: DIAGNOSIS

The gardener crumbles the soil between his fingers; he looks, listens, senses, kneeling among the plants. On the basis of his observations, he judges the garden's needs. When the plants look lush and full, he assumes conditions are right for proper growth. If the leaves are yellowed and floppy, he may see this as a sign that the soil is too damp, so the roots can't breathe. He can raise the bed and aerate the soil, permitting better drainage. If the leaves are withered, dry, and spindly, the gardener should water more frequently. When the garden grows but does not produce fruit, more nutriment has been used than has been replenished and the gardener enriches the soil with compost.

Like the gardener, the doctor observes the patient and perceives signs and symptoms to determine the nature of the problem at hand. He synthesizes all impressions to make a diagnosis. The doctor's diagnosis may sound similar to the gardener's. They use the same vocabulary. Both are concerned with the balance of heat and cold, moisture and dryness, and the excess or deficiency of these conditions. A person, like a garden, is subject to external excesses of *Heat, Cold, Wind, Dampness,* and *Dryness,* as well as to deficiencies of *Blood, Moisture,* and *Qi.*

For example, a lack of *Moisture* manifesting as cracked skin or scanty urine is a symptom of *Dryness.* This may be caused by a dry climate or may simply mean that the body is unable to properly distribute its own fluids.

In Chinese medicine the diagnosis is *Dryness* regardless of whether it originates from an external climate or an internal condition. It is the relationship between the body and water that keeps the tissues moisturized. The body must be able to absorb, store, and circulate moisture in order to adequately hydrate the cells. If any of these functions breaks down, symptoms of dehydration will appear. A person with diabetes, for instance, can drink a great deal of water and still remain very thirsty because the body is unable to retain the fluid. In fact, twice as much fluid may be lost through urination than is consumed. According to Chinese medicine, diabetes is described as severe *Dryness* or deficiency of *Moisture*. The reasoning is correlative and axiomatic: *Dryness* causes *Dryness* to manifest, *Dryness* causes deficiency of *Moisture*, a deficiency of *Moisture* may cause *Dryness*. Cause and effect are difficult to distinguish. They mutually generate each other and arise simultaneously.

The logic is one of correspondence: things that correspond to the same thing correspond with each other. To illustrate, when *Fire* burns the skin, it causes redness, swelling, and pain. When these symptoms arise spontaneously, they are considered to be due to the presence of internal *Fire* or *Heat*. The source of the *Fire* cannot be seen, only its effects. Since *Heat* produces inflammation, symptoms of inflammation are referred to as signs of *Heat*.

Similarly, a person exposed to *Cold* shivers and becomes lethargic, dull, and unresponsive. When such symptoms arise regardless of the external temperature, the person is manifesting the condition of internal *Coldness*. *Coldness* is associated with the signs and symptoms of lowered metabolic activity: depressed mental function, retarded circulation, weakness, and malaise. Again, the cause and the effect are inseparable.

This system of correspondence describes the parallelism and synchronicity of events in the inner and outer world of the human organism. All phenomena are ordered according to the *Five Phases* of *Wood*, *Fire*, *Earth*, *Metal*, and *Water*, which represent five evolutionary stages of transformation and correspond with five *Organ Networks*, five seasons, five climates, and five personality types. The workings of the body are associated with each of the seasonal cycles of birth, growth, ripening, harvest, and decay. Each of the five *Organ Networks* performs a function within the cycle. Analogous to the five climates and seasons in nature is the internal milieu generated by each of the *Organ Networks*. Disturbance of the internal milieu may provoke the *Liver* to generate *Wind*, the *Heart* to generate *Heat*, the *Spleen* to generate *Dampness*, the *Lungs* to generate *Dryness*, and the *Kidneys* to generate *Cold*.

According to this correspondence logic, various conditions of distress are linked with each *Network*. The *Network* responsible for digestion is the *Spleen*. Any problem of indigestion is related to it. This *Network* is also

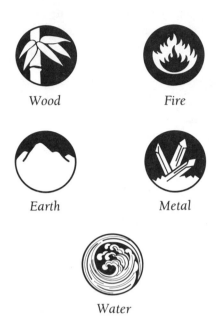

Wood   Fire

Earth   Metal

Water

The theory of correspondence describes the parallelism and synchronicity of events in the inner and outer world of the human organism. All phenomena are ordered according to *Yin Yang* and the *Five Phases* of *Wood*, *Fire*, *Earth*, *Metal*, and *Water*, which represent five sorts of fundamental process, each of which corresponds with five *Organ Networks*, five seasons, five climates, and five personality types. The workings of the body are associated with each of the seasonal cycles of evolutionary transformation: birth, growth, ripening, harvest, and decay. Each of the five *Organ Networks* performs a function within the cycle. Analogous to the five climates and seasons in nature is the internal milieu generated by each of the *Organ Networks*.

Categories

sky

time

season

temperature

humidity

spectrum

realm

solidity

texture

mass

stages

form

dimension

locale

internal organs

constituents

processes

temperature

capacity

stages

Yin-Yang Correspondences

Yin	Yang
macrocosm	
moon	sun
midnight	midday
winter	summer
cold	hot
wetness	dryness
dark	luminous
hidden	revealed
dense	porous
hard	soft
heavy	light
forming	transforming
material substance	subtle influences
human microcosm	
feelings and thoughts	response and expression
core—interior of body	surface—exterior of body
below navel	above navel
right side	left side
Liver, Heart, Spleen, Lung, Kidney	*Gall Bladder, Small Intestine, Stomach, Large Intestine, Bladder*
Blood and metabolic fluids (*Yin* essence)	*Qi* and metabolic heat (*Yang* essence)
buildup of tissue (anabolism)	breakdown of tissue (catabolism)
coldness	heat
weakness and depletion (empty)	strength and repletion (full)
decline/death/gestation	birth/growth/maturation

Categories	Wood	Fire
macrocosm		
power	expansion	completion
climate	wind	heat
season	spring	summer
direction	east	south
time	dawn	noon
stage	birth	growth
color	aquamarine	red
odor	rancid	acrid
flavor	sour	bitter
sound	crashing	roaring
human microcosm:		
faculty	active awareness (*hun*)	transcendent awareness (*shen*)
motive	self-serving	self-dissolving
quality	emotive	sensitive
activity	implementing	intuiting
expression	anger	joy
condition	arousal	excitement
voice	hollering	giggling
organ	*Liver Network*	*Heart Network*
tissue	eyes, nails, ligaments, nerves	external ear, tongue, arteries
substance	nutrified blood	oxygenated blood
essence	tears	sweat

Earth	Metal	Water
transition	contraction	consolidation
humidity	dryness	cold
late summer	autumn	winter
center	west	north
late afternoon	dusk	midnight
maturity	degeneration	death/germination
yellow-ocher	white	black/purple
fragrant	fishy	rotten
sweet	spicy	salty
humming	cracking	sucking
passive awareness (*yi*)	subliminal awareness (*po*)	primal awareness (*zhi*)
self-locating	self-defining	self-preserving
reflective	deductive	instinctive
absorbing	analyzing	scanning
rumination	sorrow	fear
poise	inhibition	withdrawal
quavering	sobbing	groaning
Spleen Network	*Lung Network*	*Kidney Network*
mouth, lips, gums, muscles, collagen, and fat	skin and pores, body hair, lymph vessels, and veins	inner ear, head and pubic hair, bones, teeth, and marrow, brain and spinal cord, anus, urethra, cervix, ovaries, and testes
chyme and chyle	lymph	cerebrospinal fluid
saliva	mucus	sexual secretions

associated with the capacity to formulate ideas and focus attention. Thus, a problem related to foggy thinking and poor concentration may also be related to excess *Dampness* affecting the *Spleen*. Similarly, the *Liver Network* regulates the smooth flow of *Qi*. Excess *Wind* affecting the *Liver* induces erratic behavior, uneven emotions, or uncoordinated movement.

In this way, Chinese medicine reveals the impact of distress upon the whole person—disease reshapes mental, emotional, and physical life. Like a weatherman, the doctor of Chinese medicine forecasts the onslaught of stormy weather and predicts who is likely to get what.

Five types of people emerge from the configurations of physique and character that correspond with the *Five Phases* and *Organ Networks*. Not by an act of will, but out of their predispositions, habits, and tendencies, these types "make their diseases," manifesting the strengths and weaknesses of their nature. Earth becomes easily oversaturated, and the *Earth* type generates phlegm, edema, and mental quagmires. Fire flares easily, and the *Fire* type produces inflammation, dehydration, and high anxiety. Wood proliferates rapidly, and the *Wood* type provokes trembling, cramping, and rage. Water hardens and freezes, and the *Water* type develops sclerosis, arthritis, and indifference. Metal cuts away and restricts, and the *Metal* type becomes breathless, stiff, and unarouseable.

PROBLEMS IN SEARCH OF A SOLUTION: TREATMENT

If the cause of disease is understood as imbalance, then the goal of treatment is to recover balance. Problems are resolved through methods of complementarity. To resolve conditions of *Cold*, apply warmth; to resolve *Heat*, apply cool. Stimulate movement to relieve stasis and astringe leakage to protect depleted reserves. Disperse excess, strengthen weakness, moisten *Dryness*, drain *Wetness*. When the *Spleen* is excessive, strengthen the *Liver* to counterbalance it, and when the *Spleen* is deficient, strengthen the *Heart* to nurture it.

Acupuncture and herbs are the primary techniques that evoke the self-regulating response of the organism to reorganize and replenish the *Qi*, *Moisture*, and *Blood*. Each method works by a different mechanism. Acupuncture adjusts the density and flow of *Qi* in the channels, which in turn affects the circulation of *Blood* and *Moisture* and the function of the internal organs. Herbs also affect the quantity and quality of *Blood*, *Moisture*, and *Qi* through their impact on the organs via the digestive and metabolic systems. Together these methods perform the therapeutic tasks of reorganizing the internal milieu, maximizing the flexibility and adaptability of the organism.

There are as many treatment approaches as there are individuals. Chinese medicine can formulate a treatment according to the particular expression of an illness. There are almost limitless combinations of acupuncture points and herbs to meet the needs of diverse patients. A given herb or acupuncture point eliminates the *Damp Heat* that may be expressed as herpes, while others relieve the *Coldness* that engenders the stiffness and spasm of arthritis. The single symptom, such as a cough, may arise as a consequence of *Wind, Cold, Heat, Dampness,* or *Dryness* affecting the *Organ Network* of the *Lung* or *Kidney.* Different herbs and acupuncture points would be selected for each different type of cough. The doctor combines patterns of points and herbs the way the gardener combines irrigation, composting, hoeing, and weeding to eliminate obstructions, nurture growth, and maintain integrity.

THE GARDENER AND THE MECHANIC

In ancient China ancestors were worshiped and revered. They were considered a more significant part of the community than the living insofar as they were thought to rule the world. The dead were not seen as separate from the living; death was an important, revered stage of life, not merely the end of it. Anatomical dissection of a dead body would have been disrespectful and, for that reason, utterly forbidden. Doctors were only allowed to study living bodies. Nonliving process could not be examined, and the whole could not be divided into parts.

In the Western scientific model, life is dissected into separable, discrete parts within the context of a fixed and stable environment that can be measured objectively. In the Chinese model, life is about the dynamic, constantly shifting relationships of one functional system with another, always within the context of the whole system. No aspects of the personality or body function as independent, discrete entities.

Interaction occurs at every level. Our emotions shape our body; our body generates feeling. The state of the *Liver* affects the function of the *Heart.* The function of the *Heart* affects the expression of the personality. The logic is circular and each person is an interconnected *Network.*

The models of East and West are different, as is the point of view, the emphasis, methods, outcomes.[4] What works in the garden may be inappropriate in the factory. Compost doesn't nourish a machine, and oil and gasoline do not enhance the soil. Chinese medicine readjusts balance, enhancing self-healing and helping chronic, long-term problems. Western medicine affects the structural components, suppressing and eliminating pathologic phenomena, intervening in life-threatening crises.

Within the vocabulary of Western medicine, disease is defined as either "organic" (that which interferes with the structure of the tissue) or "functional" (anything that is not caused by an objectively determined structural abnormality). Since disease is understood primarily as a defect of structure, there is no "real" basis for a functional disorder.

Functional problems like migraine, fatigue, mental illness, colitis, rheumatism, asthma, menstrual cramps, and so on are often referred to as "psychosomatic" since they cannot be shown to originate in the body and are therefore relegated to the mysterious realm of the psyche. A strength of Chinese medicine lies in its power to detect and meaningfully describe dysfunction even though the structure appears intact and physically sound. Rather than look for abnormalities of structure, Chinese medicine looks for disharmonies of Qi that, over time, can affect structure but may appear prior to gross manifestations of or clinically diagnosed disease.

This ability to read the body before structural damage occurs sometimes enables Chinese medicine to prevent disease before it develops, to slow down its progress, or perhaps even to halt degenerative processes such as arteriosclerosis, arthritis, and nervous and autoimmune disorders. It also enables the doctor of Chinese medicine to effectively treat problems for which Western medicine has no known treatment.

However, once structural damage has occurred, there is no pathologist to look at cells under a microscope to determine what is malignant carcinoma or what bacteria are responsible for a given infection. There is no surgeon to remove a damaged organ or liberate a healthy baby trapped in her mother's womb. Chinese medicine does not separate the problem from the person who has it—this is both its strength and weakness. Similarly, Western medicine's capacity to do just that accounts for its great technological success and also for some of its more serious limitations.

There is value in each and both. Claude Bernard, a French physician in the late nineteenth century, claimed that the *milieu intérieur*, the condition of the person, was the critical factor in health and disease. This position was overshadowed by Louis Pasteur's assertion of the germ theory, stating that external attack by microbes was more significant than the soil or climate in which disease flourished. The focus shifted from the state of the organism to the attacking pathogen, from the person to the disease. This shift has come to characterize Western medicine, regardless of whispers from Pasteur on his deathbed that Bernard was right.

Now another shift is beginning to gain momentum, thanks to a shrinking planet and an expanding paradigm. With the growing accessibility of Chinese medicine, the strengths of both medical technologies might be combined, minimizing the weaknesses of each.

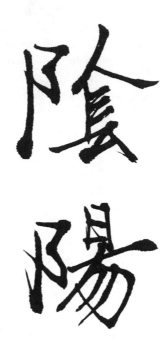

Yin-Yang

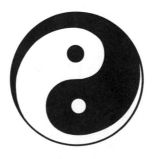

Yin-Yang Symbol

CHAPTER FOUR

CYCLES OF CIRCLES:
A THEORY OF RELATIVITY
YIN-YANG

Heaven was created by an accumulation of Yang; the Earth was created by an accumulation of Yin. Water and fire are the symbols of Yin and Yang; Yin and Yang are the source of power and the beginning of everything in creation. Yang ascends to Heaven; Yin descends to Earth. Hence the universe represents motion and rest, controlled by the wisdom of nature. Nature grants the power to beget and to grow, to harvest and to store, to finish and to begin anew.

Ilza Veith, *Nei Ching*

BEFORE LEARNING CHINESE MEDICINE, I STUDIED WITH SOCIAL THEORISTS influenced by Hegel, a German idealist philosopher. The relational, interactive, process-oriented thinking of Chinese medicine resembles Hegelian dialectics. This was not altogether coincidence since many European philosophers were affected by Eastern thought. It was this similarity that charmed me from the start. Because Chinese medicine was about interwoven relationships and continuous processes of decaying and becoming rather than a reductionist examination of things in and of themselves, I had eagerly anticipated studying it.

Dialectical logic captures *Yin-Yang* thinking. Within dialectics the whole is a contingent structure, in reciprocal interaction with its own parts and with the larger whole of which it is a part. As parts and wholes evolve as a consequence of their relationship, constants become variables, causes become effects, and systems develop that regenerate and destroy the conditions that gave rise to them.[1]

OPPOSITION AND UNITY

The Tao is an undifferentiated whole. It is both the unity of all things and the way the universe works. Out of this oneness emerges *Yin-Yang*: the world in its infinite forms. *Yin-Yang* is a symbolic representation of universal process that portrays a changing rather than static picture of reality. The *Yin-Yang* model is also used to differentiate aspects of process. Within the magnetic field of fundamental opposition and creative tension, each aspect interrelates, interpenetrates, and depends upon the other. The poles of a unified whole are characterized in relation to each other, revolving cycles of the "one" becoming the "other." *Yin-Yang* can be a difficult concept for Westerners to grasp because it escapes strict either-or categories that are fixed and concrete. Wholly relative in its designations, *Yin-Yang* depends entirely on the point of view of the observer, as this Taoist poem reflects:

> To the frogs in a temple pool
> The Lotus stems are tall;
> To the gods of Mount Everest
> An elephant is small.

All things have a polar nature: time is divided into day and night and summer and winter, gender into male and female, place into heaven and earth, temperature into hot and cold, direction into up and down, space into

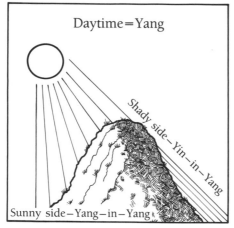
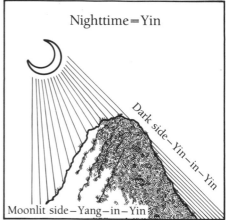

The *Yin-Yang* of the Mountain

The shady side of the mountain is *Yin* in relation to the sunny side, which is *Yang*. As the sun rises and moves across the sky, however, the warmth and light of the morning upon the one slope shifts to the other slope in the afternoon—the sunny and shady sides merge and alternate. *Yang* becomes *Yin*, and *Yin* becomes *Yang*. As the day becomes night, the entire mountain is dark, cool, and quiescent. In the night when the moon shines on the mountain, the light of the moon is *Yang* within the dark *Yin* of night.

inside and outside, and so on. But designations of *Yin* or *Yang* are made only in relation to each other. For example, the sun is bigger, brighter, hotter (*Yang*) in relation to the earth, which is smaller, darker, and cooler (*Yin*). The earth, however, is more *Yang* in relation to the moon, which is more *Yin*. *Yin* and *Yang* cannot be separated. There is no dark without light, no front without back, no up without down, no in without out, and no heat without cold. There is no space without time, no birth without death.

Yin also appears within *Yang*, and vice versa. For example, if *Yang* is considered to be warm, expanding, and light, and *Yin* is cool, contracting, and dark, then the shady side of the mountain is *Yin* in relation to the sunny side of the mountain, which is *Yang*. As the sun rises and moves across the sky in relation to the mountain, however, the warmth and light of the morning upon the one slope shifts to the other slope in the afternoon—the sunny and shady sides merge and alternate. *Yang* becomes *Yin*, and *Yin* becomes *Yang*. As the day becomes night, the entire mountain is dark, cool, and quiescent. In the night when the moon shines on the mountain, the light of the moon is *Yang* within the dark *Yin* of night.

DESIGNATIONS OF YIN-YANG

Because everything is in motion, all process is cyclic, and everything contains its opposite, the dilemma of what came first, the chicken or the egg, is transcended in Chinese philosophy by accepting them as inseparable agents of the process of creation. Chinese theory does not separate cause from effect; instead, the one invariably turns into the other in an ever-repeating cycle of metamorphosis. The day does not cause the night, birth does not cause death, summer does not cause winter, but one precedes and the other follows. Life is a game of leapfrog with events tumbling over each other in a perpetual cascade. The chicken makes the egg—*Yang* generates *Yin*—but the chicken grows out of the egg—*Yin* produces *Yang*. They are only mutually generative. Which came first (linear logic) matters less than how they interact (systems, dialectical, relational logic).

All states, events, and moments can be characterized as being *Yin* or *Yang*, relative aspects of an alternating cycle along a single continuum. *Yin* is at the core, sinking, condensed, and internal. *Yang* is at the surface, rising, dispersed, and external. The humidity of the air accumulates and condenses into clouds. This dense mass of vapor (*Yin*) builds until the moment of discharge (*Yang*), when the weight and density of the moisture transforms into thunder, lightning, and rain. Relative to each other, *Yin* is quiescent, static, and contracting, whereas *Yang* is dynamic, active, and expansive.

Yin responds to *Yang*'s stimulus, and *Yang* is supported by the solidity of *Yin*. *Yin* is dense and hidden, while *Yang* is dispersed and exposed. In a   51

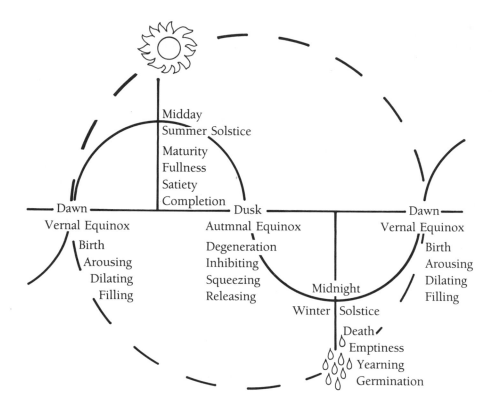

Midday
Summer Solstice

Maturity
Fullness
Satiety
Completion

Dawn
Vernal Equinox
Birth
Arousing
Dilating
Filling

Dusk
Autmnal Equinox
Degeneration
Inhibiting
Squeezing
Releasing

Midnight
Winter Solstice
Death
Emptiness
Yearning
Germination

Dawn
Vernal Equinox
Birth
Arousing
Dilating
Filling

Yin-Yang Tidal Flow of Rhythm

The processes in nature and in the life of living organisms correspond to the stages of transformation of *Yin-Yang* manifested by seasonal, diurnal, developmental, and physiological cycles of flourishing and withering, lightening and darkening, beginning and ending, expanding and contracting.

candle, the beeswax and wick are the material foundation: solid, heavy, *Yin*; the flame, which moves upward, is insubstantial in nature: bright, hot, *Yang*. The interaction of the two is what produces the useful light and heat and reflects the interaction of matter and energy. Their dependence on each other renders them inseparable. *Yang* makes things happen. It transforms. *Yin* provides the material basis for the transforming power of *Yang*. Energy—heat, activity, light—transforms matter. If *Yin* is a noun, then *Yang* is a verb, and life is a complete sentence.

52

If *Yin-Yang* is likened to a battleground, the fort represents the *Yin*. Relatively hidden and protected from threat, it shelters the noncombatants and food. The fort stores the potential or reserve energy. The field of battle is exposed, relatively unprotected, *Yang*. Upon it the precious stored-up *Yin* substance is transformed into *Yang* activity.

Health is defined as the poised balance between *Yin-Yang*, and sickness is the result of a deficiency or excess, a *Yin-Yang* disharmony. Survival is based on an organism's capacity to adapt to changing conditions and maintain equilibrium. *Yin-Yang* harmony is a metaphor for sustaining adaptability and equilibrium.

YIN-YANG AND THE HUMAN BODY

Yin-Yang also describes human process. The stages of life go from conception to birth, growth, decline, and death. Our youth (*Yang*) is like the hare— quick, capricious, erratic, and light. Our older years (*Yin*) are more like the tortoise—slow, deliberate, dense, and persevering.

When we expand and fill out chests with air, we are in the *Yang* phase of respiration; when we exhale and empty our lungs, we are in the contractive *Yin* phase. We perpetually fill and empty our stomachs, our lungs, our hearts, our minds. We are active (*Yang*) and lie quiet and rest (*Yin*).

Yin is the material basis, tissue, for the transforming power of *Yang*, which reorganizes and regenerates. Food (*Yin*) is transmuted by metabolic activity (*Yang*) into more substance (tissue) and more energy (heat and metabolic activity). The sperm (*Yang*) joins the egg (*Yin*), and new life is created by their merger and interaction. Thus the sperm mobilizes and transforms the substance provided by the egg. The sperm derives its propulsive and activating power from the male (*Yang*), and the egg derives its receptive and nurturing power from the female (*Yin*).

The internal organs of the body, hidden and protected from external influence, are *Yin* relative to the exposed skin and muscle, which are *Yang*. The lower part of the body is in contact or rooted to the ground, *Yin*, whereas the upper body is able to move freely, *Yang*, even when the legs are rigid. The front of the body is protected by folding the arms and legs to enclose the chest and abdomen, whereas the back of the body is relatively exposed. Hence the front is more *Yin* relative to the back, which is *Yang*.

Immunity functions as the first line of defense: guarding the surface protects against internal harm. Using our battle analogy, the field army wards off attacks on the fort. If they get cut off from the fort, the troops will run out of ammunition and food. If the *Yang* is weak, the body is unable to ward off attack and enemy forces penetrate the protective walls. If the *Yin* forces of the fort are not strong, supplies and food are insufficient to meet the 53 fighters' need to refuel the energy they have expended. The *Yin* fort provides the substance that sustains the *Yang* activity in the field. Without substance, activity is weakened; without activity, substance is insecure and unprotected. They mutually support each other as an interdependent and indivisible system.

The exterior surface of the human body (skin, hair, superficial nerves, and blood vessels) is exposed and therefore *Yang*. The internal structures (viscera, bones, brain, and spinal cord) are the basis of sustenance and therefore *Yin*. The internal *Organs* can be further differentiated into the "hollow" *Organs* (*Yang*), which perform functions of digestion and elimination (catabolism), and the "solid" *Organs* (*Yin*), which perform the function of assimilation and storage (anabolism). The solid *Organs* are analogous to the rock that soaks up the sunlight and stores this energy as heat for later use, much like a passive solar heater. The hollow *Organs* can be likened to a water wheel, which is capable of transforming the movement of water into energy for work. The water wheel itself cannot store up energy, and the heated rock cannot perform work directly.

Together, as *Yin* and *Yang*, a paired solid and hollow *Organ* comprise *Organ Networks* (commonly referred to by the *Yin Organ* name). The dense *Yin Organs* of the *Liver, Heart, Spleen, Lung,* and *Kidney* store the essential and potential energy derived from substances; the hollow *Yang Organs* of the *Gallbladder, Small Intestine, Stomach, Large Intestine,* and *Bladder* process the substances of the external environment. However, *Yin* and *Yang* are relative, not absolute designations: the *Heart* is a "solid" *Organ* and therefore *Yin*, yet its propulsive contraction while squeezing the blood through the vessels is *Yang*. This is what is meant by the *Yang* within the *Yin*.

QI, MOISTURE, AND BLOOD

In the human body, *Qi* and *Blood* are manifestations of *Yang* and *Yin* respectively. The concept of substance as *Yin* and activity as *Yang* is illustrated by the following: the *Blood* itself is *Yin*; the activity of the blood circulating is *Yang*. The mucus itself is *Yin*; its secretion, movement, and expectoration are *Yang*. Urine and perspiration are *Yin*; the filtration process that generates urine and the heat that promotes perspiration is *Yang*. Nutrient substances are *Yin*; the metabolic activity of digestion is *Yang*.

Water has a *Yin* nature. *Blood* has a *Yin* nature. Like water, *Blood* is a soft, yielding substance that takes on the form of its container. Moist and dense, it is the medium for the nutritive essence that feeds the tissues of the body. The *Blood* is also considered the medium of the mind insofar as it carries information (in Western terms this takes the form of chemical messengers or hormones) that regulates body function. *Blood* has the nature of

Yin, but *Yin* is not the same as *Blood*. *Yin* is a universal principle, a concept, an aspect of a dynamic process, whereas *Blood* is a substance that exists in the living body. The *Qi* (*Yang*) moves the *Blood* (*Yin*).

Fire has a *Yang* nature. *Qi* has a *Yang* nature. Like fire, *Qi* is insubstantial, mobile, changeable, a catalyst for movement and transformation. In fact, *Qi* is synonymous with movement and process. *Blood* and *Qi* are as inseparable as *Yin-Yang*. If they are separated, the *Blood* does not move and the *Qi* has no basis, so there is no life. Based on these principles, the circulation of *Blood* is induced by the sucking and squeezing action of the lung, which moves the *Qi* throughout the body. Blocking this flow of *Qi* inhibits the circulation of *Blood*. Obstructing *Blood* exhausts *Qi*. When the muscles are not active and the vessels cannot pulsate, the *Blood* will not circulate. This happens when people who are bedridden over a long period develop stasis ulcers or bed sores. Lack of activity leads to a stagnation of *Blood* and *Moisture*, which in turn leads to degeneration and death of tissue.

Yang also corresponds to the basal metabolic state. The warmth that we associate with life when a person is completely at rest (as in deep sleep or coma) belongs to *Yang*. There may be no perceptible movement or activity, yet if the body is warm with moist vapor being exhaled, then we know the person is alive. *Yang* and *Yin* are the fundament from which *Qi* and *Blood* derive their existence—just as the mother gives birth to the child, but the child grows on its own.

Moisture is the intermediate state of *Blood* generating to *Qi* and *Qi* transforming *Blood*. *Qi*, *Moisture*, and *Blood* can each be located on the *Yin-Yang* continuum as differentiated manifestations of the unitary life force, which is also *Qi*.

EVERYDAY LIFE

The course of our everyday lives requires that we balance the interior process of nurturing the self (*Yin*) with being engaged in the exterior work of the world (*Yang*). Our activity in the world fosters our productivity, then we retreat from the business of the day each evening to relax, rest, and sleep in order to accumulate and replenish our store of *Qi* for the day to follow.

Our contemporary culture encourages constant, often frenetic, activity. People are so consumed with their productivity that they often neglect allowing enough time for the self to be replenished. To overwork, overexercise, overparty, and overengage in the act of love is to overindulge in *Yang*, which leads to burnout of *Yin*. The body cannot for long tolerate consuming more than is replaced. The consequences of this may be muscle, joint, bone, heart, or kidney problems perhaps as serious and sudden as a heart attack.

On the other hand, to be preoccupied with matters of internal health and overly focused on nourishing and protecting the delicate interior of the body could mean an overemphasis on the *Yin* phase of accumulation. A collector who keeps acquiring more and more goods that have potential value is so busy amassing and storing that he has no time or energy left to put his hidden treasures to use in the productive life of the world. The *Yin* is protected, but the *Yang* is lifeless. Similarly, a person who is all mass or substance (*Yin*) and no energy (*Yang*) is lethargic, inert, and cannot work or play well. Without exercise the muscles atrophy and the cardiovascular system weakens.

The key is to achieve balance, which means being flexible, diverse, moderate, and in harmony with your own rhythms and needs. Chinese medicine makes use of acupuncture, herbs, diet, physical exercise, massage, mental discipline, and the modification of life-style habits as forms of therapy to reestablish the rhythmic swing of the *Yin-Yang* pendulum.

YIN-YANG CHARACTER PATTERNS

Some people can be characterized as being more *Yang* or *Yin*, based on their character and body structure. Yet it is common for people to manifest qualities of both, such as inhabiting a relatively *Yin* body with a more *Yang* personality.

A *Yang* body is larger, stronger, more tense, springy, and muscular, with a greater capacity for food and activity and a minimal requirement for rest. *Yang* prefers and feels comfortable in a stimulating, complex environment and acts quickly and impulsively as if endowed with an unlimited supply of stamina and invincible immunity to harm. It is a predilection of *Yang* to overindulge without severe consequences and, when sick, to suffer intensely and recover quickly.

A *Yin* body is smaller, more slender and sinewy, and soft and dense rather than tense. To be *Yin* is to enjoy quiet, calm, simple environments and possess a more limited capacity for food, work, and interaction. It is a preference of *Yin* to avoid prolonged stress and to desire regular, adequate periods for rest and rejuvenation. *Yin* illnesses develop gradually, and symptoms linger. *Yin* tends to be more conservative and efficient, again, more like the tortoise than the hare. *Yang* is not necessarily healthier than *Yin*. A person with a more *Yin* constitution may live longer and accomplish more because his or her life-style and environment are less stressful. A more *Yang* individual is likely to suffer the long-term consequences of abuse, neglect, and shortsightedness.

My father is more *Yang*, and I'm more *Yin*—he strains to sit still and relax, whereas I am content to abandon myself, reading and reflecting for hours. He drives himself hard. In 1972 a heart attack motivated him to stop smoking cigarettes or taking calls that required him to perform emergency surgery in the middle of the night. Since his heart attack seemed related to emotional stress as well, he became more conscious about his state of mind, avoiding upsets when he could. Although he didn't understand himself in *Yin-Yang* terms, through his actions he had begun to modulate his extreme *Yang* by better protecting his *Yin*. I, on the other hand, needed not to slow down my level of activity, but rather to do more physically. Jogging felt too incompatible with my nature, so I stimulate my *Yin* with *Yang* activity by swimming daily, doing t'ai chi ch'uan (Chinese movement exercise), and walking.

In our culture, the characteristics of *Yang* are often regarded as being more desirable than those of *Yin*. It is better to be a rabbit than a turtle. The aggressive, hard-driving, ambitious, upwardly mobile personality is admired and rewarded. Our cultural heroes and heroines are Paul Bunyan, John Henry, Superman, Wonder Woman, and James Bond. Great physical prowess, a certain clever cunning, and audacious savvy are *Yang* characteristics. In Asian culture the opposite is true. In the Orient it is the wise sage who is distinguished not by his physique, but by his hidden powers of wisdom and philosophy.

Cultural judgments aside, to say someone is *Yin* or *Yang* does not necessarily imply that one is strong or weak, healthy or sick, but more describes *how* someone is strong, weak, or sick. Recognition of *Yin-Yang* patterns helps us observe how we live our lives and predict the ways in which we will become ill and can be treated.

When *Yin* is overabundant, *Yang* collapses, overcome by cold, static inertia. When *Yang* is overabundant, it exhausts the *Yin*, depleting *Blood* and *Moisture*, which results in emaciation. A cold and weak (*Yin*) person needs to stay warm by dressing appropriately and eating warming foods. A hot and hyperactive (*Yang*) person needs to guard against dissipating *Qi* by overuse and abuse and by learning to relax, exercise self-restraint, and be patient.

Whereas the *Yang* type is subject to delusions of boundless, superhuman strength, the *Yin* type is subject to fears of inadequacy. Through profligacy, the *Yang* type can become weakened or deficient and therefore more *Yin*. The *Yin* type, through conservation, can acquire increased energy and expand limits, becoming more *Yang*. Each can learn from the other: *Yang* can benefit from the long-term and thrifty perspective of *Yin*; *Yin* can learn to focus, express, and actualize energy more like *Yang*. *Yang* needs *Yin* for its foundation, and *Yin* needs *Yang* for its fruition.

Yang types tend to become *Yin* deficient and *Yin* types tend to become *Yang* deficient. People who lack *Yang* have trouble rising with the dawn and kindling their morning fire. They crave sunlight, warmth, and enjoy spring and summer. Since their own fire is low, they benefit from outside stimulation that awakens, motivates, and activates them. They might be likened to snakes and lizards, which are difficult to arouse until after they have basked on a warm rock in the sun. Someone who is *Yang* deficient and lives in a cold climate will be challenged to maintain circulation, digestion, enthusiasm, and libido because their limited fire is being used to sustain basic survival.

Yang easily becomes overextended by vibrating at a high frequency, like the honeybee, engaging in incessant work and activity. Neglecting sleep and nourishment increases the probability of shortening an intense life. For someone more *Yang* who lives in a hot, dry climate, it is a challenge to avoid dehydration, restlessness, and irritability.

If *Yin* is deficient over time, *Yang* becomes deficient, and vice versa. Not only do *Yin* and *Yang* balance each other, they mutually create each other as well. When *Yin* is dissipated, *Blood* and *Moisture* are depleted and *Yang Qi* loses its source. A person becomes weak, fatigued, and has a lowered resistance to stress. When *Yang* is deficient, vital functions like respiration, digestion, and circulation are retarded, and the body is unable to generate *Blood* and tissue. Again, a person becomes weak and tired with a poor ability to heal and recover from infections or injuries. A deficiency of one ultimately becomes a deficiency of the other.

The stages of disease can also be understood according to *Yin-Yang* patterns. When a disease develops quickly, it is in the acute or *Yang* stage. As the disease becomes chronic, it passes into the *Yin* stage. Usually acute diseases affect the superficial functions or surface of the body, where they encounter the first line of defense, the *wei Qi*. If the disease overwhelms the body's resistance and penetrates to deeper, secondary layers, the disease enters a *Yin* or internal stage. Regardless of where the disease is located or how long it has existed, it can be classified according to its effects. If the symptoms are very extreme or severe, the disease is considered an excess illness, and excess belongs to *Yang*. If the symptoms are mild or diffuse, it is a deficiency syndrome, which belongs to *Yin*.

Correspondences of *Yin-Yang*

Yin	*Yang*

Universal

substantive	active
contracting	expanding
descending	ascending
cold	hot
watery	dry
forming	transforming
heavy	light
hidden	revealed
interior	exterior

Physiological

generation of: blood, lymph, hormones, mucus, urine, perspiration, nutrient substances, collagen, fat	process of: circulation, secretion, discharge, peristalsis, pulsation, metabolism, respiration

Constitutional Patterns

low energy, lethargic	high energy, hyperactive
sallow, pasty, pale complexion	ruddy, swarthy, flushed complexion
small, soft, flaccid body	large, firm, fleshy, body
delicate features	coarse features
weak soft voice	projecting loud voice
hypotensive	hypertensive
tends to feel cold	tends to feel warm
tends toward damp	tends toward dry

Diagnostic Parameters

internal	external
cold	hot
deficiency	excess
chronic	acute

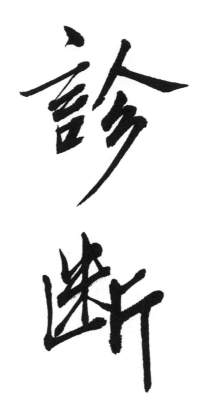

Reading the Patterns: Diagnosis

CHAPTER FIVE

READING THE PATTERNS: DIAGNOSIS THE DOCTOR AS DETECTIVE, AS ARTIST

Illnesses may be identical but the persons suffering from them are different. The . . . emotions and the . . . excesses affecting people are not the same. Some people may be strong and others weak as far as their Qi or the condition of their body is concerned. . . . One's nature may be tough or soft, one's sinews and bones may be firm or brittle . . . there are patients who suffer in their heart from grief, and others who enjoy happiness. If one treats all those patients who appear to suffer from one identical illness with one and the same therapy, one may hit the nature of the illness, but one's approach may still be exactly contraindicated by the influences of Qi that determine the condition of the individual patient's body. . . . Physicians therefore must carefully take into account the differences among the people and only then decide whether the therapeutic pattern they employ suits . . . the individual constitution on the basis of the criteria mentioned above.

> Unpublished translation of text by Hsu Ta-ch'un in 1757, translated by Paul Unschuld and presented in a lecture at the International Acupuncture Symposium, San Francisco, March 30, 1987.

DIAGNOSIS IS THE FIRST STEP IN MEDICAL PROBLEM-SOLVING. ITS TASK IS to organize a complex set of variables and interpret the relationships among them. Traditional Chinese categories, techniques, and objectives differ from what we are used to in the West. The categories are drawn from *Yin-Yang* and *Five-Phase* concepts, the techniques do not rely on technology, and the objective is to formulate a picture of healthy and distorted patterns of function rather than named diseases related to a single cause.

Like the detective, the doctor unravels mysteries and solves problems by chasing leads, following hunches, and gathering evidence. Information is collected, sifted, and classified according to relevant categories, then interpreted to formulate a hypothesis. Examination uncovers the raw data, and diagnosis explains what, how, and why events occurred in order to determine appropriate therapy.

Like the police artist who gathers bits of memory from witnesses to sketch a composite drawing, so the doctor relies on history, observation, and discussion. The artist incorporates the data into a preconceived model of human form that shows how bones, muscles, skin, and hair fit together. With each new piece of information, the drawing alters to more closely resemble the suspect. The doctor employs the intuitive skills and logical techniques of both the artist and detective, using theoretical constructs to organize and integrate information.

It usually takes more than one construct to describe reality. Diagnosis employs many distinct yet overlapping frames of reference to establish the criteria and methods of assessment. Chinese medicine, like Western medicine, searches for causes. The difference is that in Chinese medicine, causes are really descriptions of underlying relationships rather than descriptions of material agents or pathogens. The *Five Adverse Climates* and *Emotions* are often translated into English as "causative factors," yet they do not represent material things like bacteria or viruses. Instead they describe groups of symptoms and subjective states. There is no way to detect or verify these pathogenic influences except by their manifestations. These phenomena are classified within the broad parameters of *Yin-Yang* and *Five-Phase Theory*. Greater differentiation is elaborated through the more specific concepts of *Qi, Moisture*, and *Blood*, the *Eight Guiding Principles*, and the functional models of the *Five Organ Networks*.

Each set of diagnostic parameters provides one dimension of the total picture, the way cameras on a movie set record the same scene from a different angle. Each method confirms and validates the others. These points of view parallel each other and interact through their mutual correspondence to the fundamental concepts of *Yin-Yang* and *Five-Phase Theory*. Like the editing room in which the footage is spliced together, a diagnosis becomes one person's seamless moving story.

There are many possible combinations and permutations of interacting variables. This chapter illustrates methods and techniques of information gathering and the process by which a complex array of symptoms, signs, and other characteristics is interpreted.

CATEGORIES OF STRESS AND THE GENESIS OF DISEASE

Efrem studied in China at the Kunming Railway Workers Hospital in the midst of an icy winter. Because it was almost as cold indoors as out, he took notes wearing gloves, periodically wrapping his hands around a hot cup of tea. A tense and downhearted young man walked into the hospital acupuncture clinic complaining of numbness and immobility on the left side of his face. The left corner of his mouth drooped, interfering with his speech. Terse and reticent, he appeared unhappy as well as worried about his condition. He reported that he had spent much of the previous day riding his motorcycle, whipped about by the harsh cold wind. The doctor placed needles in points corresponding to the areas of paralysis, warming the area with a lighted moxa stick. She also inserted needles on the top of his feet in a point on the *Liver* meridian. Efrem asked why she included these distal points. She replied that the young man felt angry and depressed following a disagreement with his family and had torn off on his motorcycle to relieve his frustration. She felt that his emotional state had predisposed him to being injured by the cold wind. Treating the *Liver* channel would help to loosen the *Qi* that had become blocked by prolonged frustration and unhappiness.

A disturbed emotional state, harsh weather, and imprudent behavior combined to adversely affect the health of this young man in Kunming. Generally, Chinese medicine recognizes emotions, climate, and life-style as the primary sources of pathogenic stress. Sudden changes in weather or prolonged exposure can leave the body vulnerable to attack by wind, heat, dampness, dryness, and cold. Intense, persistent or suppressed emotional reactions such as anger, joy, rumination, sorrow, or fear can cause a disruption of the circulation of *Qi* and *Blood*. Misuse of the body through overwork, overuse of the senses, or prolonged sitting, lying, or standing wastes the *Qi* and injures the *Blood*. Overindulgence in or neglect of dietary and sexual needs depletes *Vital Essence*.

THE FIVE CLIMATES

The *Five Climates* correspond to the cycle of the seasons. When a person exhibits internal response patterns analogous to external climatic conditions, Chinese medicine postulates that a person has that condition: that climate exists internally. Cold, for example, makes things contract. Contracted blood vessels constrict circulation, chilling the body and producing a craving for warmth. When symptoms correspond to those produced by cold, Chinese medicine describes a person as manifesting a condition called *Cold*, regardless of whether actual exposure to external cold caused the condition. An adverse internal climate can be unrelated to outside weather. An inhabitant   63 of the Antarctic can manifest a condition of *Dampness* when the air is dry, or *Heat* in the dead of a fiercely cold winter.

Whenever specific "weather" starts to dominate the body milieu, it can become a pathogenic stress. This may be both the source and the outcome, the root and the fruit, of imbalance. Usually a multiplicity of factors contribute to the disease pattern in which one excess condition combines with another. There is not necessarily a causal chain of events, but a circle of invariable associations.

WIND

The nature of *Wind* is movement that rises and falls unpredictably, rustling and disturbing the location and direction of things. Because spring is a time of sudden and rapid change, it is considered the season of *Wind*. Both this season and climate correspond to the *Wood Phase*.

Of all the climatic forces that can engender disharmony, *Wind* is deemed the most virulent, as in "an ill wind that blows." The concept of *Wind* refers not only to the movement of air, but to the capricious, foreboding nature of shifting conditions; hence the expressions "winds of war" and "blown away." Being perched in a tree as it's shaken by gusts of gale-force wind conjures up an image of instability, disequilibrium, and fright. *Wind* can steal into the body, just as it finds its way through the cracks and crevices of doors and windows. It creates an intense draft, the nature of which is to unsettle and disrupt surface and interior circulation.

In the body, *Wind* can manifest as jerky movement, dizziness, uncoordination, or symptoms that migrate from one region of the body to another, suddenly appearing and disappearing without apparent pattern. *Wind* invading the surface of the body manifests as soreness, itching, and sensitivity of the skin and muscles. The latter occurs when circulation is obstructed by external attack. Disorders of external *Wind* are the common cold and flu, characterized by dizziness and migratory pains in the joints, muscles, and head. Diseases of internal *Wind* are characterized by labile emotions, vertigo, tremors, headaches, seizures, strokes, and the agitation of the *Liver Qi* by fever, deficiency of *Blood*, or emotional instability. Because of the ability of *Wind* to penetrate the body's defensive perimeter, *Wind* can create a portal through which the other adverse climates—*Dampness, Dryness, Cold,* and *Heat*—enter the body.

HEAT

The nature of *Heat* is to accelerate metabolic activity, dilate blood vessels, and activate circulation. *Heat* tends to rise and move out toward the surface. Summer is dominated by *Heat*, and both correspond to the *Fire Phase*.

When *Heat* becomes excessive, it generates conditions such as inflammation, rapid pulse, and fever. Inflammation is characterized by redness, swelling, and pain. Among other types of swelling and pain, *Heat* is distinguished by the appearance of redness and the feeling of increased warmth. In Chinese medicine it is not necessary to have a fever recorded on a thermometer to establish the presence of excess *Heat* somewhere in the body. Hot conditions are often associated with thirst, dryness, constipation, difficult urination, agitation, a desire for cold, and an aversion to warm foods, drinks, and climate.

The tendency for *Heat* to move toward the surface is illustrated by perspiration, the manifestation of *Yang Heat* released or discharged through the skin. This may be due to increased metabolic activity from exercise, feverish diseases, or the ingestion of warm or spicy foods. When *Heat* invades the surface, it may also show up as skin eruptions such as red rashes, welts, sores, ulcers, boils, and acne.

A reddened appearance of the face, neck, and eyes reflects the rising tendency of *Heat*, often occurring in association with intense emotional states such as anger, happiness, or embarrassment. A person "red-faced" with embarrassment, "livid [or purple] with rage," "hot under the collar," and so on manifests the ascension of internal *Heat*.

Certain B vitamins, thyroid hormone, sugar, coffee, adrenaline, spicy food, alcohol, and amphetamines all produce *Heat*. If someone already has excess *Heat*, these substances may exacerbate the condition and encourage the accompanying symptoms.

DAMPNESS

The nature of *Dampness* is to sink and accumulate, like a stagnant swamp. *Dampness* is characterized by an abnormal buildup of fluids or excess secretions. It appears as swelling and a sense of fullness and heaviness, locally or throughout the body. Because of its tendency to collect and coagulate, *Dampness* easily causes stagnation and obstruction of circulation. Late summer is dominated by humidity or *Dampness* and corresponds to the languid and sultry *Earth Phase*. During this period of relative inactivity, the air is motionless, the water is still, the atmosphere is heavy. Whether there is significant humidity in the air or not, feelings that are sluggish, apathetic, dull, or torpid provide evidence of the influence of *Dampness*.

Dampness on the surface of the body shows up as oily skin, sticky perspiration, subcutaneous edema, and swelling around the joints. Internally, *Dampness* is indicated by the appearance of phlegm, abundant discharge of mucus, water retention, and edema of the abdomen and extremities. Heaviness of the head and limbs, dull pains, and lethargy characterize *Dampness*. Dairy products, starchy and glutinous foods, steroids, birth control pills, and watery fruits and vegetables generate *Dampness*.

Dampness rarely appears by itself. It is usually accompanied by *Cold*, *Heat*, or *Wind*. When *Dampness* combines with *Cold* there is constricted   65 circulation, aversion to *Cold*, stiffness and soreness of the muscles and joints, and fatigue.

When *Dampness* combines with *Heat* there may be red, painful swellings, thick purulent discharge, blisters as in herpes or shingles, and inflammations such as cystitis, jaundice, and bronchitis. Any sore, abscess, or ulcer with pus or fluid indicates *Dampness* or *Damp Heat*. Sugar, alcohol, and fatty or fried foods create *Damp Heat*.

Dampness combined with *Wind* produces swellings that appear, disappear, and migrate (such as hives, swollen lymph nodes, accumulation of air and fluid in the stomach or intestines), bubbly phlegm, and itching, oozing sores and ulcers. In severe cases *Wind* and *Dampness* can together obstruct the brain and sense organs, producing seizures, strokes, and other neurologic disorders characterized by clumsiness, uncoordination, disequilibrium as in vertigo, and muddled, fuzzy thinking.

DRYNESS

The nature of *Dryness* is to wither and shrivel. *Dryness* damages fluids and is manifested by symptoms of dehydration. Brittle hair and nails, cracked and wrinkled skin and mucous membranes, irritated eyes, dry stool and constipation, lack of perspiration, and scanty urine occur with *Dryness*. *Dryness* dominates autumn, the season associated with the *Metal Phase*.

External Dryness usually occurs in hot or windy weather. However, internal *Dryness* occurs when body fluids are damaged or lost due to other factors. Heat, profuse perspiration, prolonged diarrhea, excessive urination, and loss of blood may all lead to *Dryness*. Hot, spicy foods, stimulants, diuretics, antihistamines, and other astringent medications that dry secretions and arrest discharges can result in *Dryness*. *Dryness* in turn can generate irritation, inflammation, and *Heat* due to a lack of lubrication and moisture. In conditions of weakness and deficiency, loss of blood and fluids will lead to internal *Dryness*. Another consequence of *Dryness* due to deficient *Blood* or *Moisture* is the appearance of internal *Wind* experienced as dizziness and disturbances of vision and hearing. This may arise in conditions like anemia.

COLD

The nature of *Cold* is to slow things down by chilling them. *Cold* depresses metabolism and retards circulation. Winter is dominated by *Cold*, and both correspond to the *Water Phase*.

When *Cold* attacks the surface, the skin and muscles contract with shivering and goose bumps. This is accompanied by fever if the body's defensive *Yang* energy is mobilized to repel the invader. This protective response may accompany any of the *Adverse Climates* that frequently appear in combination with each other.

Cold can also arise internally from either a deficiency of metabolic heat

(*Yang*) or the ingestion of an excess of food, liquid, or medicine that is considered to be *Cold*. The concept of *Cold* includes that which has been refrigerated and is thermally cold as well as foods that are categorized as having a *Cold* nature. Prolonged stress, illness, lack of proper nutrition, or repeated exposure to cold climate or substances can lead to a depletion of *Yang*. In this case, *Cold* overcomes *Heat* and *Yin* overcomes *Yang*.

Refrigerated or raw foods and chilled drinks are *Cold*. Ice cream and iced drinks are particularly damaging to the *Yang* energy. Because of their ability to counteract inflammation and fever, medicines such as antibiotics and aspirin have a *Cold* nature. Antacids counteract stomach inflammation and are also considered *Cold* medicines.

The stomach depends on the power of digestive *Fire* to break down and process food. These *Cold* medicines weaken and undermine digestive function because of their ability to dissipate heat. The repeated administration of antibiotics to children damages their already sensitive and underdeveloped digestive systems, which leads to innumerable problems in their later childhood and adulthood. The most common consequence is weakness of the immune system, manifested as allergies. The resulting deficiency and *Coldness* set the stage for disorders such as asthma, colitis, arthritis, eczema, and candidiasis.

Accompanying the aversion to cold is a desire for heat and a craving for warm foods and liquids. There is a feeling of weariness and debility as well. Retarded circulation also leads to a stagnation of *Blood* and *Moisture*, which may congeal or harden into clots, lumps, or masses associated with fixed and localized tenderness and pain.

THE FIVE EMOTIONS

Just as climates exist within the seasons, emotions are primal forces within the human psyche. All of us experience times of anger, joy, rumination, sorrow, and fear during the course of our everyday lives. These emotions are often appropriate. It is natural to feel mad when thwarted, happy when fulfilled, pensive when attention is focused inward, sad over loss, and alarmed in the face of danger. When any one state, however, dominates our internal experience or outward behavior, it interferes with the conduct of daily life and disrupts the smooth flow of *Qi*.

The *Five Emotions* are associated with the *Five Phases*. In excess, these emotions generate imbalance. *Anger* causes energy to rise—it tends to flare up and lash out with sudden explosiveness, like the windy storms of spring, unpredictable and intense. *Joy* causes energy to disperse—it tends to dissipate and be lost. Being overcome by joy can leave a person giddy and weak like the intense heat of summer, exhausted and drained. *Rumination* causes en-   67 ergy to slow down—sluggish movement tends toward stagnation, leaving one lazy and inert, like the oppressive humidity of late summer, slow and torpid. *Sorrow* causes energy to stop—it tends to constrict and close down. Imprisoned by grief, one is cut off from life; like the drying leaves of autumn, feelings wither and motivation crumples. *Fear* causes energy to sink—the bottom falls out. When survival is threatened, one becomes petrified with fright and loses control. As in the perilous cold of winter, people feel frozen with fear.

The emotions are immaterial yet palpable. Although—or because—they are experienced deeply, they are difficult to define and categorize. Nevertheless they have profound and tangible effects. In Chinese medicine they are considered one of the major influences upon health and disease. *Wind* and *Anger* particularly injure the *Liver*, *Heat* and *Joy* the *Heart*, *Dampness* and *Rumination* the *Spleen*, *Dryness* and *Sorrow* the *Lung*, and *Cold* and *Fear* the *Kidney*.

ANGER

When *Anger* predominates, a person becomes easily upset by frustrations and obstacles, unable to appropriately restrain feelings. This person is volatile, engaging in erratic and impulsive behavior. He vacillates between riveted interest and subdued indifference. These unstable emotions and unpredictable actions result in the uneven circulation of *Qi* and *Blood*, creating a generalized state of tension. This kind of person often leads a double life. Usually he exerts tremendous self-discipline in order to maintain self-control and composure. But when the stress builds, or when he relaxes and loosens his inhibitions, he is likely to explode in rage or indulge in thoughtless, rash behavior. At work he may be dedicated, outgoing, and resourceful, but on the weekends after a few drinks he may "fly off the handle" and "go through the roof." He is prone to ailments such as ulcers, hemorrhoids, and migraine headaches.

JOY

When the pleasure principle is the main focus of a person's life, she becomes unable to retain her reserve of energy. She seeks gratification at every turn and becomes jaded, driven to seek continuously more stimulation. She appears fun-loving and romantic but in fact is unable to sustain her interest and excitement without external props and other people's attention. She dislikes being alone. By herself she feels lifeless; in company she comes alive. She is prone to free-floating anxiety, insomnia, despair. Her easy excitability manifests as giggling, talkativeness, giddiness, and garrulousness. This type of person dissipates her energy by burning the candle at both ends. When she's not up, she's down. When she's not filled with excitement, she's empty and hopeless. The high level of activity causes accelerated metabolism which may take the form of hypoglycemia, anorexia, or schizophrenia. These are manifestations of *Heat*. However, the presence of *Heat* is not accompanied by light or clarity. In fact, this person is often confused, bewildered, and apprehensive.

RUMINATION

When a person is overly pensive and contemplative, he can easily become fixated on worrisome thoughts and ideas. He is often tormented by his overconcern for details and becomes caught in circular thinking from which there is no escape. His approach to life may become obsessive to the point that he is unable to have any fresh thoughts or experiences. Secure but dull, safe yet sorry, he is prone to apathy and boredom. He may be construed as a stick-in-the-mud. People can depend on this type of person because he is reliable, sympathetic, and a good caretaker. Without the demands of work or responsibility to others, he can become inert, dropping back into the well-worn trails of his own mind. In this state, his energy becomes stagnant and leads to poor digestion, heaviness, and flabbiness.

SORROW

When *Sorrow* pervades, a person insulates and defends herself from the pleasure of attachment and the pain of loss. She arranges her life for the purpose of avoiding risk and the vagaries of passion. She can become possessive, acquisitive, and domineering in an effort to control her environment. Her striving for self-protection may keep her too detached and inaccessible for true intimacy. She is pleasant but cool. She has easy disdain for people she considers sloppy and undisciplined and is uncomfortable with displays of emotion. Her life is designed to keep her feelings in. She appears tight, well mannered, and scrupulously put together. Without the ordered arrangement of her daily life, this person becomes completely vulnerable and threatened. Overcontrol is her theme and can manifest as asthma, constipation, and frigidity. She wards off excitement and feeling.

FEAR

Fear arises when survival is threatened. A man who is in the grip of *Fear* can think only of escape. His life is dominated by the expectation of threat, so he isolates himself and hides from the world. He becomes furtive and suspicious, relies on no one and prefers to be left alone. He is the hermit, drifter, and loner. He anticipates the worst, imagining calamity and disaster lurking around every corner. He lives under a cloud of doom and gloom. Critical and cynical, he believes the world is fundamentally harsh, unsafe, and unfriendly. Among other people he remains aloof. His isolation may eventually cut him off from life, leaving him cold and hard like stone, impenetrable and devoid of spirit. Because of this hardening, he is prone to develop arthritis, deafness, and senility.

METHODS OF EXAMINATION:
OBSERVATIONS, QUESTIONS, PALPATIONS

Western diagnosis often involves evaluation of a battery of laboratory tests and machine measurements. Chinese diagnosis emphasizes methods that rely solely on the practitioner's own sense perceptions, judgment, intuition, and experience. The practitioner inventories what he sees, hears, smells, and feels. He listens to the patient's feelings and complaints. He asks questions about activities and events that cannot be observed directly.

Using himself as the instrument, the doctor takes the measure of the patient: focusing mind and perception upon the gestalt of posture, stature, emotional and behavioral expression; upon specific attributes of the tongue, pulse, and complexion; and finally upon the areas and quality of pain or discomfort, restriction or freedom of movement, overall vigor and weakness.

Like the *Feng Shui* adept who divines the currents of *Wind* and *Water* that circulate through the environment to place people in a proper and beneficial alignment to them, the doctor turns himself into a divining rod that reads the movements of *Qi*, *Moisture*, and *Blood*, assessing whether the *Five Organ Networks* are working harmoniously.

The patient reports on current physical, mental, and emotional complaints, states, and attitudes. Patterns of sleeping, eating, eliminating, working, and relaxing, as well as responses to stress, needs, desires, and goals, are useful information. The doctor wants to know not only the nature of the problem, but the nature of the patient.

Patient and doctor work together, recapturing and re-creating relevant history, noting tendencies, patterns, and cycles that might be influencing the present condition. Together, family health, emotional, physical, and sexual development, childhood illness and treatment, injury, trauma and its resolution or lack thereof, and times of crisis and change all reveal the evolutionary stages leading to the present state.

Just as every cell in the human body contains in its DNA a template of the entire organism, so in Chinese medicine any part of the body (pulse, tongue, eye, ear) broadcasts information about the whole. Just as the genes contain all the information about the potential form and development of the person, any aspect of a human being can become a window or lens for revealing the state of the person. This applies not only to the physical body, but to the thinking and feeling body as well.

METHODS OF DIAGNOSIS

To observe: complexion, eyes, tongue, nails, hair, gait, stature, affect, quality of excretions, secretions

To listen and smell: sound of voice and breath; odor of breath, skin, excretions, secretions

To question: current complaints, health history, family health history, patterns of sleep, appetite, weight, elimination, menses, stress

To touch: texture, humidity, temperature, elasticity of skin; strength and tone of muscles; flexibility, range of motion of joints; sensitivity of diagnostic points; radial pulse evaluation

---

MAY I PLEASE SEE YOUR TONGUE?

Of all the possible methods of examination, two are considered most useful and reliable: inspection of the body and coating of the tongue, and palpation of the pulse at both wrists. The tongue is characterized by its color, texture, moisture, size, and shape. A healthy tongue fits comfortably in the mouth and is smooth, moist, bright, pink, and firm, with a thin white fur that covers the upper surface.

Changes in the body of the tongue generally reflect long-term dysfunction of the viscera, whereas changes in the fur reflect short-term disturbances of digestion, fluid balance, and heat regulation.

In acute conditions such as a cold or flu, the tongue may be red at the tip with a yellow or white fur that is thicker than normal. The red tip indicates *Heat* and possibly fever, and the thickened fur indicates an *Adverse Climate* such as *Cold* or *Dampness.*

An enlarged, pale, and flabby tongue with greasy or cheesy white fur is associated with deficiency and *Dampness* or excess *Moisture.* This is characteristic of illnesses such as chronic bronchitis, colitis, nephritis, or a weak and enlarged heart. The thick, wet quality of the fur is a sign of excess *Moisture* manifested as phlegm in bronchitis, loose, watery stool in colitis, and edema of the feet and hands in heart disease or nephritis.

The tongue fur primarily mirrors the *Qi* of the *Stomach.* Quite *Yang,* this *Qi* is referred to as the "digestive *Fire,*" the "smoke of the *Stomach.*" If the fur is yellow, there is an excess of *Heat* in the *Stomach,* associated with stomach pain or acidity, constipation, and a sore, dry mouth or throat. If the fur is thick and white like cottage cheese, this reflects an extreme accumulation of *Cold* and *Dampness* usually associated with marked deficiency of digestive *Fire,* manifesting in nausea, bloating, lack of appetite, and loose bowels.

The color and shape of the tongue body also reflect the intrinsic strength

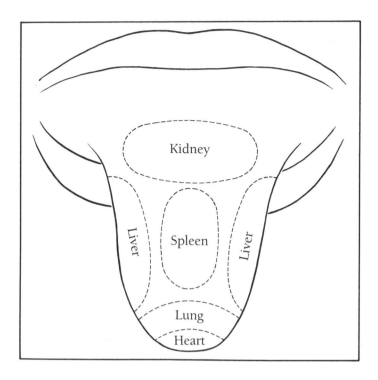

Tongue Zones

Kidney zone: organs and functions below the navel including kidneys, adrenals, large intestine, small intestine, bladder, uterus, ovaries, and testicles; reproduction, elimination, regeneration, locomotion, vegetative metabolism.

Spleen zone: organs and functions between diaphragm and navel and between right and left sides including stomach, spleen, pancreas, transverse colon, lower portion of esophagus, duodenum; digestion, assimilation, anabolic metabolism.

Liver zone: organs and functions in lateral areas of the body between diaphragm and navel including diaphragm, liver, gallbladder, spleen, hepatic and splenic flexures of large intestine; digestion, elimination, detoxification, catabolic metabolism, coordination.

Lung and *Heart* zones: organs and functions above the diaphragm including, lungs, heart, diaphragm, esophagus, trachea, bronchi, mouth, nasopharynx, nose, ears, eyes, brain; respiration, circulation, digestion, mentation, perception, communication.

and functional capacity of the individual. If the tongue is very red overall or in one area, this indicates the presence of fever or inflammation that is attacking the *Organ Networks*. The *Heart*, *Lung*, and *Liver* are most vulnerable to damage by *Heat*, which shows up as redness on the tip and edges of the tongue. In prolonged febrile or chronic inflammatory illness, the entire tongue may become deep red. In addition, if the tongue looks dry or parched, this indicates serious depletion of *Moisture*, manifested by scanty urine, constipation, thirst, and dryness of the skin and mucous membranes. In these situations the tongue may appear to be shrunken and shriveled.

Pallor of the tongue usually indicates chronic deficiency of *Qi*, *Blood*, and *Moisture*. When this is severe, the tongue may take on a purplish hue, indicating that deficiency has led to stagnation of the *Blood*. This color appears in cases where there is *Coldness* of the body and limbs, tiredness, shortness of breath, and pain in the chest, abdomen, or joints.

The progress of illness is also disclosed by the tongue. As illness improves, the quality of the fur and color of the tongue become more normal. If the illness worsens, so will the tongue and fur. Realistically it is common for individuals to have a complex tongue picture showing conflicting conditions of *Heat* and *Cold*, excess and deficiency. For example, the tongue of a person with a chronic peptic ulcer and acute influenza might appear flabby and pale, reddened at the tip, with yellow fur in the center. This indicates the intermingling of chronic interior deficiency with acute exterior excess.

Each part of the tongue corresponds to the condition or state of an *Organ Network*. To see the condition of the *Heart Network* one looks at the extreme tip of the tongue, whereas to gauge the state of the *Lung* one looks near the tip. So a very red tipped tongue indicates not only the general presence of *Heat*, but *Heat* affecting these two *Networks*. A tongue that is purplish indicates poor circulation, particularly associated with the stagnation of *Qi* or *Blood* in the *Liver*. And greasy yellow fur in the center of the tongue reports *Damp Heat* in the *Spleen* and *Stomach*.

Many external factors can also affect the appearance of the tongue, such as smoking, coffee, alcohol, and the use of pharmaceutical drugs. Under these conditions, the tongue may reflect the effect of these agents rather than give a true picture of the underlying state. This is why the practitioner never relies on only one method of diagnosis.

MAY I PLEASE FEEL YOUR PULSE?

Pulse diagnosis is based on the principle that *Qi* and *Blood* circulate as a single entity. By feeling the movement of blood in the vessels, the activity of *Qi*, *Moisture*, and *Blood* is inferred. The pulse is produced by the movement of blood in the arteries, but movement is initiated by the force of *Qi*. The Chinese saying "Where *Qi* goes, *Blood* flows" communicates this synergy

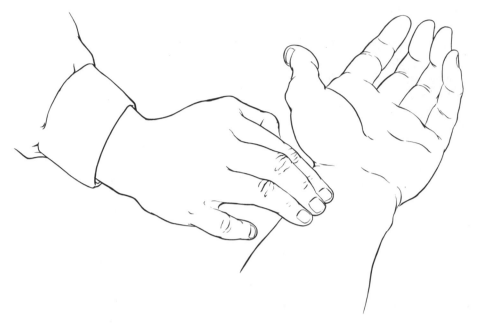

Palpating the Pulse

of *Qi* and *Blood*. When *Qi* and *Blood* are disturbed, *Moisture* may become abnormal as well.

The practitioner feels three positions on each wrist along the radial artery. These positions correspond to metabolic zones known as the *Triple-Burner* or *Three-Heater*. The position closest to the thumb corresponds to the chest and upper body (the *Heart* and *Lung*). The middle position corresponds to the upper abdomen (the *Stomach, Spleen, Gallbladder,* and *Liver*). The position farthest from the wrist corresponds to the lower abdomen (the *Kidney, Bladder, Small Intestine,* and *Large Intestine*).

The strength, rate, rhythm, and size of the pulse express the integrity of the *Qi* and *Blood* and the functional activity of the *Five Organ Networks*. A healthy pulse is regular, with four to five beats per cycle of respiration and a smooth, flowing feeling as it rises and falls. It is both elastic and resilient, evoking a sense of relaxed and vigorous rhythm and harmony.

As many as thirty-two pulse qualities are described in the classical texts, each indicating a particular type of disturbance. For example, if the pulse is "floating"—that is, it can be felt with light pressure but fades away as the pressure increases—it indicates an *Adverse Climate* (*Wind, Cold, Heat, Dampness,* or *Dryness*) has penetrated the surface from the outside. If the pulse is

Left

Heart: all organs and functions above the diaphragm, especially on the left side of the body

Liver: all organs and functions between the diaphragm and the navel especially in the lateral areas of the body

Kidney Yin: all organs and functions below the navel, especially in the pelvic region on the left side of the lower abdomen

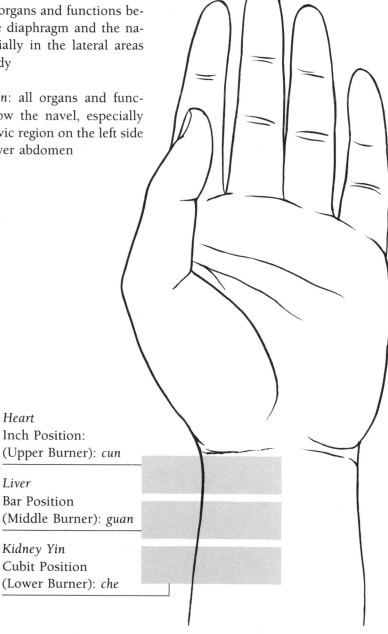

Heart
Inch Position:
(Upper Burner): *cun*

Liver
Bar Position
(Middle Burner): *guan*

Kidney Yin
Cubit Position
(Lower Burner): *che*

Right

Lung: all organs and functions above the diaphragm, especially on the right side of the body

Spleen: all organs and functions between the diaphragm and the navel, especially in the central area of the abdomen

Kidney Yang: all organs and functions below the navel, especially in the pelvic region on the right side of the lower abdomen

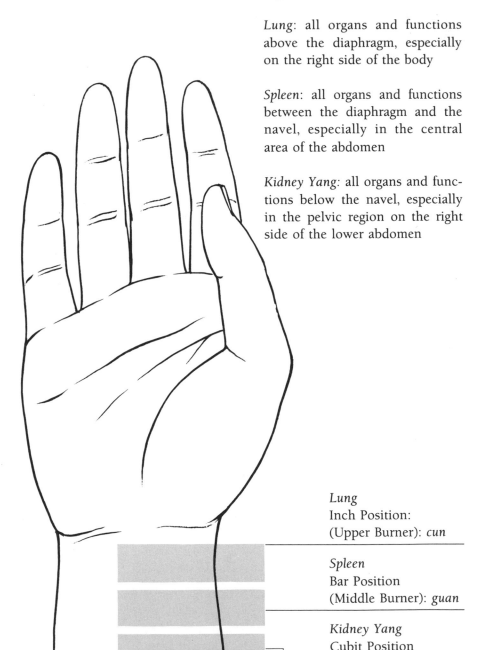

Lung
Inch Position:
(Upper Burner): *cun*

Spleen
Bar Position
(Middle Burner): *guan*

Kidney Yang
Cubit Position
(Lower Burner): *che*

floating and rapid, or floating and strong, this reflects the influence of these *Adverse Climates* in conflict with the vigorous defensive *Qi* of the body. The "sinking" pulse is its counterpart. It is perceived only with deeper pressure and feels like a stone settling in water. Since it is relatively hidden or buried, it indicates that the problem exists at the deeper internal level.

The slow pulse suggests that *Cold* is retarding movement, manifesting in a lack of warmth, whereas the rapid pulse suggests that the presence of *Heat* is accelerating movement and activity. A thin and forceless pulse is associated with weakness and a lack of sufficient *Qi* and *Blood*. A big, full pulse that "pounds" against the fingers suggests excess and may be felt when too much *Heat* is found in the *Heart, Stomach, Liver,* or *Intestines*. Generally, problems of a *Yin* nature are indicated by a frail and weak pulse, while problems of a *Yang* nature are indicated by a strong and full pulse. A given individual may exhibit a full and forceful pulse in one position and a soft and weak pulse in another, suggesting that one system is hyperactive and another is underactive. Stagnation tends to produce a tense and erratic pulse. It can be generated by both conditions of *excess* or *deficiency*. *Heat* can be generated by a lack of *Yin* as well as an excess of *Yang* or *Fire*. Most people are not diagnosed as having problems of a purely *Yin* or *Yang* nature, and often more than one *Organ Network* is involved in their disorder.

THE EIGHT GUIDING PRINCIPLES

The *Eight Principles* are four sets of polar categories that distinguish between and interpret the data gathered by examination. These include *Yin-Yang, Cold-Heat, deficiency-excess,* and *interior-exterior*. They determine the relative nature, quality, and location of the *Qi, Moisture,* and *Blood* within the body as a whole and within each of the *Five Organ Networks*.

The energetic activity of the organism is determined by qualities that distinguish between *Heat* and *Cold*. The locale of a disturbance is judged by the presence of symptoms in the *exterior* region (affecting skin, hair, muscles, tendons, joints, peripheral blood vessels, nerves, and meridians) or the *interior* region (affecting the visceral organs, deep vessels and nerves, brain, spinal cord, and bones). The virulence of a pathology is compared with the inherent strength of the body by the presence of symptoms and qualities that indicate *excess* or *deficiency*.

Excess refers to noxious pathogenic influences such as the *Adverse Climates* or *Emotions* and abnormal accumulations of *Qi, Moisture,* and *Blood*. *Deficiency* refers to a lack of the fundamental constituents, *Qi, Moisture,* and *Blood*. Any condition can then be summarized in terms of the relative dominance of *Yin* and *Yang*.

Syndromes of Distress: The Eight Guiding Principles	
Guiding Principles	*Physiological process*
Cold	retarded metabolic activity
Heat	accelerated metabolic activity
Deficiency	hypofunction or diminished capacity of any organ or physiological process; decreased resistance to stress or infection
Excess	hyperfunction or obstruction of any organ or physiological process; increased reactivity to stress or infection
Internal	affecting deeper layers of tissue and levels of function of the visceral organs, brain, spinal cord, bones, deep vessels and nerves, middle and inner ears, lining of body cavities, and internal reproductive organs
External	affecting the superficial layers of tissue and levels of function including the skin, hair, nails, peripheral vessels and nerves, muscles, tendons, ligaments, joints, eyes, external ears, nose, mouth, teeth, breasts, anus, and external genital organs
Yin	*Cold, deficient* and *internal* syndromes. This category summarizes the fundamental or composite nature of a disease process that includes *Cold, deficient,* and *internal* syndromes.
Yang	*Heat, excess,* and *external* syndromes. This category summarizes the fundamental or composite nature of a disease process that includes *Heat, excess,* and *external* syndromes.

Clinical Manifestations	Pulse and Tongue Picture
generalized or localized sensations of cold or chill; measured decrease in body temperature; pallid complexion, skin, or mucous membrane	very white tongue fur; pale or purplish tongue body; slow or tense pulse
generalized or localized sensations of heat or burning; measured increase in body temperature; reddening or flushing of complexion, skin, or mucous membrane	yellow tongue fur; reddened tongue body; rapid or bounding pulse
persistent generalized or localized feelings of fatigue, weakness, emptiness, or dull pain	scanty or absent tongue fur; pale flabby, or scalloped tongue body; weak and/or thin pulse
persistent generalized or localized feelings of fullness, tension, agitation, or intense pain	thickened, viscous tongue fur; reddened, swollen, stiff, or quivering tongue body; very strong, large, or tense pulse
no special symptoms	changes in the tongue body; changes in the pulse at the deep level
no special symptoms	changes in the tongue fur; changes in the pulse at the superficial level

Using the *Eight Principles* enables the practitioner to formulate certain therapeutic objectives. Where *Cold* predominates, the body must be warmed. Where *excess* persists, it must be dispersed. When the disease is *internal*, deep-acting remedies must be employed. Similarly, *Heat* is cooled, *deficiency* tonified, and *external* ailments are treated with remedies that act on the surface.

THE ACUPUNCTURIST AND THE HERBALIST

Just like an irrigation engineer needs different data than a soil analyst, the acupuncturist needs different information, or the same information organized differently, than the herbalist. Herbs are classified by categories describing the disruption of *Qi*, *Moisture*, and *Blood* corresponding to the *Eight Principles* and *Adverse Climates*. For example, the herb poria dispels *Dampness*; angelica nourishes deficient *Blood*; astragalus generates *Qi*; forsythia and chrysanthemum clear *Heat*.

Five-Phase Theory is more critical for acupuncture. It is not enough to know that *Dampness* or *Heat* need to be dispersed, or that deficiencies of *Qi* and *Blood* need to be tonified. The acupuncturist also needs to know which *Organ Network* assumes primary responsibility for the disruption of *Qi* in order to treat the appropriate channel. The methods of the acupuncturist emphasize the direct manipulation of *Qi* within the *Organ Networks*.

The properties of herbs are assimilated metabolically by the internal organs and then dispersed throughout the body as *Qi*, *Moisture*, and *Blood*. There are particular herbs that clear *Damp Heat* from the body. With acupuncture there is a different process—the elimination of *Damp Heat* is accomplished by adjusting the circulation of *Qi* of the *Organ Networks* responsible for distributing and transforming *Moisture* and generating heat. The *Damp Heat* is not treated directly, but rather through the functional relationship within and among *Organ Networks*. If the relationships among the *Organs* are harmonic, the pathologic condition resolves itself. *Five-Phase Theory* puts the relationship among *Organ Networks* into perspective. The doctor who practices both herbal medicine and acupuncture gathers all the evidence and synthesizes and interprets it, using both the *Eight Principles* and *Five-Phase* approaches.

SAME SYMPTOM, DIFFERENT DISORDERS

To use *Five-Phase Theory* it is necessary to identify which *Organ Network* is disturbed. The evaluation identifies where the symptom is located, when it occurs, whether anything makes it better or worse, and what other events may have occurred just prior to or at the same time as the symptom. This information is interpreted via lines of correspondence that link symptoms, timing, and circumstances with *Organ Networks*.

In the West, a symptom like a headache may be treated universally with aspirin or Tylenol. This same headache needs differentiating in Chinese medicine. It's like the many words in the Eskimo language that describe varieties of "snow." In Chinese medicine a multiplicity of disease patterns produce what in Western medicine is one named symptom or disease.

For example, disturbance of the *Liver Network* can produce migraine or bilious headaches associated with nausea, vomiting, and sensitivity to light and noise. These headaches may be provoked by anger and occur more frequently in the spring. Disturbance of the *Stomach* and *Intestines* may cause headaches associated with nasal and sinus congestion, acidity, flatulence, and constipation. This type of headache may appear in the morning and improve in the evening. Especially in hot, humid weather, disturbances of the *Spleen* and *Heart* may cause headaches associated with fatigue, dizziness, perspiration, and anxiety. In winter, headaches associated with backache, chilliness, and profuse urination may suggest a disturbance of the *Kidney*. The headache could be a simple matter of acute indigestion or related to a complex and chronic problem such as hypertension, asthma, allergies, or premenstrual syndrome. Treatment for someone's headache will differ according to which *Organ Network* is disturbed.

The same holds true for a "cough." In Chinese medicine, a cough may be a *deficiency*, *excess*, *Cold*, *Heat*, *Damp*, or *Dry* phenomenon, characterized by the amount and type of phlegm. One type can produce blood-tinged, clear, yellow, or green phlegm, another a very small amount of clear, white phlegm or no phlegm at all. A productive cough can be further differentiated by whether the phlegm is thick, sticky, and difficult to expectorate or loose, clear, and easy to expectorate. A nonproductive cough may be accompanied by a feeling of dryness and thirst or a sense of weakness and malaise.

What differentiates one cough from another is significant, alongside the idiosyncratic patterns that distinguish one person from another. One diagnostic assessment evaluates the symptoms, the other evaluates the general condition of the person who has them. The total relationship of person to symptoms forms the diagnostic pattern. Each of the children described below complains of a different type of cough:

Becca is hot and feverish, has difficulty sleeping at night, and craves lots of cold liquids. At night her head becomes damp with perspiration and she throws off her covers. Her cough is characterized by thick, dry, tenacious green phlegm. She has to cough a lot to bring it up.

David appears pale and listless. His hands and feet are cold and clammy, and his arms and legs are sore. He craves warmth, wants to be covered by lots of blankets, and desires warm drinks. He sleeps a lot during the day and   81 at night. His cough is characterized by easy expectoration with large amounts of clear, colorless phlegm.

Jenny no longer has a fever, but for several weeks she's had a hacking cough at night and seems tired and restless during the day. She complains that her throat is dry and scratchy, and her lips are red and parched. Offered drinks, she shows no interest. When she does cough, there is little phlegm and it is sometimes tinged with blood.

Alex had a cold several weeks earlier without a fever. He recovered from the cold, but in the last few days he has a morning cough with a rattle in his chest and loose bowel movements. He seems sensitive to the cold, getting goose bumps easily, and he requests an extra sweater. He has also lost his appetite. He easily expectorates a lot of frothy gelatinous mucus, especially in the morning.

Here's how a doctor of Chinese medicine would interpret the condition and treat each of the four "coughs":

Becca's condition is generally characterized by *Heat* (fever, night sweats, restlessness, and green phlegm) and *excess* (thick phlegm, high fever, restlessness). Her diagnosis is an acute cough of the *Heat* type. This requires a therapy that clears *Heat*, relieves thirst, calms coughing, and loosens phlegm. Since Becca has an *excess* condition, she can tolerate a strong treatment, and it's unnecessary to attend to strengthening the body (tonification). The primary goal for Becca is to treat the symptoms.

Along with David's acute illness, his general condition is one of weakness and fatigue. His cough is diagnosed as a *Cold* type (chilliness, clear phlegm, craves warmth) accompanied by the underlying condition of *deficiency*. In general, *Cold* types of cough are treated by methods that stimulate circulation, perspiration, and expectoration. Because of the signs of weakness, however, the treatment should avoid overstimulation and be complemented by strengthening or tonifying therapy to replenish the *Qi*.

Jenny's cough is the kind that develops from a prolonged recovery from an acute illness. Her lips are red and her throat is dry, suggesting that her fever consumed essential body fluids. Yet she is not thirsty. This lack of thirst, combined with the presence of fatigue, indicates that her body has been weakened and that she does not have the energy to recover. Her cough is the *deficient-Heat* type. The *Heat* is no longer due to fever, but rather to dehydration, deficiency of *Moisture*, and the dissipation of *Qi*. Therapy for Jenny will be directed primarily at restoring *Moisture* and increasing *Qi*.

Alex's cough appeared after apparent recovery from a cold. This suggests that in fact the cold was not completely cured, but rather that the illness had penetrated to a deeper level in the body. The combined symptoms of chilliness, loose stool, and loss of appetite indicate weakened metabolism and resistance. When the metabolic *Fire* is deficient, the interior becomes *Cold* and *Moisture* tends to congeal. Alex's phlegm appears in the morning upon awakening, the time of day the body's metabolism is at its lowest ebb and the external environment is the coolest. Treatment for Alex emphasizes warming the body and stimulating metabolism in order to eliminate the *Cold* and dissipate the phlegm. Whereas for Becca and David the treatment is directed primarily at eliminating the symptoms, for Jenny and Alex the treatment is directed at restoring *Qi* and strengthening the body.

Diagnosis is thus the process of determining what, how, and why particular events occur so that we're informed about what to do. It is a process of discovery in which decisions are made according to different frames of reference and orders of complexity, from the most general parameters of *Yin-Yang* and *Five Phases* down to the very specific ones of *Qi*, *Moisture*, *Blood*, *Eight Guiding Principles*, and *Five Organ Networks*: Is the condition one of *Heat* or *Cold*, belonging to *Metal* or *Fire*, affecting the *Qi* or the *Blood*, of the *Spleen* or the *Liver*? The craft of the clinician, like the detective and artist, is in capturing the essence of the person and the nature of the disease within the net of these descriptive and interpretive criteria.

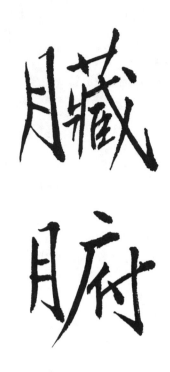

Five Organ Networks:
Traditional Chinese Physiology

CHAPTER SIX

FIVE-PHASE THEORY:
EVOLUTIONARY STAGES
OF TRANSFORMATION

As a microcosm, human beings embody all the phases within themselves. Within each thing is contained all things. In the seed is the tree; in the tree is the forest. . . . Life forms are stations for the reception and transmission of forces, through which all are nourished. Each thing exists to nourish all others and, in return, to be nourished itself. In this manner, each kingdom of nature serves to receive and transmit life. . . . These forces are not all material, but include subtle energies of . . . a spiritual nature. . . . In the inner world, a central sun is also the source of life. The inner sun is our true self. . . .

Vasant Lad and David Frawley
The Yoga of Herbs

THE URGE TO ORDER OUR PERCEPTIONS AND DEFINE THE WORLD IS AS old as humankind itself. From observation and contemplation, we generate symbols that reflect our experience back to us, demystifying existence by discovering and deciding how reality is organized. Chinese philosophy does this through the notions of Tao, *Yin-Yang*, and the *Five Phases*.

Tao is a composite of everything, the intrinsic order of all things. The way we interact with Tao, with nature, is described by *Yin-Yang* and the *Five Phases*. Chinese cosmology suggests that life's movement is like a spinning ball on a flowing river, a tide of wind and water, a vortex revolving while rhythmically contracting and expanding (*Yin-Yang*) as we are carried along by the currents of Tao.

The *Yin-Yang* model symbolizes the creation process through the interaction of bipolar forces. *Five-Phase Theory** further differentiates this dynamic into the relationship between five fundamental powers, partitioning the continuum of movement into identifiable stages. *Five-Phase* thinking pro-

---

*Five Phases is a translation of the Chinese phrase *Wu Xing*, meaning five (*wu*) fundamental processes, agents, interactive phases, movements, transformations, or powers (*xing*).

vides the basis for describing the development of forms, systems, and events. It postulates that everything in creation can be categorized within these basic parameters: *Wood, Fire, Earth, Metal,* and *Water.*[1]

If *Yin-Yang* is like shadow and sun in varying proportions, *Five-Phase* is like the rainbow spectrum. Shades of darkness and light create the drama and intensity, and the *Five Phases* provide the shape, character, and hue. *Green, Red, Yellow, White,* and *Black* correspond to each of the *Phases.*

Five affords a more complex description of phenomena than two. Combining *Yin-Yang* and *Five-Phase* generates an even more intricate system of two times five, or ten. Any process that can be described in terms of *Yin-Yang* can be further differentiated into *Five-Phase.* Any of the *Five Phases* can be further differentiated into *Yin-Yang.* Each of the five colors can be distinguished as bright and intense, *Yang,* or pale and diffuse, *Yin.*

Just as *Yin-Yang* can be used to describe the alternation between sun

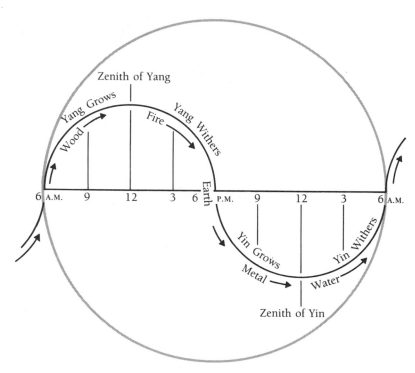

Five-Phase Yin-Yang Rhythms

The stages of transformation that define all processes in nature can be similarly described by the two interpenetrating paradigms of *Yin-Yang* and *Five Phases.*

and shade, heat and cold, dry and wet, so the *Five Phases* represent the seasons of the earth, the stages of human life, the waxing and waning of *Yin* and *Yang*. Just as day is *Yang* and night *Yin*, so the dawn is *Wood*, midday *Fire*, afternoon *Earth*, evening *Metal*, and nighttime *Water*. *Five-Phase* and *Yin-Yang* concepts always illuminate and cast shadows upon each other.

FIVE-PHASE THEORY: A HOLOGRAPHIC MAP

The underlying assumption of Chinese philosophy is that the forces that govern the cycles of change occurring in the external world are duplicated within our human bodies and minds. Patterns in nature are recapitulated at every level of organization—from the rotation of the planets to the behavior of our internal organs. These ancient Oriental ideas conform to what some modern thinkers call the "holographic paradigm": the organization of the whole (nature) is reflected by each and every part (plants, animals, human beings).[2]

Within the human being, the same forces that organize the physical, sensory, and perceptual life of the organism (soma) affect the emotional, intellectual, and spiritual life of the person (psyche). Within this framework, the *Five-Phase* model has a diverse range of application. Using anthropologist Gregory Bateson's phrase, it is a "pattern which connects."[3]

A complex web of relationships was spun between the *Five Phases* and human culture. Affairs of state and society were conducted according to these principles. Proper times to plant and harvest, advance and retreat in battle, wed and procreate, and the methods of preserving health were prescribed by this system. The *Five Phases* are an almanac of the human cycles of momentary and lifelong change, a map that charts the course of process, a guide for comprehending our unfolding.

PHASES AS TRANSFORMATIVE STAGES

The *Five Phases* identify stages of transformation, patterns of expansion and contraction, proliferation and withering. Each *Phase* has an intrinsic primal energy, an ontological influence that shapes events. For example, human beings go through cycles in their lives similar to the seasons in nature—beginning in birth and ending in death, with stages of growth, maturity, and decay in between. Within the life cycle, the power of each *Phase* can be observed.

The *Wood Phase* is seen in birth, new life bursting forth. The newborn, at first small and fragile like a tender green shoot, mobilizes tremendous energy for swift growth. The baby moves from the *Yin* phase of gestation, 87

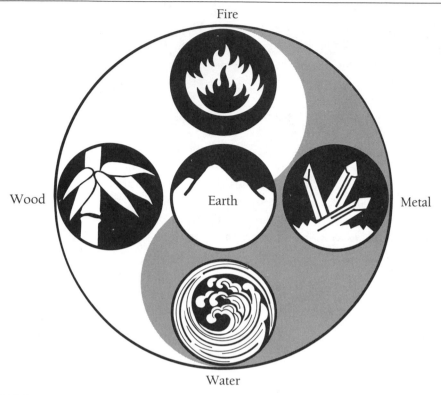

Fire

Wood

Earth

Metal

Water

WOOD	FIRE	EARTH	WATER	METAL
East	South	Center	North	West
Dawn	Midday	Late afternoon	Midnight	Dusk
Awakening	Wakefulness	Transition	Slumber	Quieting
Spring	Summer	Late summer	Winter	Autumn

Five Phases With Earth in the Center

One representation of *Earth* within the *Five-Phase* model is as the center or axis, the point of reference of the four cardinal directions, the middle of the Middle Kingdom that was ancient China. Later on, in an effort to align *Yin-Yang* and *Five-Phase Theory*, *Earth* came to represent the time and space of transition from one stage to another, particularly the passage between the apex of *Yang* (*Fire*) and ascendance of *Yin* (*Metal*). For example, between summer and autumn is late summer, between noon and dusk is late afternoon. Within this logic, *Earth* was placed schematically along the circular continuum between *Fire* and *Metal*. This diagram has become the one conventionally used to describe the *Five-Phase* relationships in Chinese medicine.

corresponding to *Water*, to the *Yang* phase of growth, corresponding to *Wood*. The peak of this *Yang* phase is reached in adulthood when we are in our prime. This corresponds to *Fire*. Our "ripening," the stage during which we luxuriate in our maturity, corresponds to the *Earth Phase*. We revisit *Yin* through degeneration and aging, which corresponds to *Metal*. In our dying we return to the *Yin* state of dissolution, the *Water Phase*, and the emptiness from which we emerged.

Just as the *Five Phases* delineate transformations of the life cycle, they also describe the process of our daily existence. Our awakening is associated with *Wood*, and our movement toward a state of complete wakefulness corresponds to *Fire*. Becoming sleepy represents *Metal*, and the state of sleep itself corresponds to *Water*. *Earth* represents the still point, the balance between the polar movements, when neither one nor the other ascends. Our integrity is based on the proportion and rhythm of each of the *Five Phases* within us, regulating our waking and sleeping, activity and rest, arousal and inhibition.

PHASES OF PULSATION

The power, quality, and direction of each *Phase* can be observed in any given internal process. In expanding the chest, for example, we move out into our world, and in contracting we gather our resources, experiencing ourselves as contained within our own boundaries. *Wood* is the *Phase* of expansion, culminating in the *Phase* of *Fire*, which spreads energy across and away from the surface (*Yang*). *Metal* is the *Phase* of contraction, culminating in the *Phase* of *Water*, which consolidates energy at the core (*Yin*). Our *Wood* aspect leads us outward toward *Fire*, where we feel at one, a part of it all; our *Metal* aspect leads us inward toward *Water*, where we recognize our separate and historical self. Our *Earth Phase* stabilizes us so that we can handle the gyrations of our oscillating process. Consciousness that exists beyond time, in the realm of space, belongs to *Fire*. Our bodies, lineage, genes, and will to pass from generation to generation through time belongs to *Water*. The realm of action belongs to *Wood*, definition to *Metal*, and balance to *Earth*. Familiarity with each of the *Five Phases* acquaints us with the individual waves within the common sea of our being.

In tension with the great *Yin Phase*, *Water*, is the great *Yang*, *Fire*. *Water* gives rise to the germination of substance, and *Fire* gives rise to the completion of materialized form. The latent power of the apple seed in the creation of the apple tree derives from *Water*. The manifest power of the tree to mature and bear shiny red apples, completing and fulfilling its potential, derives from *Fire*. Whereas *Metal* and *Wood* represent stages of expansion and contraction, *Water* and *Fire* represent stages of generation and completion.

The lines of correspondence between the *Five Phases* and human experience divide the body into *Five Organ Networks*, each of which corresponds to one *Phase*. These *Organ Networks*, echoing the nature of each *Phase*, describe the physiology and psychology of the organism. By extrapolation people can be generally classified into five character types by matching healthy and distorted expressions of the soma and psyche with the characteristics of each of the *Five Phases* and *Organ Networks*.

Five-Phase Theory is like a fugue, with ascending and descending rhythms and recapitulations, repetitions, echoes, and variations on a theme. Each

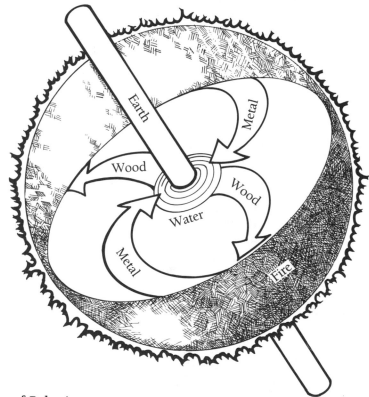

Phases of Pulsation

Symbolizing the organism as a sphere: *Metal* (*Yin*) represents contraction, movement inward toward the core. *Water* (extreme *Yin*) represents the core, the site of germination and creation. *Wood* (*Yang*) represents expansion, movement outward toward the surface. *Fire* (extreme *Yang*) represents the surface, the site of culmination and completion. *Earth* represents the axis, the point of balance, around which the forces of *Yin-Yang* revolve and spin.

Organ Network is a living system, a melody, expressed through the instrument of the soma and psyche. In the body, dissonance manifests as physical symptoms and patterns of dysfunction. In the psyche, bothersome traits, fixations, and dilemmas manifest as distortions of character and patterns of distress. The function and interaction of the *Five Organ Networks* establish the basis for understanding the five character types.

FIVE ORGAN NETWORKS: TRADITIONAL CHINESE PHYSIOLOGY

To maintain the abundant circulation of *Qi* and *Blood* is to sustain the material life of the organism, the integrity of mind and tissue. Each *Organ Network* refers to a complete set of functions—physiological and psychological—rather than to a specific and discrete physical structure fixed in an anatomical location. For this reason they are referred to as *Organ Networks* rather than simply organs. Identified by the names of the *Yin Organs*, each paired system consists of *Liver-Gallbladder, Heart-Small Intestine, Spleen-Stomach, Lung-Large Intestine,* and *Kidney-Bladder.* *

Yin corresponds to organs that store *Qi*. Here *Qi* means *Essence*—the most refined state of material substance. The *Yin* organs are more stable and constant, representing the more homeostatic mechanisms that regulate pressure, temperature, distribution, and metabolism. Constituting the body's foundation, they're both more consequential and more vulnerable. Disease of these organs is considered deeper and more critical. *Yang* corresponds to the organs that transform matter. They are more active and unstable in character because of their participation in the process of digestion and elimination.

As an aggregate of organs, tissues, channels, and physiologic functions, each *Network* is critical for the sustenance of life. Each embodies a distinctive intellectual, emotional, and behavioral style as well as physiological corre-

---

*Although there are five *Organ Networks* and ten viscera, there are twelve channels. Two functional entities called the *Pericardium* and *Triple-Burner* have no corresponding visceral structures yet have acupuncture channels associated with them. The *Triple-Burner* is viewed as an integrating function that ties together and harmonizes the physiologic processes of the primary *Organ Networks*. It regulates the metabolism and the distribution of body fluids other than *Blood*. The *Triple-Burner* is represented by the three cavities of the body: the chest, abdomen, and pelvis. The *Pericardium*, or *Heart Protector*, is viewed as the active mechanism of the *Heart*, whereas the *Heart* itself is accorded the role of harboring the spirit and maintaining conscious awareness.

In the historical development of Chinese medical theory, the existence of other organs such as the brain and uterus were defined as "strange organs" outside of *Five-Phase* or *Yin-Yang* theory. These "strange organs" such as the uterus, brain, *Pericardium*, and *Triple-Burner* do not fit neatly into the *Five-Phase* model. For our purposes, the *Pericardium* and *Triple-Burner* can be subsumed within the *Phases* of *Fire* and *Water* respectively. Although they are anatomically distinct structures, the brain and uterus are not understood as functionally separate from the *Organ Networks* of the *Kidney, Heart, Liver,* and *Spleen*, and neither do they have their own distinct channels.

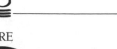

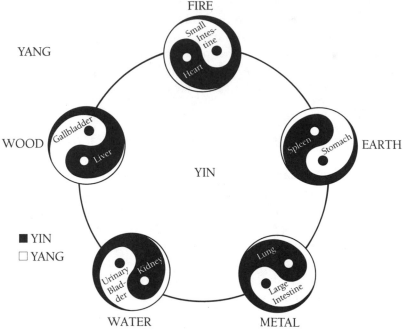

FIRE

YANG

WOOD

EARTH

YIN

■ YIN
□ YANG

WATER   METAL

Five-Phase Organ Network Correspondences

Each *Organ Network* refers to a complete set of functions—physiological and psychological—rather than to a specific and discrete physical structure fixed in an anatomical location. For this reason they are referred to as *Organ Networks* rather than simply organs. Each paired system is identified by the names of the *Yin Organs*.

---

spondences. Each has its own responsibilities (a job to do), a strategy (how to do the job), and a character (a way of being, a personality) that reflect the power of each *Phase*.

The *Liver* stores the *Blood* and regulates the even movement of *Qi*. The *Heart* propels the *Blood* and is the seat of consciousness. The *Spleen* generates and distributes nourishment. The *Lung* receives and disperses *Qi*. And the *Kidney* stores the *Vital Essence*. Together the *Organ Networks* comprise the team that gets the work of the body done. Through the division of labor, all tasks are accomplished.

CIRCULATION OF QI FROM DAY THROUGH NIGHT

Qi and *Blood* circulate continuously in an orderly sequence from one *Organ Network* to the next throughout the day and night, accounting for maximum

Our Functional Shape: A Continuum of *Organ Networks* as *Yin-Yang* Protoplasm

Our inner and outer shape is defined not only by cavities and structures, but also by an alchemy of processes governed by the functions of the *Organ Networks* impelled by the inexorable ebb and flow of *Yin* (*Jing*) and *Yang* (*Shen*) as *Qi* and *Blood* pulse and stream through the organism.

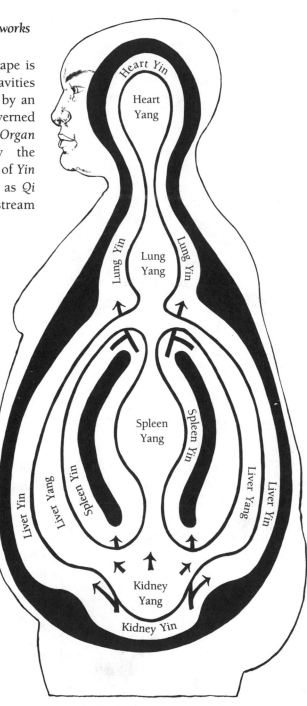

and minimum periods of function. During the day, *Qi* expands outward toward the surface of the body (*Yang*) and during the night *Qi* retreats into the body's core (*Yin*). *Yang* peaks at midday, *Yin* at midnight. Every two-hour period during the day and night clocks an alternating ebb and flow of *Qi*. One *Organ* and its associated channel fills, while another empties. For example, from three to five A.M., the *Qi* of the *Lung* reaches its peak, while the *Bladder* is at its lowest ebb. At noon the *Heart* reaches its peak and the *Gallbladder* its ebb.

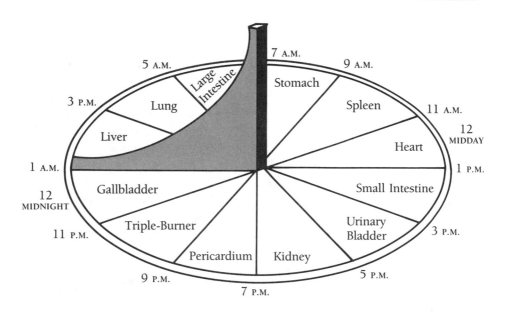

The Rhythmic Circulation of Qi from Day through Night

Stomach peaks 7 A.M.–9 A.M.	Pericardium peaks 7 P.M.–9 P.M.
Spleen peaks 9 A.M.–11 A.M.	Triple-Burner peaks 9 P.M.–11 P.M.
Heart peaks 11 A.M.–1 P.M.	Gallbladder peaks 11 P.M.–1 A.M.
Small Intestine peaks 1 P.M.–3 P.M.	Liver peaks 1 A.M.–3 A.M.
Urinary Bladder peaks 3 P.M.–5 P.M.	Lung peaks 3 A.M.–5 A.M.
Kidney peaks 5 P.M.–7 P.M.	Large Intestine peaks 5 A.M.–7 A.M.

The *Stomach* and *Spleen* are at their peak function between seven and eleven A.M. This is the time of optimal digestion and assimilation and helps to explain why the first meal of the day is so important for maintaining adequate energy. The time of peak function for the *Large Intestine* occurs at five to seven A.M., just prior to that of the *Stomach*. This suggests that the natural rhythm is to empty in preparation for receiving. During sleep, the anabolic or regenerative phase is at its maximum. The time of awakening is the beginning of the catabolic phase, when energy is liberated for the purpose of doing work. Symptoms that appear and disappear regularly during different times of the day correspond directly to this ebb and flow of *Qi*.

Symptoms of *excess* appear during peak hours, those of *deficiency* during the ebb tides of *Qi*. Symptoms of *Kidney deficiency* often manifest between five and seven A.M. This accounts for the difficulty some people have in awakening with vigor and enthusiasm. Conversely, excessive *Kidney Qi* may manifest as increased stiffness and pain in the lower back during the peak hours of *Bladder* and *Kidney* function, between three and seven P.M. Heart disease has particular hours of aggravation: heart attacks occur more frequently around midday and heart failure at midnight. People subject to migraines often awaken during the peak function of the *Liver*, between one and three A.M., with a severe headache. These same people may experience fatigue, mental lethargy, and perhaps even a weakening of vision between one and three in the afternoon, following lunch.

According to the classical theory, the most opportune time to intensify the *Qi* of any channel is just after it peaks, when it has the greatest momentum. The best time to disperse *Qi* is prior to the peak period, before it gathers full strength. This same dynamic applies to the seasonal rhythms of ebb and flow. The best time to strengthen the *Lung* is during the fall, which also subdues and restrains *excesses* of the *Liver* and *Gallbladder* (*Metal* controls *Wood*). *Kidney Essence* and *Fire* are best supplemented in the winter; this is a time when elder Chinese men and women drink their ginseng tonic. The *Liver* is nourished in the spring, the *Heart* during summer, and the *Spleen* in late summer. The Chinese classics also say it is important to treat a disease in the time and season of its origin. Allergies that arise in the spring are treated in the same season to achieve the greatest results. Rheumatism that occurs after exposure to the cold of winter may become full blown in spring, yet it must be treated during the season of its origin, winter, and may only be palliated in spring, summer, and fall. Patience becomes practical virtue since it is often necessary to return full cycle and wait for the most propitious time to resolve a dysfunctional pattern.

INTERACTION OF THE FIVE PHASES: SHENG AND KE SEQUENCES

The *Five Phases* interact according to patterns of generation and restraint. Along the *sheng* sequence the *Phases* generate, nourish, and support each other, counterbalanced by the *ke* sequence, which represents the dynamic of restraint, inhibition, and control. Equilibrium is maintained by these contrary patterns of proliferation and limitation.

These relationships are like those between parents and children. In the *sheng* sequence one *Phase* gives birth to the next, and in the *ke* sequence   95

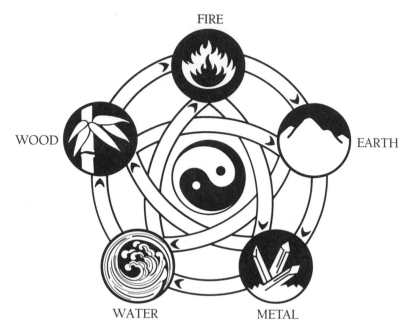

The Pattern of Five-Phase Relationships

The *Five Phases* interact according to patterns of generation and restraint. Equilibrium is maintained by these contrary patterns of proliferation and limitation. In the *sheng* sequence one *Phase* gives birth to the next, and in the *ke* sequence each *Phase* sets limits, insuring that no *Phase* oversteps its bounds.

---

each *Phase* sets limits, insuring that no *Phase* oversteps its bounds. Metaphorically this can be understood as follows: *Water* nourishes *Wood* by moistening it and restrains *Fire* by quenching it. *Wood* generates *Fire* by providing fuel for combustion and inhibits *Earth* by covering it. *Fire* generates *Earth* by reducing matter to ash that forms soil; *Fire* restrains *Metal* by burning and melting it. *Earth* supports *Metal* by forming minerals and bringing them to the surface but controls *Water* by damming and absorbing it. *Metal* vitalizes *Water* by permeating it with refined substances that enhance its life-giving properties. *Metal* restrains and inhibits *Wood* by cutting it.

Just as *Water* nourishes *Wood*, within the body, the *Kidney Essence* can be understood to generate the *Blood* stored by the *Liver*. As *Wood* feeds *Fire*, the *Blood* of the *Liver* can be said to nurture the spirit of the *Heart* by providing the mind with its basis. As *Fire* generates *Earth*, the *Heart* supports the *Spleen* by providing the warmth and metabolic energy (oxygenated blood) necessary for the transformation and assimilation of food. As *Earth* gives rise

Supporting Sequence: *Sheng*

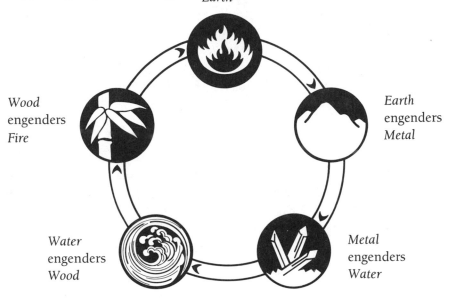

*Fire
engenders
Earth*

*Wood
engenders
Fire*

*Earth
engenders
Metal*

*Water
engenders
Wood*

*Metal
engenders
Water*

Restraining Sequence: *Ke*

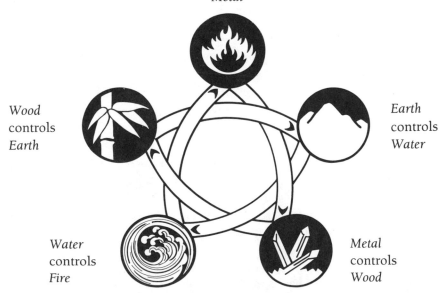

*Fire
controls
Metal*

*Wood
controls
Earth*

*Earth
controls
Water*

*Water
controls
Fire*

*Metal
controls
Wood*

to *Metal*, the *Spleen* supports the *Lung* by raising *Food Essence* upward to be combined with *Air Essence*, forming the pure *Qi* that circulates in the channels. And just as *Metal* vitalizes *Water*, the *Lung* nurtures the *Kidney* by precipitating its moist *Qi* downward to be collected and stored as *Essence* by the *Kidney*.

Sheng and *ke* define the relationships between the *Organ Networks*. In correspondence with the *ke* sequence, as *Water* controls *Fire*, so the *Yin* moisture of the *Kidney* counterbalances the *Yang* fire of the *Heart*. As *Fire* controls *Metal*, so the *Heart*'s capacity to rule the *Blood* complements the *Lung*'s capacity to govern the *Qi*. As *Metal* restrains *Wood*, so the *Lung*'s power to mobilize *Qi* counteracts the *Liver*'s power to gather the *Blood*. As *Wood* dominates *Earth*, so the activating power of the *Liver Qi* awakens the transformative function of the *Spleen*. And since *Earth* dams *Water*, the *Spleen*'s ability to absorb and distribute *Moisture* counterbalances the *Kidney*'s ability to concentrate *Essence* and excrete fluid.

An *Organ Network* overly restrained *collapses* and, if not kept within proper limits, becomes *exaggerated*. Overly restrained, its force and influence dissipate and diminish, becoming passive and impotent. Inadequately restrained, it magnifies, becoming bound up, intensified, and oppressive. When prolonged, either situation will transform into the other and lead ultimately to the attrition of the power and potential of the person.

Five-Phase Theory explains the interaction of the *Organ Networks* in a broad and general way. Descriptions of physiologic processes in Chinese medicine can become very complex, just as they do in Western medicine. For our purposes it is sufficient to have a circumscribed understanding of the *Organ Networks* and their correspondences within the *Five-Phase* model.

THE CONSEQUENCES OF DISSONANCE

All the *Organ Networks* are interconnected and interdependent. If the behavior of one becomes *exaggerated*, this results in the depletion of some and the hyperactivity of others. An overly brawny *Liver* depletes the *Kidney*, destabilizes the *Heart*, oppresses the *Spleen*, and obstructs the *Lung*.

If an *Organ Network* becomes undermined through stress and *collapses*, this triggers a different pattern of depletion and overactivity. If the *Liver collapses*, the *Spleen* and *Lung* become overly strong, the *Kidney* and *Heart* become vulnerable and exhausted. A simple excess or *deficiency* of one *Organ Network* persisting over time devolves into complex patterns of disharmony and disease.

Diseases of *excess* often migrate from one *Organ Network* to another along the *ke* sequence. That is, a disharmony of the *Liver* may afflict the *Spleen*. If this is not corrected, the *Spleen* passes this problem on to the

Kidney, the *Kidney* to the *Heart*, the *Heart* to the *Lung*. Finally, the disease comes home to roost in the *Liver*.

Deficiency diseases often develop along the *sheng* sequence. Weakness is transmitted from parent to child: from *Kidney* to *Liver*, *Liver* to *Heart*, and so forth until the disease returns to its point of origin. The gravity of a disease can be assessed by determining how far along the sequence it has progressed and how many *Networks* are seriously affected.

Wood: Liver Patterns

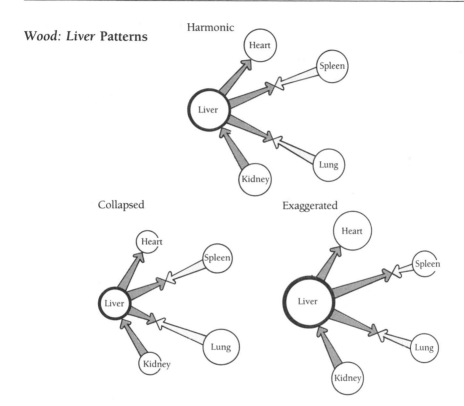

Harmonic and Dissonant Patterns

A simple *excess* or *deficiency* of one *Organ Network* persisting over time devolves into complex patterns of disharmony and disease. Diseases of *excess* often migrate along the *ke* sequence, whereas *deficiency* diseases often develop along the *sheng* sequence. The harmonic pattern depicts the predominant *Organ Network* in relative equilibrium with the other *Networks*. The *exaggerated* pattern represents the predominant *Organ Network* oppressing the *Organ Networks* along the *ke* sequence. The *collapsed* pattern shows the depletion not only of the predominant *Organ Network*, but of those along the *sheng* sequence with encroachment of those *Networks* along the *ke* sequence.

Fire: Heart **Patterns**

Harmonic

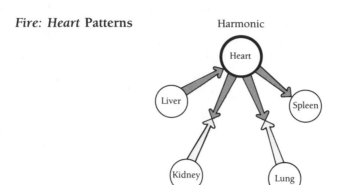

Collapsed

Exaggerated

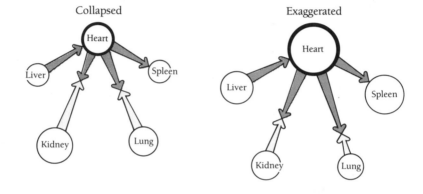

Earth: *Spleen* Patterns

Harmonic

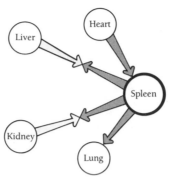

Collapsed

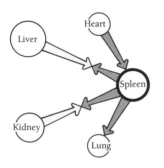

Exaggerated

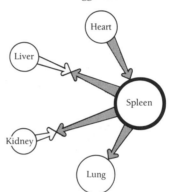

Metal: Lung Patterns

Harmonic

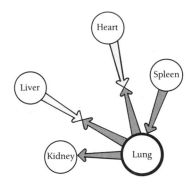

Collapsed

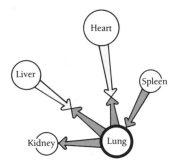

Exaggerated

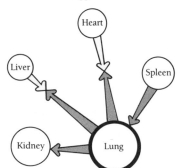

Water: *Kidney* Patterns

Harmonic

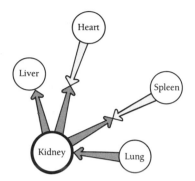

Collapsed

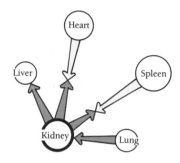

Exaggerated

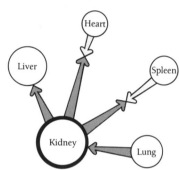

FOR EXAMPLE, THE LIVER PATTERN

Disease patterns usually involve two or three *Organ Networks* in addition to the one primarily disturbed. For example, the *Organs* most affected by the *Liver* are the *Organ* it controls (*Spleen*), the one that is its controller (*Lung*), and the one that is its parent (*Kidney*).

If an *Organ* is strong, the pattern is different than if it's weak. When an *Organ* is powerful, the origin of the complaints usually involves *Organs* under attack or being drained. When the *Organ* is feeble, primary complaints usually involve the *Organ* itself and sometimes the one succeeding it in the *sheng* sequence. For example, if the *Liver* is weak and the *Lung* is strong, the person will contract symptoms associated with an attack on the *Liver* by the *Lung*, such as depression, irritability, pain in the groin or genital organ, and tiredness. The symptoms result from the *Lung* literally suppressing *Liver Qi*, preventing its ascension and expansion.

Since the *Lung* dominates the *Qi*, it can inhibit the free flow of *Liver Qi* and the easy expression of feelings, thoughts, and desires. This shows as a flatness and dullness of response and sensation—depression. The contractive or *Yin* nature of the *Lung* is constricting the expansive *Yang* nature of the *Liver*. When this occurs, peristalsis is also affected because the *Liver* cannot regulate the smooth flow of *Qi* within the *Spleen* and *Stomach*. Symptoms of poor digestion occur, such as flatulence and constipation, because tension in the stomach and intestines causes a lack of motility.

If the *Liver* is hardy and the *Spleen* is frail, symptoms manifest that emerge from *Stomach* and *Spleen* dysfunction: pain and cramping in the stomach and intestines, bloating, erratic appetite, nausea, loose stools, and a feeling of weakness in the limbs. This is due to the harsh energy of the *Liver* invading and restricting the performance of the *Spleen* and *Stomach*.

If the *Liver* is powerful and the *Lung* is delicate, symptoms of distress will be manifest in the function of the *Lung* such as coughing, asthmatic breathing, difficult urination, rashes, itching, redness of the eyes, and dryness of the skin and mucous membranes. These symptoms are a manifestation of the uprising hot *Qi* of the *Liver* invading and restricting the moistening, dispersing, and descending function of the *Lung*.

If the *Liver's* strength causes *deficiency* of the *Kidney*, a reversal of the natural relationship may occur whereby the child (*Liver*) goes against the parent (*Kidney*). This may result in hip and low back pain, herniated disk, inflammation of the reproductive organs or dysfunctions such as infertility, impotence, excessive libido, inflammation of the genitourinary system, or the formation of cysts and tumors, including those of the prostate, uterus, ovaries, and bladder.

When one *Organ* affects another, those adjacent to it suffer. Generally, the generative *sheng* sequence, also referred to as the parent-child relationship, is more stable than the restraining *ke* relationship. Since the *Lung* is child to the *Spleen*, it becomes distressed when the parent is. When the *Spleen*'s function of generating *Qi* and *Blood* from the transformation of nutrients is suppressed by the *Liver*, it is unable to nurture the *Lung*. The *Lung*'s ability to disperse and move the *Qi* becomes impaired. This manifests as fatigue, shortness of breath, susceptibility to colds and flus, and the appearance of excessive phlegm in the nose, mouth, throat, and chest.

Parent to the *Spleen* is the *Heart*. When the child suffers, so does the parent; hence the *Heart* is also troubled when the *Spleen* becomes disturbed. Since the *Spleen* cannot efficiently nourish the blood, the *Blood* of the *Heart* becomes *deficient* (which may or may not include actual anemia), leading to instability of the *Heart Qi*. This manifests as disturbances of sleep, emotions, circulation, and an irregular pulse. The *Spleen* cannot properly restrain the *Kidney*, and the infirm *Lung* cannot adequately nurture the *Kidney*. The manifestations of this are seen at a later stage as weakness of the back, knees, and ankles and a tendency toward water retention in the hands, feet, and face.

Chinese medicine identifies disease as disorders of relationship, not as a singular, unvarying entity. Problems recognized early on can be dealt with before they develop into complex, deep-seated, chronic sickness. From the above example and the kind of widespread derangement that arises, one can imagine how disease progresses from its place of origin in the *Liver Network* and spreads throughout the body as a whole. This sort of analysis is the basis of diagnosis and prognosis in Chinese medicine.

ORGAN NETWORKS

WOOD: THE LIVER

Like a military commander who formulates strategy and tactics, the *Liver* exercises authority in collecting and directing the *Blood*. Since *Blood* is never stationary but constantly circulating, and since *Qi* courses inseparably through the body with the *Blood*, the *Liver* equitably distributes all resources, assuring the maintenance of smooth flow.

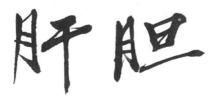

Liver-Gallbladder 105

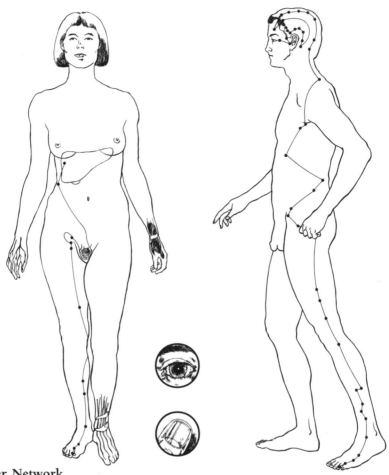

Liver Network

Role:	Viscera:	Tissues:	Fluids and Secretions:
stores and releases *Blood* spreads *Qi* raises *Qi* and *Blood*	liver gallbladder	tendons ligaments small muscles that move joints peripheral nerves iris of the eyes and eyebrows external genitalia: vagina and labia, penis and scrotum nails	bile tears

STORING AND RELEASING BLOOD

The *Liver* bears the *Yin* responsibility of storing and the *Yang* role of distributing the *Blood*. This process of regulation determines the quantity and pressure of *Blood* in the physical body and the evenness of emotion and consistency of behavior in the feeling body. The force of the *Liver* moves upward and outward, lifting *Blood* and *Qi* toward the far reaches of the head and limbs. Through this action, the *Liver* facilitates the work of the *Heart* and *Spleen* to adequately nourish the body with *Blood* and *Nutritive Essence*. The healthy sexual and procreative role of the genital organs also depends on the capacity of the *Liver*—to transmit the power of our *Essence* to another person.

SPREADING QI

The *Blood* nourishes the tissue of the body and is the source, or "mother," of *Qi*. Through the task of holding and releasing the *Blood*, the *Liver* spreads the *Qi*. The *Liver* governs the tendons, ligaments, small muscles, and nerves, motivating and regulating all body movement. In Western terms, the *Liver's* function bears resemblance to the sympathetic nervous system insofar as it is the mechanism of excitation and arousal. This movement of *Blood* and *Qi*, of muscles, joints, limbs, and viscera, constitutes the active life of the body. When movement is steady and tissue resilient, it means the *Liver* is functioning in accord with its character and responsibility.

Inability to evenly spread the *Qi* arises from a disturbance of the *Liver's* power to store and release *Blood*. This manifests as erratic activity in the body and a volatile temperament. For example, migraines occur when the *Liver* is not able to properly store, discharge, and distribute the blood to the eyes, ears, and brain: the head becomes hot and congested while the hands and feet become cold. A similar thing happens with painful menstruation: as the discharge of blood begins, if the *Liver* cannot release easily and evenly, the uterus will cramp. This same pattern of poor circulation also causes spasm in the muscles. Problems of irregularity as diverse as disturbed sugar metabolism, sudden outbursts of emotion, uncoordinated movement, blurry vision, indigestion, and constipation, or difficulty unwinding after working hard, may all occur as a result of the *Liver's* inability to maintain the smooth flow of *Qi* and *Blood*.

MATE TO THE LIVER: THE GALLBLADDER

The *Gallbladder* is the paired *Yang* organ of the *Liver Network*, which executes a part of the *Qi*-regulating role. Unlike the other *Yang* organs, which only transform and transmit matter but do not store it, the *Gallbladder* stores and secretes the bile, a pure and essential substance that stimulates peristalsis in the *Stomach* and *Intestines*, aiding assimilation and elimination.

The *Gallbladder* imparts the power of decision and the *Liver* the power   107 of action. The purity of the bile assures pure and proper judgment, clarity of vision, thought, and decision making. If the *Liver* and *Gallbladder* are dissonant, action occurs without judgment, decisions go unactualized, or a Hamlet-like paralysis of decision and action persists. Metaphorically, the *Gallbladder* and bile form a liquid crystal like the lens of the eye through which we perceive existent and anticipated, inner and outer, reality. Our prescience and foresight arise from this faculty. With a deterioration in function of the *Liver Network*, a veil obstructs vision and thought. Cataracts, glaucoma, and other deformities of the eye that diminish vision may arise.

STAGNATION OF QI AND BLOOD

Poor *Liver* function can lead to stagnation of *Qi* and eventually *Blood*. Stagnation of *Qi* is experienced in the body as a feeling of fullness, discomfort, or pain in the chest, belly, or head; in the psyche it manifests as agitation, nervous tension, suppressed emotion, and frustration. Stagnation of *Blood* is experienced as a localized stabbing or cutting pain. If this stasis of *Blood* persists for too long, it gives rise to hard lumps, masses, tumors, or chronic inflammation in the chest, abdominal, and pelvic region. A mass or lump may come and go unpredictably, like an intestinal spasm when *Qi* is obstructed, or may become a benign or malignant tumor in the final stages when *Blood* becomes "congealed." This situation is often the case in women who develop uterine fibroids, uterine hemorrhage with large clots, irregular, scanty, or suppressed menstruation, cervical dysplasia, or ovarian cysts or tumors.

Stagnant *Qi* can also obstruct the *Spleen*, affecting its ability to generate and distribute *Moisture* and *Nutritive Essence* in the body. This impairment of *Spleen* function results in the accumulation of *Dampness* and an attrition of vitality. The fluid excess itself then may become a secondary source of stagnation since it impedes the flow of *Qi*. The body often generates *Heat* to counteract this fluid excess by drying it. This *Heat* then accumulates and intermingles with the *Dampness*. *Damp Heat* can settle in the pelvis, where it damages and obstructs the *Blood*. Over time this will lead to coagulation and deficiency of *Blood*. *Damp Heat* in the *Liver* also sets the stage for problems such as genital and perianal herpes, jaundice, and hepatitis. In men the manifestations of stagnated *Liver Qi* with *Damp Heat* are prostatitis, epididymitis, urethritis, and painful ejaculation.

BLOOD OF THE LIVER

The *Blood* stored by the *Liver* is responsible for nourishing the tendons, ligaments, muscles, joints, and eyes. When the *Liver* cannot properly store the *Blood*, symptoms such as muscle spasm, dizziness, numbness of the limbs, and dry eyes occur. If the flow of *Blood* is poorly regulated, muscles and nerves become easily fatigued, and metabolic waste products are not efficiently eliminated. Stagnation of *Qi* and *Blood* in the *Liver* leads to pain and sensitivity in the muscles, eyes, and glands (such as breasts, thyroid, prostate, testes, and ovaries) and tiredness, especially fatigue that is worse after rest.

JUDICIOUS GRACE

In short, the job of the *Liver Network* is to monitor flow, maintaining evenness of emotions and clarity of judgment, giving grace and flexibility to the physical and mental body. When the *Liver* is healthy, judgment and decision making are sound, vision is clear, and action is resolute. Strengthening the *Liver* develops drive and adaptability, enhancing our capacity to cope with the vicissitudes of life.

FIRE: THE HEART

The *Heart* is considered the ruler because like a benevolent and enlightened monarch, it is all-knowing and ever-present, sharing its wisdom unconditionally for the good of the whole. Our *Fire* aspect represents fulfillment: the total expression and integration of our being, the full extent of our expansion, maturation, and development.

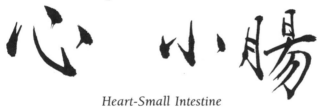

Heart-Small Intestine

PROPELS BLOOD, ENFOLDS SPIRIT

The *Heart* propels the *Blood* through the body and enfolds the *Spirit*, maintaining awareness. This continuous flow of *Blood* through the vessels both nurtures the body and serves as a vehicle for communication. The *Blood* communes with each and every cell, pervading all regions of the soma. It also "houses the mind," serving as the material matrix of the psyche.

Just as the sun provides warmth and light for all of creation, so the *Heart* suffuses and permeates the body with consciousness, sensation, and feeling. The *Heart* maintains awareness by integrating and communicating experience, establishing an interconnectedness between our inner life and external universe. The *Heart* holds and envelops the *Spirit*. In Chinese medicine, the *Shen*, or *Spirit*, does not refer to an independent, discarnate entity and is not to be confused with Western religious ideas about the soul or immortal aspects of human identity.

Spirit in Chinese medicine connotes the totality of the person's life force   109

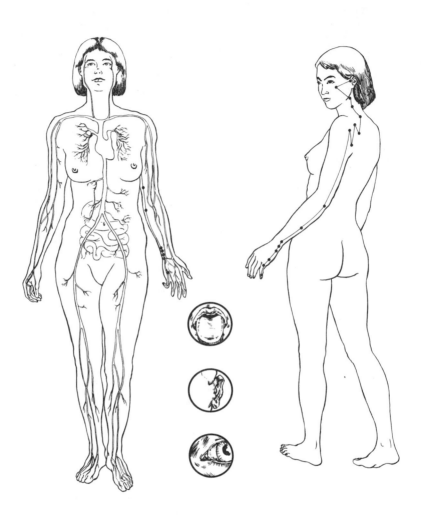

Heart Network

Role:	Viscera:	Tissue:	Fluids and Secretions:
propels the *Blood* enfolds the *Spirit* maintains awareness	heart small intestine	arteries and arterioles complexion tongue external ear corners of the eye	blood perspiration

at any given moment and represents the complete outward expression of the *Qi* through the personality. When the *Spirit* is strong, it means that the soma, psyche, and personality are well blended. This is reflected by aliveness of emotional expression, presence of mind, bright eyes, and a lustrous complexion. The *Spirit* is also the realm of the higher moral and spiritual faculties. Conscious identification with nature and humanity and the compassion that accompanies those sentiments emanate from the *Heart*.

A sense of individualized being and at the same time a sense of union with others is the power of the *Heart*. The *Heart* as the foundation of the mind in Western terms resembles the integrative function of the cerebral cortex, which gives rise to the capacity for thought, perception, sensation, speech, communication, and memory. What the *Kidney* receives through the sense organs, the *Heart* expresses through speech, the resonance of the voice, and the radiance of the complexion and eyes.

MATE TO THE HEART: THE SMALL INTESTINE

The paired *Yang* organ of the *Heart Network* is the *Small Intestine*, which separates out the useful constituents of digested food, conducting fluid waste to the *Kidney* and solid waste to the *Large Intestine*. This function permits the *Essence* of food to be assimilated by the *Spleen* and extracted into the *Blood*, which flows to the *Liver*. The *Small Intestine* assists the *Heart* in communication by the purification and transportation of fluids and substances that enter the *Blood*.

By separating the purer from coarser elements physically and psychically, the *Small Intestine* protects the *Spirit* by filtering out negative input. Pathologies of the *Heart* often manifest in inflammatory disorders of the *Small Intestine*. This occurs when overactivity of the *Heart* produces *Heat* that is transmitted to the *Small Intestine* and conducted downward and outward through the *Bladder* and *Large Intestine*. Urethritis, cystitis, ileitis, duodenal ulcers, and enteritis can be precipitated by anxiety states associated with agitation of the *Spirit*.

DISTURBANCES OF THE HEART

Shocking surprise, inordinate sorrow, or overwhelming joy can obstruct the *Heart*'s function and disrupt the perfusion of *Blood* and the continuity of consciousness. An individual whose *Heart* has been overwhelmed by emotional trauma may suffer a "break with reality," a heart attack, or stroke. If the *Blood* of the *Heart* is insufficient, even without emotional trauma, the mind will have no house in which to dwell, and the *Spirit* will "wander and roam." This *deficiency* is experienced as forgetfulness, distraction, restlessness, and disturbed sleep. The *Heart* becomes overheated and overactive when the *Yin* or *Blood* becomes *deficient*. This *Heat* manifests as incessant talking, disturbing dreams, aberrations of behavior, disjointed thinking, or blood in the urine, stool, or sputum.

In order for the *Heart Network* to function well, it must remain peaceful and protected. When there is agitation and unrest, it is difficult for the *Heart* to respond appropriately to sensory input. This makes the *Heart* insecure and generates a feeling of anxiety. Under stress, circulation is abnormal and thinking becomes disordered and confused.

When the *Qi* of the *Heart* dissipates, a healthy pink complexion can alternate between gray pallor and a scarlet veil. The person may experience sudden exhaustion and feel either too hot or too cold. Enthusiasm for life can be overcome by periods of withdrawal and melancholy. This person may have difficulty finding words and suffer short-term memory loss, shortness of breath, and perspire with slight exertion.

When the *Heart* cannot perform its job properly, arterial circulation becomes impaired: blood pressure lowers, the limbs become cool, the heart skips beats, and the person feels tired, swollen, and breathless. These are the symptoms associated with heart failure. As the *Qi* dissipates, the tendency is for the *Blood* to become sluggish and stagnant. The extremities may become numb, and the lips, nose, and fingers take on a purplish hue. As a result of this *Blood* stasis obstructing the *Heart*, angina or chest pain may occur.

FULL-BODIED SPIRIT

The *Heart* has the pure nature of *Fire*. It exudes warmth and light: the warmth of good circulation and the light of consciousness. Under stress, the warmth can either dissipate or turn to flames and the light may become cloudy. When the *Heart Network* functions properly, a person has a tranquil mind, good memory, clear senses, restful sleep, and a robust complexion. It is the nature of the *Heart* to be accessible, responsive, and serene, like a monarch who rules not by force, but by spreading joy, maintaining peace, and establishing communication.

EARTH: THE SPLEEN

As a minister of agriculture oversees the production and distribution of farm resources, the *Spleen* supplies the nourishment that sustains the organism. The raw material of food and experience is ingested, digested, and assimilated to fuel the life of the body and mind. This fuel, called *Nutritive Essence*, is extracted and converted into an abundance of *Qi* and *Blood*. Gathering and holding together is the dominion of *Earth*. Like Mother Earth, the *Spleen* is the constant provider, the hearth around which the body gathers to renew itself.

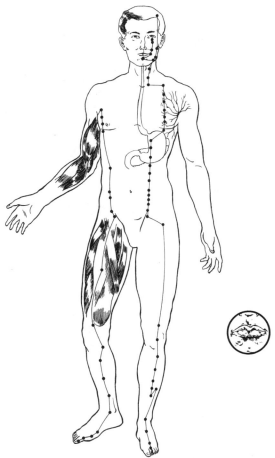

Spleen Network

Role:	Viscera:	Tissue:	Fluids and Secretions:
extracts and converts nutrients into *Qi* and *Blood* distributes *Moisture* and *Nutritive Essence* contains *Qi* and *Blood* within their conduits upholds muscles, flesh, and viscera	spleen stomach	large muscles and flesh lips mouth eyelids	lymph saliva chyle

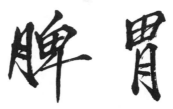

Spleen-Stomach

EXTRACT, CONVERT, SUPPLY, CONTAIN, LIFT

By providing nourishment, *Qi*, and *Blood*, the *Spleen* holds the fabric of the body together and upright, maintaining the integrity and position of flesh, blood vessels, and organs. The *Spleen* "governs the *Blood*" by keeping it within the arteries and veins and "uplifts the *Qi*," counteracting gravity, by holding the viscera and muscles in their proper place, preventing prolapse.

METABOLIC FUEL

The *Spleen* regulates metabolism. It adjusts the quantity of the pure fluid *Essence* that is refined from digestion and released into circulation. As a hydroelectric dam assures a reliable power output by controlling the amount of water flowing through the turbines, the *Spleen* regulates how much *Essence* is transformed into *Qi* and *Blood*—that is, the quantity of fuel metabolized determines how much energy is produced.

MOISTURE AND DENSITY

The distribution of *Moisture* is another function of the *Spleen*. Through the process of accumulating and releasing *Moisture*, the *Spleen* adjusts the viscosity of blood and fluids circulating through the vascular and lymphatic systems, the density of the flesh, and the total mass of the body. The dissemination of *Moisture* affects the weight, shape, and tone of tissue and the lubrication of joints and mucous membranes.

ASSIMILATION

The *Spleen* governs the physical extraction of nutrients from food and the incorporation of ideas and information by the mind. The faculties of concentration, ideation, recollection, and reflection emanate from the *Spleen*, which focuses the mind and bestows the power of intention. Intention is a means of gathering the momentum necessary to transform will, the impulse of the *Kidney*, into action, the drive of the *Liver*. Maintaining the motivation necessary to sustain effort over time arises from the *Spleen*. Regulating metabolism, adjusting the distribution of *Moisture*, holding tissue together, preserving the uprightness of muscles and viscera, and facilitating higher mental processes constitute the means by which the *Spleen* maintains homeostasis and assures adaptation and equilibrium.

CONSTANCY

The *Spleen* occupies the position of the fulcrum, the balance point through which transition occurs. By means of a fulcrum, a lever transfers energy and mass from one site to another. The *Spleen* transports *Nutritive Essence*—the basis of *Qi* and *Blood*—throughout the organism, forming and re-forming self and tissue, imparting to us a sense of substantiality and terrain. Just as a heavy keel assures the stability of a sailboat, the *Spleen* provides ballast. Body weight, size, and shape remain virtually the same from day to day. To accommodate fluctuating conditions, the *Spleen* shifts fluid and mass from place to place, retaining the body's center of gravity. By promoting continuity of mental orientation and psychological perspective, the *Spleen* preserves a sense of continuous identity in relationship to place, people, and values. Such constancy supports adaptability, the capacity to endure stress without harm.

As a strategy for counterbalancing extreme deviation, the *Spleen* alters its density to cope with stress. Shifting the mass of the body facilitates ease of movement or reinforces remaining still and unperturbed. When the *Spleen* metabolically liberates energy and fluids from tissue, relieving pressure and enhancing circulation, the flesh becomes less dense and the body becomes lighter and more mobile. When matter and fluids accumulate, flesh increases and the body becomes heavier and more stationary. The *Spleen* attempts to master disequilibrium by slowing down or speeding up the conversion of nourishment to *Blood* and *Qi*. When the *Spleen* thickens fluids and tissue, it produces stagnation and adhesion, retarding movement and weighing down the body.

OVERWHELMED

When overburdened by excessive input, either food or information, the *Spleen* cannot transform or transport what it receives, and it produces congestion instead of providing nourishment. This congestion is experienced as distension, fullness, and lethargy accompanied by ponderous, obsessive, and muddy thinking. Movement of mind and body is lugubrious and effortful. When the *Spleen* is exhausted, the mind becomes disoriented, easily distracted by scattered, superficial, and elusive thoughts. The body feels fatigue, a lack of energy and strength.

The *Spleen* "supervises" the *Blood* by keeping it within the vessels. Normally through its function of digestion and assimilation, the *Spleen* supplies the nourishment to maintain the tone and elasticity of the blood vessel walls. If the *Spleen* cannot perform this role, the blood vessel walls grow fragile and may even collapse—the basis of bruising, varicosities, chronic bleeding, and hemorrhage.

Since the *Spleen* is the source of the juices of the body that circulate in the media of blood, lymph, and saliva, it is vulnerable to problems of *Damp-* 115 *ness.* Surplus fluid spills over into the tissue. After tissue becomes saturated, fluid is shunted into joints, sinuses, abdomen, lungs, and the space between skin and muscle. This *excess* is experienced as spongy tender flesh, swelling of the belly, joints, and lymph nodes, edema under the skin, painful swellings of the breast or reproductive organs, and copious or sticky discharges from the nose, throat, mouth, and other mucous membranes. The texture of secretions is determined by the interaction of *Dampness* with *Heat* or *Cold*. Clear and fluent discharges are a product of *Cold* affecting the *Spleen*; thick and sticky discharges occur when *Heat* becomes entangled with *Moisture*.

Phlegm is congealed fluid that arises from accumulated *Dampness* and obstructs the free flow of *Qi* and *Blood*, producing stagnation. Phlegm in the respiratory tract is associated with coughing, wheezing, and expectoration of sputum. Phlegm affecting the joints, muscles, and nerves is felt but not seen— this "invisible phlegm" creates arthritic and rheumatic pain, dizziness, seizures, even paralysis.

MATE OF THE SPLEEN: THE STOMACH

The *Yang* partner within the *Spleen Network* is the *Stomach*, which "rots and ripens" food by moistening and decomposing it. In contrast with the *Spleen*, the *Stomach* needs fluids to execute its duty. Yet excessive wetness makes the *Spleen's* job of absorbing and distributing fluids more difficult. Since the *Stomach* is *Yang*, its nature is warmer and drier and therefore needs the balance of *Yin* moisture; since the *Spleen* is cooler and damper, *Yin*, it needs the balance of *Yang* dryness.

Normally the *Spleen Qi* moves up, bringing pure *Essence* to the *Lung*, and the *Stomach Qi* descends, bringing impure matter and liquid to the *Intestines*. If instead the *Stomach Qi* rebels and moves upward, belching, hiccups, nausea, regurgitation, and inflamed gums can occur. It is the *Spleen's* upward-moving *Qi* that maintains organs, vessels, and tissues in their proper place. If *Spleen Qi* sinks downward, diarrhea and prolapse of organs and veins occurs, especially of the stomach, intestines, uterus, and rectum, causing hernias and hemorrhoids.

WEAK SPLEEN: DEPLETED QI AND BLOOD

Just as *Spleen* weakness leads to *deficiency* of *Qi*, it also leads to a *deficiency* of *Blood*. Symptoms of this are anemia, dry skin and hair, blurry vision, pale lips and nails, dizziness, and fatigue (muscle atrophy, weakness, and emaciation). The *Heart* depends on the *Blood* formed by the *Spleen*, the lack of which leads to symptoms like palpitations and insomnia. Similarly, without having adequate *Blood* to store, the *Liver* will become unstable, unable to properly regulate the *Qi*. This in turn causes disruption to the digestive function of the *Spleen*. For the *Lung*, when the moist *Essence* generated by the *Spleen* is insufficient, its delicate lining, plus that of the nose and large intestine, becomes dry and fragile. This hinders the blending of *Essence* (*Food* and *Air*), leading to a loss of vitality and weakening of body defenses.

GREAT SUSTAINER

Thus the *Spleen* assists the *Liver* and *Heart* by maintaining the integrity of the blood vessels, nourishing the *Blood*, and maintaining its proper viscosity so that it flows smoothly. This helps to preserve the stability of the mind and emotions. It assists the *Lung* and the *Kidney* by generating *Essence* and distributing adequate *Moisture* and lubrication for skin and mucous membrane.

METAL: THE LUNG

In the *Lung*, the *Qi* of Heaven (air) joins with the *Qi* of Earth (nutrition), forming the *Qi* that vitalizes human life. Like a minister who conducts affairs of state and determines territorial borders, the *Lung* governs the relationship between the inside and the outside, setting limits and protecting boundaries. With restraint and delicacy, expanding and contracting, the *Lung* collects, mixes, and scatters the *Qi*, instilling rhythm and order.

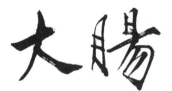

Lung-Large Intestine

ESTABLISHING THE CADENCE OF QI

The newborn's first breath ushers in its separate, individual existence. The activity of respiration drives the *Qi* throughout the body. This continuous bellowslike pulsation of the chest and abdomen sets the basic rhythmic pattern of all functions in the organism. To receive air, the *Lung* empties, slowing the movement of *Qi*, and when the chest fills, the movement of *Qi* accelerates. In Western terms, the function of the parasympathetic nervous system is analogous to that of the *Lung* insofar as it is a mechanism for inhibiting and quieting activity.

Many physical and spiritual self-mastery systems adhere to the premise that by controlling the breath one can achieve and preserve mental clarity, emotional tranquillity, and physical vigor. Accordingly, Taoist adepts developed a practical discipline of breath called *Qi Gong* to cultivate vitality and prevent disease.

As in the alchemical process of transmuting the base metals of lead and   117

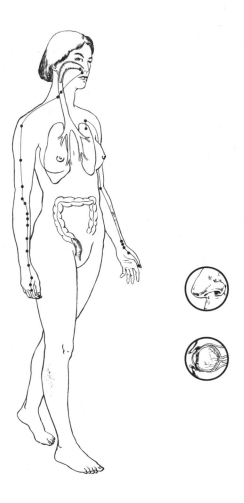

Lung Network

Role:	Viscera:	Tissues:	Fluids and
refines the *Qi*	lung	nose	Secretions:
establishes	large intestine	sinuses	mucus
rhythm		nasopharynx	secretions
maintains		bronchi	
boundaries		skin and mucous	
and defenses		membranes	
		body hair	
		sclera of the eye	

mercury into gold, the *Lung* extracts the *Essence* from *Air*, combining it with the *Essence* from *Food* sent by the *Spleen*, distilling it into the pure, correct *Qi* of bodily life. The *Lung* then guides this refined essence downward from the head into the chest and abdomen and outward toward the muscles, skin, and extremities. Through exhalation, the *Lung* eliminates the by-products of its alchemical work by expelling the turbid, used air. If this descending and dispersing cadence is thwarted, an uprising of rebellious *Qi* causes coarse breathing, headaches, tightness of the chest and shoulders, and mental distress.

EXTERNAL SECURITY

As the interface between our inner and outer world, the *Lung* manages external security. Sometimes referred to as the "third *Lung*," the skin is the outermost surface of the self, providing an elastic envelope that contains us, shielding against intrusion. The *Lung* transpires across the dermal layer: through perspiration, plus opening and closing the pores, it constantly adjusts the moisture and temperature of the body. Like a screen of variable porosity, the *Lung* tightens and thickens the skin to ward off undesirable influences and seal in valuable internal resources, or it loosens and thins the skin to release unwanted internal substances or feelings and permit penetration of desirable influences. Often the first strategy for treating acute illness is to drive the pathogenic influences of *Cold*, *Heat*, and *Wind* out through the skin by using methods that stimulate peripheral circulation and open the pores. The *Lung* mobilizes the periphery, called the *wei Qi*, or first line of defense, which enables the body to adapt to its environment and resist adversity. If the *Lung Qi* is weak, our physical and emotional protection is reduced, making us vulnerable to infectious diseases as well as to the negative thoughts and feelings of other people.

DISPERSION OF MOISTURE

The smooth dispersion of *Moisture* to all parts of the body is also a task of the *Lung*. It collects the *Fluid Essence* transported upward from the *Spleen* and moisture from the air and "precipitates" it downward, like mist, to the *Kidney* and *Bladder* as well as releasing it as sweat. Thus the *Lungs* serve to regulate urine output. If the *Lung Qi* is prevented from properly descending, *Moisture* accumulates in the upper body, causing facial edema above and scanty urinary output below. If, on the other hand, the *Lung Qi* is severely weakened, *Moisture* and vitality may leak away from the body through excessive sweating (perspiration at rest) or uncontrolled urination (incontinence), because the *Lung Yang* can no longer vaporize the *Qi* upward. Since *Moisture* is generated by the *Spleen* and transported to the *Lung*, if there is a *Spleen* problem, there will be a buildup of *Moisture*, or *Dampness*. This *Dampness* in the *Lung* can congeal into phlegm, which obstructs the bronchi,   119 throat, and nose, impairing respiration, causing coughing, asthma, and nasal congestion. The *Lung* is the upper source that accepts the *Qi*, and the *Kidney* is the lower source that grasps and anchors the *Qi*. Shortness of breath can occur when the *Kidney* cannot store the *Qi* that the *Lung* receives.

THE LUNG-HEART CONNECTION

Since the *Lung* commands the *Qi* and the *Heart* rules the *Blood*, the *Lung* and *Heart* depend upon each other. The axiom "Where *Qi* goes, *Blood* flows" means that the movement of *Qi* governs the flow of *Blood*. The beat of the heart keeps pace with the breath, and the *Blood* follows the *Qi* on its return to the *Heart*. A congestion of *Lung Qi* impedes the circulation of *Blood*, causing palpitations and fullness in the chest. A *deficiency* of *Heart* function impairs respiration, causing shortness of breath and easy sweating. Other disturbances of the *Lung* manifest as disorders of the skin, mucous membrane, and venous circulation. Manifestations of this include dry and wrinkled skin, allergic dermatitis, loss of body hair, varicose veins, sensitivity to drafts and changes in temperature, and diminished immunity to colds, flus, and other infectious microbes.

MATE OF THE LUNG: THE LARGE INTESTINE

The *Large Intestine* is the *Yang* partner of the *Lung Network*. It amasses and discharges the refuse of digestion and metabolism, continuing the process of refining that begins in the *Lung*. By dispelling stale air and excreting turbid matter, the *Lung* and *Large Intestine* separate out that which we no longer desire or need.

Generally, the *Large Intestine* delineates and shapes that which we no longer want and that which is not us—creating the space for recognition of what we do want and who we are. It helps us to concretely distinguish between what is useful and useless, beneficial and harmful, right and wrong, self and nonself.

When the *Large Intestine* is not functioning properly, distinctions become vague and ambiguous, and the mind becomes unclear and cluttered. Failure to eliminate the old leaves no room to take in what is fresh and new, leaving an unpleasant feeling of stuffiness, staleness, and lifelessness. Conversely, being unable to extract and retain the good leaves a person weak, empty, and withered. The *Large Intestine*, together with the *Lung*, promotes the processes of separation, distillation, individuation, and elimination, engendering a distinct sense of form and value.

The ease with which we are able to let go of unnecessary thoughts, feelings, and attachments is facilitated by the function of this *Network*. Letting go can be experienced in the extreme as a loss of control, provoking an urgent desire to exercise stricter self-regulation. For the sake of security, relaxation and flexibility may be sacrificed. This reluctance to easily release impulses and express feelings develops into a posture of rigidity and with-holding. Suppressing physical and emotional responsiveness is a way of ar-moring oneself, stiffening and hardening the protective envelope of the psyche and soma. The skin and superficial musculature become rigid, the deeper muscles of the diaphragm and intestines become spastic and tense. Asthma, constipation, stiffness of the spine and neck, and spastic colon are the consequences of this overrestraint of *Lung* and *Large Intestine*. Mental fixation and emotional inhibition limit the range of response, restricting creativity and the adaptability of the organism.

INSPIRATION, FORM

With inspiration and expiration the body inflates and shrinks, defining the margins of contraction and expansion, the fundamental polarities of *Yin* and *Yang*. Breathing is separated into inhalation and exhalation—between the two there is a brief interval, a moment of stillness that partitions events, marking beginnings and endings. The *Lung* is sensitive, tender, yielding, open, and refined as it directs the *Qi*, providing form, structure, and definition. When the *Lung* is vigorous and strong, the skin is smooth, supple, and vibrant, the body has abundant physical power, an even tempo, and superior immunity. The *Lung* is the source of inspiration—it creates the open space, the empti-ness within which new ideas and emotions take shape.

WATER: THE KIDNEY

The *Kidney* consolidates and stores the *Qi* that initiates and keeps life grow-ing. Like a minister of interior who conserves natural resources, stockpiling essential raw materials for use in times of growth, crisis, or transition, the *Kidney* preserves what is essential, the *Essence*, of human life. As the well of vitality and endurance, the *Kidney* is the germ of intellect, creativity, and houses our instinct to procreate and survive.

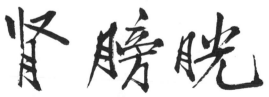

Kidney-Bladder

HARBORS THE GERM

Before we are born our parents endow us with *Essence Qi*, which following birth is fortified by *Air Qi* from the *Lungs* and *Food Qi* from the *Spleen*. Both inherited and acquired *Qi* is collected within the reservoir of the *Kidney* to 121

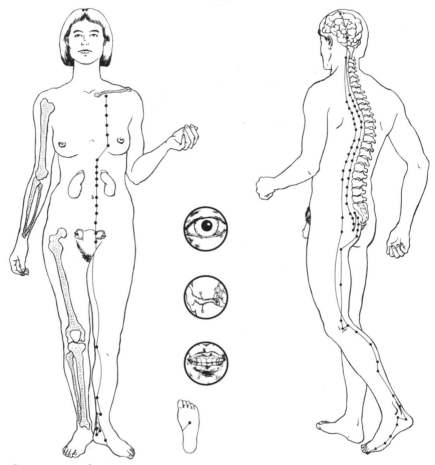

Kidney Network

Role:	Viscera:	Tissues:	Fluids and Secretions:
generates and stores *Essence*	kidney	ovaries	sexual secretions
governs reproduction and growth	bladder	testes	cerebrospinal fluid
balances fluids		brain	
anchors *Qi*		spinal cord	
		spinal column	
		bones	
		bone marrow	
		teeth	
		pubic and head hair	
		inner ear	
		pupil of the eye	
		anus and urethra	

be dispensed as needed. To say the *Kidney* holds the *Essence* means it generates and warehouses the original material substance that forms the basis of all other tissues—it grasps the kernel from which all life springs. *Kidney Essence* can be likened to the genetic information encoded in DNA, the template of biological destiny, which along with basic structural proteins forms hormones and enzymes that direct cellular metabolism. The *Kidney* is the fundament that upholds our continuous regeneration, the link in our chain of being. Responsible for procreation, the *Kidney* transmits our physical and cultural inheritance as a species from millions of years of evolution. It is the source of our imagination, enabling us to look backward at our ancestral origins, our heritage, and look forward to envision our future and create our progeny.

As the deep-reaching roots of a sapling suck the juices of the earth while its leafy branches imbibe sunlight and air, so the *Kidney* secures essential sap (*Yin*) while imparting essential heat (*Yang*). *Kidney Yin*, like the root system, nourishes and moisturizes, whereas *Kidney Yang* warms and activates. Even though the *Kidney* is the most *Yin* organ, it contains within it the *Yang* seed of its opposite, *Fire*. The rudimentary vegetative mechanisms that sustain the organism—analogous to the integrated function of the hypothalamus, pituitary, and adrenal glands in Western terms—are governed by the *Kidney*. The primary catalytic substance, *Kidney Essence (Jing)*, enables the *Spirit (Shen)* to express itself. *Jing* and *Shen* interact to create the soma and the psyche, the *Water* and *Fire*, the *Yin* and *Yang*. The presence (*Shen*) that animates the being is required to humanize its vessel, the body. The vessel (*Jing*) is necessary to give mindful existence its form.

REGENERATION

The *Kidney* supports the reproductive organs (ovaries, uterus, testicles, prostate), the reproductive material (sperm and ovum), and reproductive activity (sexual impulse, ovulation, ejaculation, fertilization, gestation). When the *Kidney Qi* is abundant, sexual and reproductive life is vigorous and lasting. The supply of inherited *Essence* is finite—our lifespan is demarcated by its ultimate diminution.

GROWTH

The *Kidney* engenders the structural elements of the body and regulates growth. The proper unfolding of mental and physical maturation depends upon the adequate supply of *Essence*, which gives rise to the marrow, which in turn produces the brain and spinal cord, bones, teeth, blood, and hair. The brain is called the "sea of marrow," meaning that the cleverness and acuity of the mind and senses are subsidized by the *Kidney*, as is the timely appearance of teeth, secondary sexual characteristics, the ability to store calcium in the bones, inscribe experience in the memory, and accelerate the manufacture of red blood cells.   123

When *Essence* is plentiful, the life force and the ability to resist disease and adapt to change are strong. Poor health, developmental deformities, mental retardation, fragility of bone, and premature aging signify insufficiency of *Essence*. Withering of the skin, deterioration of the joints, fading of mental faculties, stiffness of the spine, loss or graying of hair, dimness of vision and hearing, loss of teeth, impotence, and infertility betray its decline. Ample stamina, luxuriant hair, perennial vigor, sound teeth, and agility of thinking evidence flourishing *Essence*.

FLUID METABOLISM

Kidney Yin is the basis of all liquid substances in the body, and *Kidney Yang* regulates the balance and circulation of these constituents. All internal secretions and interstitial fluids are derived from the synthesis of inherited and acquired *Yin Essence*, including tears, saliva, mucus, urine, sweat, cerebrospinal fluid, synovial fluid, plasma, and semen. The *Yin* aspect of the *Kidney* accepts and stores the *Qi* that precipitates downward from the *Lung* and the surplus *Qi* from the *Spleen* and *Stomach*, transmitted by the *Small Intestine*. By sucking in the descending *Qi* from the *Lung* and holding on to it, the *Kidney* anchors the *Qi* like a root, permitting deep inhalation and perfusion of oxygen (*Air Qi*). The *Kidney* in the lower body and the *Lung* in the upper body act upon the *Qi* as the moving coil within a magnetic chamber generates an oscillating electrical field. The *Qi* constantly moves downward and upward between the poles of the pelvis and chest.

If too much fluid condenses in the lower body, it stagnates, producing lower abdominal bloating, swelling of the knees and ankles, and puffiness beneath the eyes. Water retention represents either the inability of the *Kidney* to discharge turbid fluid or the excessive accumulation of surplus energy in the form of *Moisture*. In either case, the buildup of interstitial fluid can interfere with the circulation of *Qi* and *Blood*, affecting primarily the *Lungs* and *Heart*. Excessive *Moisture* in the *Lung* becomes phlegm and is manifested by puffiness of the face and skin between the eyebrows and upper eyelids. In the *Heart Network* excess *Moisture* shows as edema within the chest and upper abdomen and swelling of the hands and tongue.

MATE OF THE KIDNEY: THE BLADDER

As the *Kidney* filters pure from turbid fluid to produce urine, vaporizing *Moisture* upward and recycling nutrient and lubricating fluids, the *Bladder* holds and releases the unneeded fluid. Through its *Yang* partner, the *Bladder*, the *Kidney* controls the urethral sphincter, regulating the discharge of urine and semen. Through the other lower sphincters of the anus and cervix the *Kidney* regulates the retention and release of stool and menstrual blood.

BASAL METABOLISM

Just as an ember hiding its dense heat within a dark husk of charred wood ignites new fuel, so *Kidney Yang* kindles metabolic process. Whereas the bright flashing *Yang* of the *Heart* shimmers across the surface through the eyes, the *Yang* of the *Kidney* is buried below the navel, where warmth is felt but not seen, like the molten core of our planet. *Kidney Yang* supplies the necessary spark that stirs the organism, warms the body, animates the *Spirit*, activates the *Spleen* and *Liver*, assists the *Lung* in mobilizing *Qi*, instigates reproduction, regulates water metabolism, and oversees the *Bladder* in the storage and discharge of urine. If *Kidney Yang* is exceptionally robust, one has superior resistance to cold, reliable digestive power, and lifelong sexual potency.

When the circulation of fluids is not regulated, it is often a problem of *Kidney Yang* not controlling *Kidney Yin*. Essential heat must not cease; if it does, the body cannot remain warm, respiration falters, and food cannot be digested. With a *deficiency* of *Kidney Yang*, the person feels cold and is cold to the touch, and symptoms manifest such as diarrhea, frequent or incontinent urine, infertility, impotence, premature ejaculation, loss of hearing, ringing in the ears, dizziness from fatigue, and weakness and pain in the knees, lower legs, and low back.

Kidney Yang is vulnerable to damage by exposure to physical cold—cold weather or air conditioning—and by the ingestion of iced or refrigerated foods and beverages. *Kidney Yin* is subject to damage by chemical agents, such as antibiotics, analgesics, tranquilizers, food additives, air pollutants, and recreational drugs. It may also be harmed by inadequate intake of water and too much bitter, salty, or hot, spicy food. The *Kidney* is generally undermined by inadequate sleep, excessive exercise, sexual activity, or work.

THE ORIGINAL SOURCE

All other *Organs* depend on the *Kidney* for moistening and regeneration (*Yin*) and for animation and warmth (*Yang*). The *Kidney* enables the *Spleen* to lubricate and nourish tissue and supplies the *Heat* essential for digestion; the *Heart* relies upon *Kidney Yang* to exert the force required for systole; the *Lung* requires the vaporizing, moistening, and anchoring power of the *Kidney*. The *Liver* needs the moistening of *Kidney Yin* to nourish the *Blood* and subdue the *Fire* of the *Liver*, and it requires the mobilizing function of *Kidney Yang* to regulate and distribute the *Blood*. A *deficiency* in another *Organ Network* adversely affects the *Kidney* by draining its reserves of *Essence*.

Together the *Yin* and *Yang* of the *Kidney* construct the substance and stimulate the function of the soma and psyche. The *Kidney* is like an inland sea: on the surface languid and serene, fed by seasonal rains and crystal-pure underground rivers, with warm mineral-rich vapors bubbling up from beneath its floor, breathing renewal into salty waters that teem with primordial marine life. Submerged within us, the *Kidney* envelops the hidden, quintessential treasure house of life's potentiating power.   125

Typical Disease Patterns		
Wood	*Fire*	*Earth*
Syndromes		
Disturbances of peripheral nerves and circulation	Cardiovascular diseases	Disturbances of digestion and absorption
Disturbances of equilibrium, coordination, locomotion	Disturbances of speech, thinking, emotional expression	Disorders of lymphatic circulation
Migratory pain or swelling	Sleep disturbances	Disorders of fluid distribution or viscosity (lymphatic circulation)
Tension, cramps, and spasms of muscles, nerves, and organs	Collagen deterioration (lupus, rheumatoid arthritis, marfan)	Diseases of the muscles
Disorders characterized by erratic and irregular function	Dysfunctions of integrative function (psychosis, schizophrenia)	Disorders of blood and veins
Complaints		
Irritability	Irregular rate and rhythm of heart	Indigestion
Pain under the ribs	Pain in the chest	Abdominal distension and flatulence
Nausea	Sweating	Poor appetite or overeating
Bitter taste in mouth	Restlessness	Loose bowels
Short temper		Anemia due to malnutrition or malabsorption
Pain in lower abdomen and groin		Hemorrhoids
Irregular menses		Bruising
Abnormalities of the fingers and toenails		
Pain in the eyes and ears		

Metal	Water
	Syndromes
Pulmonary and upper-respiratory disorders Disorders of the skin and mucous membrane Airborne allergies Disorders of fluid circulation Disorders of venous circulation	Disorders of growth and development including problems of fertility, conception, and pregnancy Disorders of central nervous system (multiple sclerosis, muscular dystrophy, cerebral palsy) Diseases of spinal column, bones, teeth, and joints Disorders of fluid metabolism
	Complaints
Shortness of breath Coughing Excess of phlegm Vulnerability to colds and flus Varicose veins Slow healing of skin	Soreness and pain of lumbosacral region Loose teeth Deafness and tinnitus Thinning or loss of head hair Weakness and pain of ankles, knees, hips Weakness of hearing and vision Impotence, infertility, habitual miscarriage, genetic impairments

II
TYPES

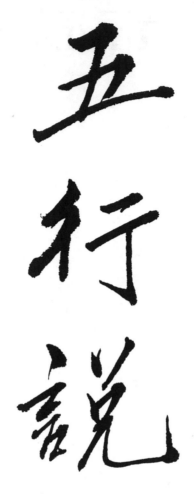

Five-Phase Theory: Who Am I?

CHAPTER SEVEN

WHO AM I:
FIVE-PHASE
ARCHETYPES

Every life is a point of view directed upon the universe. Strictly
speaking, what one life sees no other can. Every individual, whether
person, nation, or epoch, is an organ, for which there can be no
substitute, constructed for the apprehension of truth. . . . Without
the development, the perpetual change and the inexhaustible series
of adventures which constitute life, the universe, or absolutely valid
truth, would remain unknown. . . . Reality happens to be, like a
landscape, possessed of an infinite number of perspectives, all
equally veracious and authentic. The sole false perspective is that
which claims to be the only one there is.

José Ortega y Gasset
"The Doctrine of the Point of View,"
The Modern Theme

JUST AS NATIVE FLORA TRANSPLANTED TO ANOTHER REGION ADAPTS TO
the new environment in order to survive, so theories conform to cultural
settings and historical ages in order to remain relevant. Translating age-old
concepts from one culture to another in itself alters them. But in these next
chapters we have gone a step further by exercising our imaginations and
daring ourselves to cut a new trail through the old territory of *Five-Phase*
thinking.

We are reinventing as well as recapitulating classical concepts in order
to address the concerns of the people who walk through our clinic doors.
On the one hand, they just want their troubles to disappear, they want to
be "fixed" so that they can go on with their lives unimpeded. On the other,
they are curious about the origin and meaning of their difficulties and discomforts, suspecting that greater insight will enable them to avoid future
problems. People want to know: "How come I have the trouble that I do?
Where does it come from? How can I understand it? What can I do about
it? How can I prevent it in from recurring?"

Five-Phase Theory affords a particularly comprehensive, complex, yet manageable schema for self-understanding. It is an enduring conceptual system, as worthwhile to us today in America, modified and developed to conform to our culture, as it was in early China.

It is a tool to aid us in the observation of what is otherwise too hidden, too blurred, or too beyond reach: the inner, the social, and the transcendental. As a microscope brings the invisible world into view, this thinking is a lens through which we can behold the workings of our internal process. As a pair of reading glasses clarifies what is in front of our noses, these five patterns of movement bring into focus our relationships—our way of interacting with the world. As a telescope magnifies the constellations, this paradigm helps us grasp the vast scheme of the universe, aiding us in the divination of our certain place between heaven and earth.

FIVE PHASES DISTINGUISH FIVE TYPES OF PEOPLE

Our rendering of *Five-Phase Theory* postulates that we have styles of being in the world, inclinations, and gifts akin to the five seasons and powers. We are characterized by a hidden and ineffable organizing force through which all of our experience is incorporated and expressed.

Within each of us there is a particular *Phase* around which the others spin, the source from which our deepest impulses issue forth. This *Phase* is our type, the primal ontological matrix that initiates and governs the forming of our unique existence. We can distinguish five types—each of which possesses an inner landscape as distinct as the desert is from the jungle, as different as the pale dry leaves of autumn are from the flaming red dahlias of summer.

By learning how we are "put together"—how our soma and psyche are organized—our nature is revealed. When we know ourselves, we can behave accordingly. Self-recognition is a prerequisite for self-mastery. By applying the language of *Five-Phase Theory*, we can wrestle with the existential issues of identity (Who am I—how am I put together?), of purpose (What am I here to do?), and of destiny (Who will I become, and how can I make the best of it?).

Five-Phase analysis can inform us about our virtues and frailties, helping us to be wiser in our choices about what to pursue and what to avoid. Unearthing the archetypal roots of our character provides insight into our aptitudes, relationships, desires, and dreams as well as our health ailments, emotional fixations, mental doubts, and spiritual dilemmas.

Although *Five-Phase Theory* is old, the idea of *Five-Phase* "types" is our effort at grafting a Western psychospiritual branch onto the trunk of traditional Chinese medical thought. By fusing Chinese traditional meanings with Western cultural metaphors, we are expanding the ancient *Five-Phase* constructs into a phenomenological[1] model that unifies physical, emotional, and mythical realms of human experience and behavior.[2] We offer this version of *Five-Phase* thinking as our attempt at bridging Eastern and Western ideas about medicine and human process.[3]

INDIVIDUAL PSYCHOLOGY IN CHINESE MEDICINE

Psychology as we know it has not existed in classical Chinese medical thinking and remains of little importance in contemporary Chinese culture. Rather, Confucianism, with its emphatic focus on the social order, has dominated Chinese medical philosophy, ethics, and practice. In China today, individual development and welfare remain secondary to the good of society as a whole. Within this context, the psychology of individual personality has not matured beyond the somatic-psychic correspondences articulated during the Han dynasty (200 B.C.–A.D. 200).

This cultural history has translated into medical values: a healthy person is defined as a productive person, sufficiently adjusted so as not to threaten the status quo. A sound mind is assumed to be the natural outcome of a fit body and a correct relationship with family and society. This is the distance that individual psychology travels. The logic is that if people are in harmony with others in their family and society, they are presumed to be happy within themselves. The biological striving for self-determination is molded within a relatively rigid and static social model of a contented individual who exists to serve the family, the clan, and the state.[4]

In the West this set of assumptions is reversed. Individualism and personal development are elevated and rewarded as primary values. Within the social order, the common good is expected to be the natural outcome of individual freedom and fulfillment. The logic is that if people are satisfied with themselves, they will be productive and cooperative members of society. In this context, the psychology of personality assumes great significance. We strive vigorously toward self-development, always testing the constraints imposed by the need for social stability. Society in our culture is supposed to serve the individual.

Even though in China's history there has been greater concern with social role than with the issues of inner life and self-identity, generally Chinese philosophy claims that the basis for human evolution, freedom, and strength derives from harmony with nature, being familiar with and knowledgeable about the life process. Because Chinese medicine conceptually denies the division between soma and psyche, affirming the unity of body and mind, this lays the groundwork for us to use the thinking of Chinese medicine in ways the Chinese themselves have not pursued.

FIVE-PHASE THEORY FOR SELF-UNDERSTANDING

The *Five Phases* are not "things," but rather descriptions of primal forces within a universe of larger and smaller, contracting and expanding, interacting and cogenerating systems. This relational continuum is bounded at one end by more dense and tangible forms *(Yin)* and at the other by less tangible, more amorphous and diffuse forms *(Yang)*. These five forces trace process—from its inception through the *Phases*: consolidation and potentiation belongs to *Water*, expansion and initiation to *Wood*, completion and fulfillment to *Fire*, contraction and release to *Metal*, and stability and poise to *Earth*. The cosmos embodies all the *Phases*, as does each human being and process. Every individual swirls like a planet, enveloping a hidden core and displaying a surface terrain, represented by the poles of *Water* and *Fire*, *Kidney* and *Heart*. Rotational movement occurs within the context of opposition between the centripetal (contractive) and centrifugal (expansive) forces of *Metal* and *Wood*, *Lung* and *Liver*. The axis of revolution and the center of gravity and mass is represented by *Earth*, the *Spleen*, holding all other forces in harmonic tension.

This energetic model describes interaction, how the life force pulsates, inspiring and expiring, generating and degenerating, charging and discharging. Just as the magnetic needle of a compass always represents north and south, so *Water* always represents the force that stores, accumulates, and generates charge, that restores after release; and *Fire* always symbolizes the end point of expansion, consummation. Lines of correspondence between the energies of the *Five Phases* and individual structure and process establish "character types."[5]

Carl Jung established "archetypes" to describe recurring themes of universal significance, synthesizing the insights of psychoanalytic thought and Eastern mysticism. Following Jung's example, we've named five archetypes to represent the anthropomorphic qualities of each *Phase*, joining the insights of Western psychology with Chinese correspondence thinking.[6] One *Phase* predominates, shaping and defining us as well as creating the most meaningful context for our evolution to unfold. The existential issues and questions central to our life are embodied in the symbolic archetypal figures associated with each *Phase*.

To say a person leads his or her life as a *Pioneer, Philosopher, Peacemaker, Alchemist,* or *Wizard* is to evoke an image of the most affirming context within which an individual achieves self-expression. For example, the *Pio-*

neer personifies *Wood*, striking into the wilderness with a bold, adventurous spirit to break new ground, face challenges, overcome difficulty, and conquer the unknown. The *Pioneer* is action-oriented, whereas the *Philosopher*, who characterizes *Water*, is preoccupied with seeking truth and exploring the hidden mysteries through the medium of his own imaginative mind. The *Peacemaker*, stable, centered, and relaxed, personifies *Earth*, drawn toward being a mediator in the service of harmony and unity. The *Wizard*, embodying *Fire*, is magnetic and exciting, inspiring faith that dreams can be realized and desires fulfilled. The *Alchemist*, who personifies *Metal*, observes, studies, and analyzes phenomena to extract fundamental laws and principles in the service of a universal order.

The rocks in the river can shift, redirecting the water's course, altering the shape of the riverbanks, but inexorably the river, twisting and turning, follows the gravitational pull from the mountains to the sea. In that sense the river, like our identity, does not change its fundamental direction of flow. How we live out our lives may shift and vary, but the primacy of one *Phase* as our organizing force remains; we change, but our type does not. One *Phase* fashions the context within which we evolve and acts as our primary frame of reference, guiding our instincts and how we live them.

Knowing whether the power of *Wood*, *Fire*, *Earth*, *Metal*, or *Water* is preeminent sheds light on the goals we set, the risks we take, the competence we manifest, the postures we adopt toward people and projects, the expectations we have, the things that most threaten us, and the satisfactions from which we derive the greatest rewards. Our pattern also explains the otherwise mysterious configuration of our particular symptoms, why our stress manifests as sinus congestion, our friend's as fits of irritability with neck tension, and our child's as lethargy and a stomachache. It reveals under what circumstances we feel conflict and why we prefer certain solutions, where there is resistance and bound-up energy and where there is collapse and emptiness. Which of our talents and faculties are most developed and which remain stunted and neglected? In what context do we flourish, and in what context do we suffer, experiencing frustration and disappointment?

For example, *Wood* does well under the intense competitive pressure that upsets *Earth* and paralyzes *Water*. *Water* prefers to have time to think things through, and *Earth* feels most comfortable when people are working together cheerfully. So *Wood* thrives on the challenge and fast pace that threatens *Water* and *Earth*. *Metal* appreciates the same order that can hastily be cast aside by the impulsiveness of *Wood* and the excitability of *Fire*. *Earth* can be hurt and discouraged in attempts to be warm and friendly with *Metal* and *Water* types who remain detached and withdrawn. Yet *Earth* may also be just the animated, imposing social force these types need to be included in events that would otherwise pass them by.

We gravitate toward an environment that suits our character; similarly, it's easiest to develop in areas where we have natural talent. Maslow's phrase "When the only tool you have is a hammer, you treat everything as if it were a nail" describes typical fixations of character. For *Wood* it is easy to interpret any circumstance as requiring audacious action. *Fire* might perceive gratification as the end goal of any situation. *Metal* adheres to rules and protocols even when these have become a hindrance. *Water* may prefer to cogitate, perhaps losing the opportunity to realize or fulfill those visions. And *Earth* may be so concerned with establishing balance and harmony that the dynamic tension essential for movement and change is neutralized.

The *Five Phases*, corresponding to the five seasons, can be portrayed as five people. Composite characters for each *Phase*—Sally, Hector, Dorothy, Louis, and Kate—act out each archetypal destiny. Since our English language is gender specific, each type is alternately male and female. Yet the qualities and characteristics of each type appear in male and female alike. The distinguishing features of each of the *Organ Networks* are embodied in each of the five character types.

Although one *Phase* predominates as our organizing force, we exist as a complex amalgam of all the *Phases* in continuous interplay—so all *Five Phases* exist within every person. Like our DNA, the pattern of these relationships is the tao of our individualized process, the template that molds our internal and external behavior.[7] When action is demanded, our *Wood* kicks into gear. When it is time to take pleasure in the achievement of our goals, the *Fire* aspect takes charge. When we let go of old habits and values to prepare for a new stage of our life, the power of *Metal* enables us to sigh deeply and release. When our labors demand that we stop, rest, take stock of what we have done, and rededicate ourselves to a fresh purpose, our *Water* aspect gives us the renewed vitality and will to carry on. When the vicissitudes of our lives threaten to overturn or deflect us from our path, our *Earth* aspect returns us to an even keel.

TYPOLOGY IS NOT EQUIVALENT TO PATHOLOGY

Our patterns of disease and health both correspond to the *Phase* that typifies us. That is why the *Five-Phase* system can be used to simultaneously examine not only the process of sickness, but also the process of health. Pathology and ontogeny are both expressions of our instrinsic self-organizing process—one undermining, fragmenting, overwhelming, devolving, and the other affirming, integrating, enlivening, and evolving.

One way of applying *Five-Phase Theory* has been simply to equate pathology with typology—ailments alone are then the basis of typing. Within this reasoning, the *Organ Network* in which you have the most symptoms becomes synonymous with your type. For example, if your symptoms are puffy eyes, backache, chilly hands and feet, and paralysis of motivation, all these problems are associated with the *Kidney Network*, so you are considered a *Water* type. However, the *Phase* corresponding to the greatest number of our symptoms is not necessarily the one that organizes us. Symptoms often appear not only in our primary *Phase*, but in those in conflict with or being dominated by it.

Each *Phase* and *Organ Network* is like a political leader who can be benevolent and socially responsible or greedy and self-aggrandizing: each one can serve the greater good of the body as a whole or its own narrower self-interest.[8] We can think of the body as a political entity in which each *Network* functions like a Department of State. The *Liver* is like a strategic minister of defense, the *Heart* the royal monarch, the *Spleen* a minister of agriculture and trade, the *Lung* a minister of justice and secretary of state, and the *Kidney* a minister of interior and natural resources. Each of these has a political role to play in serving the state of the organism, as well as an individual need for maintaining its own existence.

Each primary *Phase* can subjugate or inhibit parts of ourselves that are less developed. Our core *Phase* can be a bully, injuring other *Phases* by its domination. Or it can become weak, neglecting to provide the leadership we rely upon for direction and guidance, and in turn be encroached upon by the *Phase* that controls it. We can be thwarted as well as served by our core *Phase*.

The *Phases* that restrain or are restrained by our primary *Phase* are the ones likely to manifest the gross distortions of our structure and character. Often our most obvious and dramatic symptoms are located in the two *Phases* along the control or *ke* sequence.

For example, for an *Earth* type, disturbances are likely to show up in *Water* (restrained by *Earth*) and in *Wood* (which restrains *Earth*). *Exaggerated Earth* oppresses *Water* and antagonizes *Wood*. When the *Spleen* is dominant, *Dampness* and the stagnation that occurs with it inhibit the function of the *Kidney* and *Liver*. An *Earth* type might experience a sore lower back, swollen ankles, and premenstrual water retention, all indications of *Kidney* disturbances, along with fullness in the head and pressure behind the eyes, which reflect *Liver* disturbance. When *Dampness* in the *Spleen* hampers the capacity of the *Liver* to make decisions and initiate action, a person feels obsessed with small changes and decisions and reluctant to commit to big decisions and their consequences. The effect on the *Kidney* is to create an unsettling feeling of doubt and insecurity, as if one's source or identity is never firmly grasped. Thus the characteristic affability and gregariousness of the *Earth* type may be hemmed in by an undercurrent of irritability and vulnerability.

When difficulty or trauma distort our true nature, disharmony manifests as aberrations of character, disturbances of physiologic function, and deformations of physical structure. This means that the behavior of an *exaggerated Organ Network* has overwhelmed and oppressed others or that it has *collapsed*, its force dissipated, creating an unstable vacuum. Signs of conflict are likely to appear along the *ke* sequence in *exaggerated* patterns and within the predominant *Organ Network* and its "mother" and "child" along the *sheng* sequence in *collapsed* patterns. If the predominant *Organ Network* is *exaggerated*, it needs to be subdued; if it is *collapsed*, it needs to be nourished. *Exaggerated* and *collapsed* patterns can and often do coexist, as do *excess* and *deficiency*, *Heat* and *Cold*. Harmony is restored when appropriate therapeutic measures of tonifying or purging, consolidating or dispersing, restore stability by easing conflict and correcting inequities. The strategy of caring only for the leader is not enough when the followers are in distress, nor is aiding the followers enough to guarantee the prudent behavior of the leader. Both must be supported or limited according to their need and their role.

When our motion is disturbed by external forces or internal upheaval, our path becomes crooked and our movement wobbly. Allied with our organizing force, we navigate smoothly along our path, our inner gyroscope unperturbed. Spinning freely, we feel aligned, at home in our body and right with the world. This comfortable sense of fit and freedom is what we recognize as health.

Five Phases within Each Phase

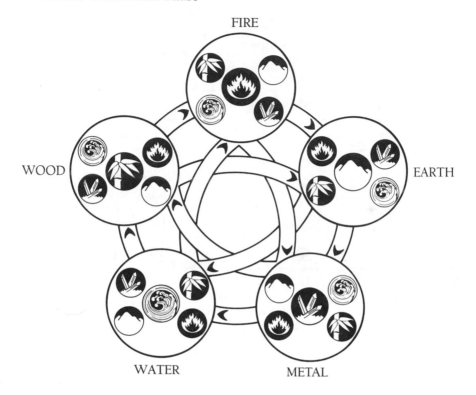

Powers of the Five Archetypes

	WOOD	FIRE
Power	Expansion	Fusion
Archetype	Pioneer	Wizard
Organized Around	Metamorphosis	Realization
Desires	Purpose	Fulfillment
Context	Challenge	Intimacy
Virtue	Fervor	Charisma
Path	Action	Compassion
Values	Utility	Intuition
Talent	Initiative	Communication
Existential Issue	Goals: What to do? Strategy: How to do it?	Dimension: How broad is my scope?
Dimensions	Movement	Space
Nourished by	Water	Wood
Nourishes	Fire	Earth
Restrains	Earth	Metal
Restrained by	Metal	Water
Subject to Injury from	Wind	Heat
Injury Enters at	Head, neck, upper back	Head, upper back, nose, mouth, throat
Sexual Values	more better longer	orgasm merging

EARTH	METAL	WATER
Moderation	Contraction	Consolidation
Peacemaker	Alchemist	Philosopher
Unification	Transmutation	Revelation
Connectedness	Order	Truth
Community	Organization	Mystery
Loyalty	Righteousness	Honesty
Service	Mastery	Knowledge
Harmony	Purity	Durability
Negotiation	Discrimination	Imagination
Orientation: What's my role? Where am I?	Boundaries: What I am and am not.	Origins/Destiny: What is my past, my future?
Location in time and space	Shape	Time
Fire	Earth	Metal
Metal	Water	Wood
Water	Wood	Fire
Wood	Fire	Earth
Damp	Dry	Cold
Head, joints, lower back, lower abdomen	Head, skin, mouth, throat, nose	Head, upper back, lower back, hips, legs
embracing connectedness	sacred ritual ceremony	penetration uncovering hidden mystery

Distortions of Five Powers

	WOOD	FIRE
Exaggerated Power	Domination	Immolation
Collapsed Power	Compression	Disintegration
Preoccupation	Work	Stimulation
Compelled to	Win	Consume
Dreads	Confinement	Gravity
Seeks the Perfect	Cause	Lover
Dislikes Conflicting	Purposes Choices Impulses	Needs Desires Attractions
Obsessed with	Solutions Change Independence	Pleasure Intimacy Seeking the Divine
Aversion to	Powerlessness Bondage Dependency	Separation Boredom Pain
Somatic Poles	Tension—Relaxation Starting—Stopping Accelerated— Retarded	Containment— Dissipation Embodied— Disembodied Active—Reactive
Tends to	Risk Stay Busy	Seek Excitement Make Contact
Existential Doubt	What Is the Purpose?	How to Express Myself?
Emotional Addiction	To Be Aroused	To Be in Love
Spiritual Fear	To Be Helpless	To Be Cut Off

EARTH	METAL	WATER
Obstruction	Restriction	Negation
Stagnation	Constriction	Petrification
Details	Rituals	Secrets
Interfere	Control	Criticize
Torpidity	Crowding	Invasion
Family	System	Teacher
Roles Loyalties Frames of Reference	Mores Standards Rewards	Visions Stories Expectations
Manipulation Pleasing Others Security	Perfection Order Differences	Mysteries Facing Death Facts
Change Dislocation Independence	Spontaneity Pollution Decrepitude	Exposure Distraction Dissolution
Dense—Porous Active—Passive Filling—Emptying	Tight—Loose Closed—Open Thick—Thin	Hard—Soft Cold—Warm Retaining—Releasing
Seek Comfort Avoid Isolation	Follow Higher Order Make Judgments	Seek Solitude Avoid Exposure
What Is My Role?	What Is Right?	Where Do I Come From?
To Be Needed	To Be Right	To Be Protected
To Be Lost	To Be Corrupt	To Be Extinct

Five Types: Affinities and Aversions

Affinities: Desires and Values

Wood	Fire	Earth	Metal	Water
Struggle	Excitement	Relationships	Order	Solitude
Action	Intimacy	Stability	Purity	Mystery
Arousal	Sensuality	Family	Reason	Continuity
Practicality	Spontaneity	Sharing	Aesthetics	Originality
Uniqueness	Expression	Harmony	Definition	Toughness
Challenge	Yielding	Loyalty	Simplicity	Self-sufficiency
Achievement	Merging	Commitment	Quality	Privacy
Agility	Passion	Diplomacy	Correctness	Anonymity
Independence	Self-exposure	Involvement	Standards	Caution
Contest	Performing	Inter-dependence	Precision	Conservation

Aversions: Fears and Difficulties

Slowness	Inactivity	Separateness	Intimacy	Sharing
Clumsiness	Separation	Disloyalty	Complexity	Rashness
Ambiguity	Confusion	Conflict	Chaos	Vulner-ability
Interference	Roughness	Change	Nonsense	Ignorance
Authority	Boundaries	Aloneness	Spontaneity	Dishonesty
Compromise	Deliberation	Impermanence	Carelessness	Super-ficiality
Frustration	Dullness	Greediness	Impropriety	Faith
Constancy	Ordinariness	Insecurity	Intemperance	Exposure
Submitting	Conservation	Emptiness	Vagueness	Waste
Confinement	Suspicion	Displacement	Shapelessness	Softness

Five Types: Challenges, Contradictions, Knots

Earth:

> Being at the still point—feeling stuck
> Wanting to be full—feeling weighted down, overstuffed, and overwhelmed
> Seeking emptiness—fearing that there is nothing at the core
> Desiring change—wanting things to stay the same
> Wanting to be needed—wary of being absorbed, losing the self

Water:

> Yearns for truth—fears exposure
> Yearns for connection—intolerant of contact
> Likes to be squeezed—scared of being squashed
> Wants to penetrate inside—detests being absorbed
> Enjoys being left alone—dreads being abandoned

Wood:

> Wants to be in charge—misses the companionship of equals
> Yearns to do, to act—subject to uncontrollable impulse
> Makes rules—likes to break them
> Demands freedom—needs to struggle
> Feels invincible—fears vulnerability and loss of control

Fire:

> Desires contact, intimacy—needs solitude
> Loves sensation and feeling—fears being overwhelmed by intensity
> Loves to say yes—can't say no
> Yearns for fusion—dreads dissolution
> Lives in the moment—dreads the future

Metal:

> Wants relationship—needs distance
> Knows what is right—accepts what is safe
> Aspires toward beauty—settles for utility
> Wants joy—fears spontaneity
> Likes creativity, ingenuity—intolerant of disorder, dissonance

SELF-ASSESSMENT QUESTIONNAIRE

The following questionnaire is designed to help you map how the *Five Phases* act and interact within you. The letters (A–E) at the end of each statement refer to each of the *Five Phases*. Mark the space at the beginning of each statement according to the strength of your response. If it strongly typifies you, place a "3" in the space; if it characterizes you somewhat, put a "1"; if you feel ambivalent or indifferent toward it, put a "0." If you have a definite negative response ("I'm not at all like this!"), put a "−2."

When you are finished, total up the number of positive (+) and negative (−) responses for each section according to the letter code: total score for "A," "B," and so on. Do this before you look at the code key so that you are not biased in your responses. Record the number of positive and negative responses on the *Five-Phase* diagram at the end of the questionnaire to plot your particular patterns.

Look at the *Phases* with the highest positive scores and see whether they are opposite or adjacent to each other: *Wood* and *Fire* and *Earth* are adjacent, whereas *Wood* and *Metal*, *Fire* and *Water*, are opposite. Adjacent *Phases* with high scores reflect a strong supporting ("*sheng* sequence") relationship. Opposite *Phases* with high scores reflect a strong conflicting ("*ke* sequence") relationship. Negative scores also suggest conflict with an opposing *Phase*. In this context, conflict is not necessarily good or bad—it represents the potential for movement and change as well as instability.

If all the scores on the diagram look pretty much the same—that is, if they differ by a value of only 1–3, you may need to go back to the questionnaire, review your responses, and eliminate those that are only a "+1." This will help to accentuate the numerical contrast between *Phases*. If there are still no significant differences, refer to the charts at the end of each chapter on the five types to determine the set of characteristics with which you identify most strongly. How do these reactions compare with your responses to the questionnaire? Also, answer the questions at the end of the questionnaire and see if you can classify your answers as belonging more to one *Phase* than another.

Whether or not the pattern that emerges now reflects your primary type is a question that you may need to answer upon further consideration. Eventually a pattern will reveal itself so that you feel you have a sense of who you are within this paradigm.

PSYCHOLOGICAL

It is typical of me (+) or unlike me (−) to:

___ be honest, even blunt, though not necessarily tactful or diplomatic A
___ be cautious and sensible A
___ enjoy frequent periods of solitude and introspection A
___ enjoy indulging my imagination and curiosity A
___ keep my feelings, thoughts, and opinions to myself A
___ be content being anonymous or on the periphery of social events A
___ be considered unusual or eccentric A
___ be involved in intellectual pursuits A
___ be content with a few good friends and minimal social activities A
___ be content figuring things out for myself A
___ be careful about what I reveal to other people A
___ be a stubborn defender of the truth as I see it A
___ be patient and persevering in spite of defeats or dead ends A
___ be objective and dispassionate A
___ feel self-sufficient in or out of a relationship A
___ choose privacy over intimacy, solitude over socializing A
___ be critical and skeptical while observing people and events from a distance A
___ pursue my own interests regardless of what others consider important A
___ enjoy projects that don't involve other people A
___ remove myself from everyday affairs and turn inward to quietly reflect upon the place of my life in the grand scheme of things A

___ feel confident and act assertively B
___ enjoy being competitive and ambitious B
___ feel powerful and invulnerable B
___ reluctantly acknowledge other people as my equals B
___ openly discuss my abilities and achievements with others B
___ be comfortable with conflict or pressure B
___ enjoy being first, best, unique, or even outlandish B
___ act with confidence and assurance regardless of what others may think or feel B
___ make quick decisions and commit myself to a course of action even if the odds are not in my favor B
___ be comfortable with difficult tasks or emergencies that demand "thinking on my feet" B
___ feel that I'm right even if others strongly disagree with or disapprove of me B
___ feel good about following my instincts and satisfying my impulses B   147

_____ be direct or provocative even if it causes discomfort or embarrassment to others B

_____ take pleasure in public recognition and admiration of my talents and achievements B

_____ be comfortable leading or directing others B

_____ follow my own hunches about what is right or wrong B

_____ to take the lead when it is necessary to get things done quickly and effectively B

_____ act boldly and decisively even if I don't have all the expertise or information that I need B

_____ enjoy the process of striving against the odds for its own sake B

_____ to want to reject or argue with other people's appraisals of me B

_____ be animated and enthusiastic C

_____ enjoy the pleasure of my senses C

_____ easily know what another thinks and feels C

_____ enjoy physical contact and emotional intimacy C

_____ be comfortable in a very stimulating environment C

_____ openly share my innermost feelings and desires C

_____ live in the here and now and not worry about the future or dwell on the past C

_____ see the humorous side of life C

_____ thoroughly enjoy getting what I want and need C

_____ be tender, intimate, and vulnerable with another person C

_____ be comfortable receiving and showing affection and pleasure C

_____ enjoy being moved emotionally C

_____ easily become completely involved in the events going on around me C

_____ become deeply identified with the feelings, thoughts, and experiences of another C

_____ be emotionally sensitive, responsive, and intuitive C

_____ remain optimistic and hopeful in spite of what others may say or believe C

_____ be completely open and exposed C

_____ identify and empathize with another's joy or pain C

_____ be unabashed in showing enthusiasm and excitement C

_____ enjoy being attractive and magnetic C

_____ be nurturing and supportive D

_____ put the needs of others before my own D

_____ enjoy frequent socializing with friends and family D

_____ care for others and try to satisfy their needs D

_____ enjoy being relied upon for reassurance and help D

_____ enjoy being the hub of my social and family network D

_____ be agreeable and accommodating D

_____ enjoy settling disputes so that all parties are satisfied D

_____ help people work together in a harmonious manner D

_____ create a relaxed and comfortable environment in which very different people can enjoy being together D

_____ be loyal and accessible to the people who are my friends, relations, or in some important way involved in my life and work D

_____ get involved in other people's lives D

_____ enjoy maintaining many diverse, even conflicting, relationships D

_____ be diplomatic and tactful D

_____ rely on the skill and intelligence of others D

_____ accept other people's characterizations of who I am D

_____ enjoy just being in the company of other people D

_____ sympathize with the circumstances of others D

_____ find ways to resolve conflict and bring about agreement D

_____ get close enough to need another person D

_____ be comfortable and sociable with people I don't know well D

_____ maintain a neat and orderly personal life-style E

_____ enjoy a convivial but undemanding social life E

_____ be in control of my environment and the way I do things E

_____ be strongly committed to my moral principles and standards of conduct E

_____ feel secure and confident in my work when I know that everyone is following proper procedures E

_____ enjoy tasks that require logical, analytical, and systematic approaches to problem-solving E

_____ appreciate being thought of as meticulous and discriminating E

_____ think of myself as being impeccable and above reproach E

_____ be self-contained and not overly involved in other people's affairs E

_____ work easily and efficiently in situations where goals and guidelines are well defined E

_____ be appreciated or admired for my skill and expertise rather than my personality or emotional enthusiasm E

_____ be judged or evaluated according to objective criteria rather than personal biases or intuitions E

_____ accept the authority of those with more competence E

_____ be systematic and methodical in my work E

_____ enjoy the process of solving puzzles and mysteries E

_____ be content with few close attachments or demanding relationships E

_____ put virtue and principles before pleasure and fulfillment E

_____ restrain myself in expressing my feelings or opinions E
_____ enjoy temperance and moderation E
_____ be tasteful and discriminating E

PHYSIOLOGICAL

I am frequently (+) or rarely (−) bothered by:

_____ lack of semen or other sexual secretions A
_____ infertility, impotence, or lack of libido A
_____ depression or weariness following sex A
_____ diminished recall of recent information or events A
_____ diminished acuity of vision or hearing A
_____ swelling or pain at the inner corners of the eyes A
_____ pain in the arches, heels, or soles of the feet A
_____ hypersensitive vision and hearing A
_____ stiffness or aching of joints or spine A
_____ unusual or painful bony protuberances A
_____ frequent, slow, or suppressed urination A
_____ incontinence of semen, urine, or stool A
_____ loss of pubic or head hair A
_____ pimples on the chin or between the nose and the upper lip A
_____ fatigue or listlessness following prolonged mental effort A
_____ stiffness or pain when bending over or standing up A
_____ dark brown, purple, or black circles around the eyes A
_____ aching in the bones from fatigue, standing, or overwork A
_____ tenderness and hardness of prostate, testes, ovaries, or cervix A
_____ diminished acuity of vision or hearing A

_____ pain at the temples, sides, back, or top of the head B
_____ vertigo and nausea B
_____ sudden blurring of vision or ringing in the ears B
_____ dry eyes B
_____ headache, earache, or eye ache from exposure to wind B
_____ difficulty swallowing or tightness of the throat B
_____ sharp pain in the eyes, ears, nose, or throat, especially during the night B
_____ a feeling of fullness or soreness beneath the ribs B
_____ sudden sharp or sticking pains in the breasts, between the ribs, in the armpits, or in any of the internal or genital organs B
_____ frequent sensitivity to bright light or loud noise B
_____ split, hardened, or thickened nails B
_____ oily skin, especially of the face, nose, and scalp B
150 _____ frequent tension in the neck and across the shoulders B

___ premenstrual grouchiness and depression B
___ irritability following sex B
___ excessive libido or frequent, uncomfortable sexual arousal B
___ boils or painful nodes in the armpits or groin B
___ severe cramps at the start of menstruation B
___ cramping or twitching of the muscles in the eyes, face, ears, calves, or feet B
___ eyes that tear a lot B

___ excessive perspiration C
___ being flushed or overheated C
___ craving or thirst for cold liquids and foods C
___ rapid or irregular heartbeat C
___ sores in the mouth or on the tongue C
___ burning sensation in the mouth, urethra, rectum, or vagina C
___ easy or uncontrollable excitability C
___ feeling faint, dizzy, or disoriented when startled or excited C
___ diminished long-term memory C
___ stuttering or talking too fast C
___ nervous giggling or talkativeness C
___ premature ejaculation or orgasm C
___ insomnia when anxious or excited C
___ anxiety or dread at dusk C
___ disturbing or very vivid dreams C
___ awakening anxious or with a racing heart C
___ blushing when startled, nervous, or upset C
___ dry, red, itchy rashes or eczema, especially in the hollow of the elbows, behind the knees, or on the palms or soles of the feet C
___ distorted perceptions or mental images C
___ inflammation of the blood vessels, tongue, outer ears, or corners of the eyes C

___ rapid weight gain and difficulty losing weight D
___ obsessive desire for or avoidance of food D
___ frequent bloating of the abdomen, especially in the evening D
___ fleshy and tender muscles especially of the upper arms and thighs D
___ weakness of the neck, wrists, ankles, and low back D
___ inflamed eyelids that tend to stick together D
___ frequent cravings for sweet, glutinous, starchy foods D
___ swollen, sore, or bleeding gums D
___ misshapen nails that tear easily D
___ cuticles that erode or become inflamed easily D

_____ swollen muscles and joints D

_____ generalized puffiness or edema D

_____ easy or frequent bruising D

_____ feeling full, heavy, and lethargic D

_____ feeling dry but not thirsty D

_____ lack of stamina D

_____ premenstrual lethargy, bloating, and water retention D

_____ pimples on the scalp, eyelids (sties), nose, or around the mouth D

_____ headaches from prolonged thinking, excessive worrying, conflict, or disappointment D

_____ prolapse of the veins in the rectum (hemorrhoids) or legs (varicosities) D

_____ dryness of the nose, throat, skin, or hair E

_____ dry, scaly pimples, especially on the cheeks, beside the nose, or on the upper back E

_____ lack of perspiration even when hot E

_____ itching from dryness E

_____ scanty urine E

_____ lack of mucus secretions E

_____ many enlarged or hard lymph nodes, especially along the sides of the neck or under the jaw E

_____ large pores on the face, nose, and upper back E

_____ many moles or warts E

_____ frequent sneezing or coughing due to changes in air temperature or moisture E

_____ wrinkling or shrinking of the skin or mucous membranes E

_____ skin that feels tight or cracks easily E

_____ congestion of the nose, sinuses, or larynx E

_____ frontal headaches due to dryness or congestion with mucus E

_____ pain in the head or chest due to disappointment or loss E

_____ shallow breathing E

_____ many small varicose veins E

_____ nasal or intestinal polyps E

_____ thin, delicate skin E

_____ dry, painful, fissures or cracks of the nostrils, lips, or corners of the mouth E

Use these questions _and/or_ the statements on the questionnaire to make _five_ statements about yourself that you feel are accurate in describing who you are. These statements, along with the map, can be used to identify yourself according to the _Five-Phase_ model.

1. What concept, metaphor, or principle is at the center of your life, and how does it motivate you?

2. What do you desire from life, and what are you seeking to accomplish, create, assist, and support?

3. What circumstances would provide you with the optimum conditions for satisfying your needs and fulfilling your expectations?

4. What values and virtues do you admire and strive to engender in yourself and others?

5. What are the fundamental activities and behaviors that express your deepest intentions?

6. What do you feel is the particular talent and perspective that you bring to any relationship or endeavor?

7. What do you want from other people and from yourself?

8. What is it about your work or job that is most satisfying, most frustrating, most difficult, most easy?

9. What are your most trying dilemmas, conflicts, and contradictions?

Self-Assessment Profile

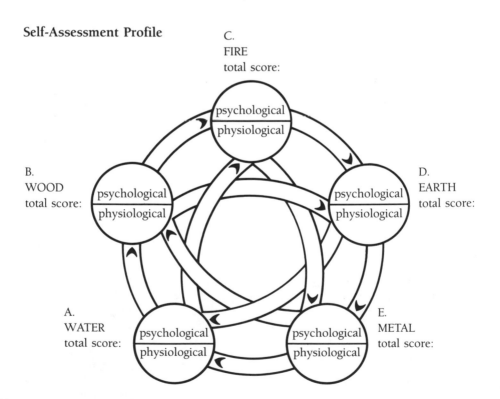

DETERMINING YOUR TYPE

Some people rightly identify with the characteristics of many types. But the object of this self-assessment process is to differentiate and make choices. When deciding which clothes to wear, you usually have many garments to choose from but select one outfit based on how it fits and whether it truly suits you. Similarly, you have to try on different archetypes to see if they fit.

But unlike clothing, you can no more change your type than you can your parents. Your organizing force, like your blood type, is with you for life. You can alter your hair color and your weight, but not your height or chromosomes. You can raise your hemoglobin, but it is to no avail to wish your blood were AB-positive when you were born O-negative.

In deliberating upon your type, it's not what you do that matters, but how and why you do it. Evie, Ed, and Susanne all spend a great deal of time cooking. Evie manages a restaurant, Ed teaches cooking classes and writes cookbooks, and Susanne frequently feeds her large extended family, inviting close friends for dinners.

Evie describes her attraction to this work: "I thrive on the challenge of getting my staff to function at a hum—everything planned just right so that the energy and the product are in a flow. I enjoy the constant demand for problem-solving—when it gets too easy, I get bored."

When Ed is asked what he likes about food, he offers a frugal, droll reply: "I like eating it." Then he continues to say that what concerns him is the form: "People seem to think I cut vegetables in interesting ways. I like to take ingredients and combine them in just the right way. I don't really care whether anybody else likes it or not. It's important to me to have room to move around and a clean and orderly space in which to work."

Susanne, on the other hand, cooks specifically to please her diners: "What I love is looking down a long table full of people I care about and having them feel good about eating food I've prepared specially for them."

Evie is a *Wood* type, Ed is *Metal*, and Susanne is *Earth*. Evie is also a perfectionist (a *Metal* characteristic) and often feeds her friends *(Earth)*; Ed takes pleasure in getting things done *(Wood)*; and Susanne works as a graphic designer, spending most of her time doing solitary, creative work *(Water)*. Each embodies traits of all the *Phases* but is most motivated and characterized by one.

YEARNING TO BE ANOTHER

Kosta is a large, friendly, fleshy philosophy professor who is extremely nurturing, sometimes to the point of neglecting his own needs. At times dissatisfied with his *Earth* nature, he wishes he were more like Achilles, the mythical warrior, rather than Ferdinand the Bull, who is content to sit quietly and smell the flowers. He struggles to bolster the rude will and determination needed for him to fight for himself and what he cares about.

Madeline is an intense doctor, a self-directed loner, a *Water* type who wishes she were more like Kosta, soft, connected, communal, and easy to know and love. She would like to change her nature in order to escape her limitations and fulfill her longings.

Some of you will be sure of your type, others will resist identification, especially with that which most represents you. Often this is because you are attempting to develop neglected aspects of your character. It is appropriate for you to want to cultivate the power of polar *Phases* that will give you greater scope and stability. During times of growth or stress it is possible to confuse that which you are striving for with that which you are. In these examples it is the *ke* relationships that are at play—Kosta is seeking to develop his *Wood* aspect to compensate for the overbearing influence of *Earth*, while Madeline needs to cultivate *Earth* to expand her *Water* nature. Kosta and Madeline demonstrate the inclination to reach for and embody what counterbalances them. It is the stabilizing power of the *ke* relationships that restrains and counterbalances us.

UNDERSTANDING SHENG AND KE

When Murray, a strident and assertive *Wood* type, needs to restore himself, he retreats from projects and commitments like a reclusive *Water* type, preferring to spend hours in solitary reading, studying, and going to the movies. When he is feeling at his peak, he burns hot like a flamboyant *Fire* type, open, charismatic, demonstrative, and exciting, a magical communicator and teacher. Murray illustrates how when the organizing *Phase (Wood)* is in *collapse*, it gravitates toward its parent *(Water)*, and in *exaggeration,* it becomes like its child *(Fire)*. In times of vulnerability as well as in times of being overcharged, it can be a *Phase* on the *sheng* sequence that masquerades as our type.

Ke implies tension, while *sheng* implies capacity. The *sheng* triad maintains our resources, our potential. Without tension, potential has no spring, no motivating impulse, no egress; and without potential, motivation has no foundation, no source, no utility. Equilibrium is the outcome of poise between opposing forces as well as sustenance of vital reserves. When the organizing pattern we call our type is harmonic, there is a satisfying complementarity between the nurturance of our potential and the intensity that brings it forth. Tension without adequate potential (reserve) leads to exhaustion, and potential without the essential ignition of intensity and striving (tension) leads to stultification and inertia.

Usually the first problems people experience are a result of *ke* sequence conflict, which is an escalation of tension between the primary *Phase*, the one it controls, and the one that controls it. This is how the *exaggerated* pattern develops. When the equilibrating mechanism of the organism has been overwhelmed by *exaggeration*, *collapse* ensues, and problems along the *sheng* sequence tend to become more apparent.

We tend to define each type in terms of the *ke* triad. For this reason we see harmonizing the relationships between *Earth* and *Water* (*Spleen-Kidney*), *Wood* and *Earth* (*Liver-Spleen*), *Metal* and *Wood* (*Lung-Liver*), *Fire* and *Metal* (*Heart-Lung*), and *Water* and *Fire* (*Kidney-Heart*) as essential in reconciling conflict and regaining stability.

STEPS TO SOLVING THE PUZZLE

Solving the puzzle of which type you are involves several steps, but not necessarily in a predetermined order. After reading the descriptions of each *Phase*, pick one that you identify with most strongly. You can also flip to the ends of the chapters and review the charts that summarize the mental faculties, emotional qualities, physical features, and problem areas of each type. Once having decided, look at the pattern of interactions between *Phases*.

Suppose you feel the greatest affinity with *Fire*. Do you also have strong responses—either positive or negative—with *Metal* or *Water*? Use this strong response along the *ke* sequence to confirm or cast doubt on your hypothetical type designation. The triad of *Metal-Wood-Earth* characterizes the dynamic of the *Wood* type, whereas the triad of *Water-Fire-Metal* characterizes the *Fire* type. Both types share tension with *Metal*, so what can help you distinguish between being a *Wood* or *Fire* type will be evaluating whether there is greater tension for you with *Water* if you are a *Fire* type or tension with *Earth* if you are a *Wood* type.

This example emphasizes that in determining what type you are, it is central to look at the interactions and relationships of the *Phases* within you. So, if you suspect that you are a *Metal* type, your pattern of affinities, aversions, symptoms, and emotional styles should reflect stronger interactions with *Wood* and *Fire* than with *Earth* and *Water*.

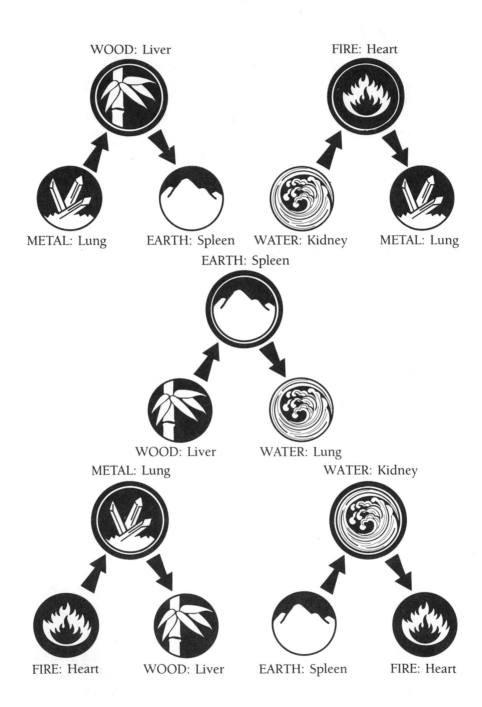

The *Ke* Relationships

FROM THEORY TO PRACTICE

Recognizing who you are and how you function within the *Five-Phase* paradigm provides a starting point from which to gain access to the practical benefits that Chinese medicine offers. It is a starting point from which to acquire the means to preserve or recover health. *Five-Phase* thinking can not only help you evaluate your personal strengths and weaknesses and forecast future difficulties, it can also guide you in the use of therapies such as acupuncture, medicinal herb formulas, and food recipes.

CHAPTER EIGHT
WOOD

Spring

The water murmurs
In the old stone well,
And, a rippling mirror,
Gives back the clear blue sky.
The river roars,
Swollen with the late rains of spring.
On the cool, jade-green grass
The golden sunshine
Splashes.

Sometimes, at early dawn,
I climb
Even as far as Lien Shan Temple.
In the spring
I plow the thirsty field,
That it may drink new life.
I eat a little,
I work a little,
Each day my hair grows thinner,
And, it seems,
I lean ever a bit more heavily
On my old thornwood cane.
      Liu Tzu-Hui
      Sung dynasty, A.D. 960–1278

WOOD IS AS FORCEFUL AND DETERMINED AS THE WIND, AS SUPPLE AS A spreading aspen stretching into a bright, cloudless sky. Spring, a time of rebirth, sudden growth, and rapid expansion, marks the ascendance of this power. Movement surges to the surface, bursting through the confinement of winter. A crescendo of excitement builds as the life process reawakens. One day the forest appears gray and lifeless, the next day sunbeams cast warm light upon branches brimming with buds. This burgeoning of activity stirs tumultuous feeling. The change is expected yet unpredictable—like the birth of a child, the precise day or moment remains a mystery; we know spring will come but not exactly when. Anticipation foments tension as well as the promise of release.

The *Liver*, whose *Qi* is akin to the phase of *Wood*, instigates movement and arouses the mind by allowing tension and pressure to build. As spring initiates the rising of sap in the trees, so the *Liver* lifts the *Blood* and *Qi*. Alternately gathering and releasing the *Blood*, the *Liver* modulates the intensity and force of all motion and process.

THE ARCHETYPE FOR WOOD: THE PIONEER

Metamorphosis is the organizing principle for the *Pioneer*. Driven by the adventure of penetrating the unknown, she contends with fate, deliberately battling adversity to tame the wilderness. Adaptive, cunning, and fiercely independent, she strikes out on her own, striving constantly to surpass her limits. Carving a broad expanse in which movement and vision are free and unfettered takes a multiplicity of forms. Inexorably drawn to travel roads not yet mapped, she treks wild mountain ridges, explores star-clustered heavens in an astronaut's suit, launches a business from scratch, or embarks upon research in yet unrecognized fields. Infatuated with what is new, curious about what is untried, she is eager to innovate, reform, and revolutionize.

Action compels the *Pioneer*. She vanquishes resistance with the thrust of a warrior's determination. Like a locomotive that gathers momentum and speed as it hurtles down the track, the *Pioneer* steers an awesome power.

SALLY: EXEMPLAR OF WOOD

Assertive in forging plans and implementing them, Sally maneuvers easily and gets things done. Highly motivated, she pursues projects with outright zeal, shifting into gear with a strategic sense of opportunity. Sally moves with nimble elegance, fully inhabiting her body. She drives herself hard, works well under pressure, and meets deadlines. Resourceful and ingenious, she excels at managing conflict and producing solutions. Her strength is not as a visionary, but as an implementer. Sally takes the ball and runs with it. Once she sets her goal, she brooks no interference to achieve it. Wielding power and influence comes naturally.

Sally's audacity bolsters her inclination to take the risks necessary to initiate change. She is willing to forfeit comfort, break with tradition, and endure hardship, perceiving the sacrifice of contentment and convention not as loss, but as liberation from the constraints of obligation and rules. With certainty and self-confidence, Sally galvanizes others, infusing them with her own ambition and optimism. With the conviction that her purpose is worthy, she expects that all obstacles can be overcome.

Impatient with sitting still, Sally can be quiet but never completely relaxed. Comfortable with perpetual motion, she is wary and alert, like a cougar stalking the forest with muscular grace, ready to react, confront, or change course. Her objective is her prey, which she hunts with craft and passion. It is no strain for Sally to sublimate other pleasures for the sake of accomplishment. She thrives within American culture, where ambition, achievement, and single-mindedness are handsomely rewarded.

Sally's confidence is matched by her commitment. Once she has decided that she wants to do something, she keeps at it until it is done, working long and hard if necessary. Once the end is in sight, she is ready to move on, to meet the next test. Others may have trouble keeping up with Sally's pace. After an arduous hike up a mountain, when the rest of her group is ready to sit and fish by the creek, Sally is off scaling another peak. She feels most herself striving, advancing, contending: grappling with a problem, initiating events, figuring out novel strategies, and pitting her competence against the odds. With a passion for the race, the gamble, and the victory, she is willing to do anything and risk everything—sink or swim, do or die. Sally is courageous, assuming tasks and undertaking courses of action that others would fear or deride. She prefers being the first, the best, or just one of a kind.

Protective and supportive of her family, Sally prides herself on being a competent provider. She does not relish hanging out idly at home, so she keeps busy. Sometimes equating domesticity with tameness and predictability, she is wary of the constraints that constant closeness require, like compromising for the sake of others' needs. She savors being wanted more than being needed. The dependency of the family can strain her yearning for freedom of movement and action.

Sally's perspective is that there is "one way, my way, the right way." She doesn't question her own judgment and authority and resists the idea that someone else may. When Sally's self-assurance becomes inflated, she stubbornly thrusts her chin and shoulders forward, assuming a provocative stance. Her momentum snowballs beyond her capacity for self-control. She keeps pushing when she should back off, tightening up when she should relax, barreling ahead when she should pause and reflect. Ignoring considerations that may cast reasonable doubt upon her choices, she bolts like a racehorse wearing blinders. Rushing ahead impetuously and defiantly, she becomes accident-prone, tripping over unseen hazards, a disaster waiting to happen, injuring herself or others unintentionally. Feeling invincible and unassailable, she indulges her impulses as if nothing can or should stop her. This insistence upon following her own lead contributes to her triumphs and her defeats.

When Sally is in the throes of struggle, the muscles of her neck and shoulders compress into a vise at the base of her skull, while the pulsing of blood in her head crests into a throbbing pain in her temples. Feverish activity inflames her eyes, tightens her chest, strains her lower back, and turns her body odor into the smell of sour milk. At these times she needs to open the valve on her pressure cooker and discharge pent-up steam. Sympathetic attempts to console her are spurned until after she finds release. A hard game of racquetball, a fierce argument, a solitary workout, or pre-vailing over a demanding piece of music help her to dispel tension, relieve bottled-up feelings, and soften her disposition.

To regulate her internal state so that it doesn't interfere with her agenda, Sally finds it expedient to rely on coffee to get her going and alcohol to slow her down. Often in a hurry, she grabs quick meals on the run, starving herself one day, overeating the next, continually overcompensating for her extremism and appetite for novelty. Intolerant of limitation, Sally tends to believe that if a little is good, more is better—her impulse is always to go farther. She dreads boredom and stays occupied with a vengeance. One month she wakes early and jogs, the next she stays up late and sleeps in. Consistently inconsistent, she pays the price of a careless life-style in the form of indigestion, pain in her joints and muscles, erratic energy, and un-predictable moods.

When Sally runs out of steam, she becomes indecisive, scattered, and distracted. Rather than encouraging relaxation, fatigue makes her feel ner-vous and uptight. The thought of resting when tired contradicts her propen-sity to push herself. Instead she tries to reinvigorate herself through stimulation, by working harder, exercising, or eating sugary, fatty, and spicy foods. This constant prodding creates more agitation and tension, which makes her feel hot, dry, and volatile. Too much heat and lack of moisture make Sally brittle and inflexible like an unwatered sapling. Losing softness and resiliency, she snaps at the slightest provocation, her good humor aban-doned. Irritable and depressed, jittery and exhausted, she is overtaken by a sullen pessimism. Easily frustrated, she begins projects that she cannot fin-ish, no longer having the zest for sustained effort. When no longer buoyed by the feeling of pressure and intensity that she identifies as the source of her strength and drive, she feels frightened, humiliated, and disabled, as if her body has betrayed her.

Sally is at her best when the pace of her life keeps her engaged but not exhausted, defined by a clear purpose but not confined to an inflexible pro-gram. Permitting herself to moderate extremism and accept structure and discipline helps her to harness her drive. This optimum functioning reflects the harmony between *Wood* (*Liver*), *Earth* (*Spleen*), and *Metal* (*Lung*). *Earth* modulates the variability of *Wood*, while *Metal* subdues and diffuses its force. *Wood* keeps *Earth* from becoming stagnant and inert and *Metal* from being vacuous and stifled.

Just as the *Liver* governs movement and pressure by regulating the flow of *Qi*, storing and releasing the *Blood*, Sally develops the power in her body and psyche by "pumping up" her emotions and fluids so that she is always primed and ready. In generating power to run a turbine or mill, a river is dammed so the momentum of falling water channels into smaller and smaller conduits, which increase its pressure and force. Self-generated pressure and tension supply Sally with the steam necessary for her to put her projects into motion. Without adequate avenues for channeling this internal force, she can develop high blood pressure, muscles locked in spasm, and emotional lability. She needs adequate mechanisms for release as well as buildup. When the *Qi* in the *Liver* is obstructed or depleted, the *Blood* cannot nourish the *Heart*, eyes, and muscles. This leads to problems like insomnia or anxiety, photophobia or blurred vision, cramps or tremors, hypersensitivity, and fatigue. When Sally is thwarted, she becomes agitated and erratic, loses foresight, and becomes awkward and uncoordinated.

Sally may also experience trouble with her menstrual cycle, another process characterized by rhythmic buildup and release. Before her period, fluid and blood accumulate in Sally's breasts and abdomen, making her feel stretched and tender. This uncomfortable strain against her tissue translates into mental and emotional urgency in her psyche. Goaded by this oppressive fullness, Sally gets cantankerous, overwrought, and eruptive, losing her judgment and perspective. She feels assaulted by noise, yet she herself tends to be loud and prone to sudden outbursts of tears, peevishness, and temper. Knotted up and restless, she sleeps poorly, anxiously anticipating the decompression and relief that accompanies the onset of her period. Sally lives two personalities, one premenstrual and the other post-. Her period behind her, she recovers her composure, once again in charge of herself.

Sally has the strength of a tiger. When she handles herself well she is capable of tremendous work—provoked and unrestrained, she can wreak havoc. Like the archetype whose nature she shares, she is a productive dynamo when conditions are right. The urge to get things moving, make things happen, and voyage onward typifies the *Pioneer*.

How We Recognize Sally As a Wood Type

At her best, Sally expresses her true nature: she is bold, decisive, clear, relishing work and performing well under pressure. On the other hand, because she is driven by a tendency to overdo, overperform, and overdirect, what was once a gratifying challenge can turn the corner into an aggravating distress. It is then difficult for her to retreat and recover a hedonic state. Boldness can become aggressive and hostile, decisiveness can become impulsive and unyielding, and clarity can escalate into fanatical adherence.

Sally can become a tyrant. When *Wood* is unbridled, it can run wild, inflicting emotional and physical trauma. When Sally's desire to remain even-tempered is confounded, her muscles swell and tighten, and her focus of attention narrows. This restricts her capacity for sustained arousal and appropriate release, making her feel shackled and compressed.

Exaggerated, inflated, or "bound" *Liver Qi* expresses itself by a propensity toward tension headaches; a drive to discharge pent-up energy in noisy, emotional outbursts; nervous, erratic behavior like eating on the run and inconsistent exercise; intolerance, indulgence, obstinence, strong body odor, a compulsion to work, and the need for sedatives to slow down.

Collapsed, deflated, or "exhausted" *Liver Qi* is characterized by irritability, indecisiveness, a sensitivity to noise, a loss of judgment and perspective, a need for stimulants, and feeling overwrought, overwhelmed, uptight, and tired. These reactions are linked to the *deficiency* and stagnation of *Liver Qi* and *Blood*. In periods of *deficiency* or *excess*, the *Liver* is unable to maintain the equanimity of the mind and emotions. In Sally, as in us all, her true nature coexists with states of *exaggeration* and *collapse*.

THE EVOLUTION OF DISTORTED PATTERNS OF WOOD

Understanding the interdependent dynamic between *Wood-Earth* (*Liver-Spleen*) and *Wood-Metal* (*Liver-Lung*) gives us insight into people like Sally. When the relationship between these forces and functions is disturbed, distortions evolve in predictable patterns. Corresponding to the arousing power of *Wood* in nature, the *Liver* awakens, mobilizes, and coordinates human process. Sally's difficulties mirror aberrant activity of the *Liver*.

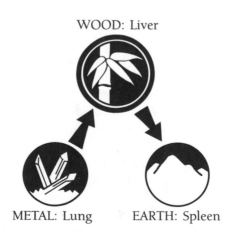

WOOD: Liver

METAL: Lung   EARTH: Spleen

The *Liver* activates the process of digestion and assimilation and, by regulating the flow (volume and pressure) of *Blood*, helps the *Spleen* disseminate nutrition. The *Blood*, enriched by the *Nutritive Essence* of the *Spleen*, is stored and released by the *Liver*. Together the *Spleen* and *Liver* distribute nutrients and *Blood*.

Together, the *Lung* and *Liver* govern the circulation of *Qi*. The *Liver*'s capacity to elevate, accelerate, and expand is matched by the *Lung*'s ability to descend, retard, and constrict. The even, rhythmic pulsation of the diaphragm, digestive tube, heart, and blood vessels is governed by this interaction.

The *Liver* restrains the *Spleen*, and the *Lung* restrains the *Liver*. When the *Liver* becomes overly strong, it oppresses the *Spleen* and antagonizes the *Lung*. Unbridled *Liver Qi* interrupts the smooth upward and downward movement of *Spleen* and *Stomach Qi*, upsetting digestion. This results in erratic appetite, irregular elimination, heartburn, gas, and spasmodic pain of the stomach and intestines. Volatile *Liver Qi* rushes up against the descending *Lung Qi*, jamming movement in the throat, chest, and diaphragm. This results in tightness of the larynx and esophagus, pain between the ribs, and shallow breathing or wheezing.

When *Liver Qi* is exhausted, movement, excitation, and pulsation dwindle. *Spleen Qi* sinks and stagnates. *Lung Qi* tightens and shrinks. Without the mobilizing force of the *Liver*, the *Moisture* of the *Spleen* collects, turning into edema, and the *Moisture* of the *Lung* congeals and turns into phlegm. The muscles become heavy and stiff, circulation becomes sluggish, and *Cold* and *Wind* penetrate easily, leading to aches and pains of the joints and tendons.

In the psyche, a distorted *Liver-Spleen* relationship engenders conflict around the need for change and stability, adventure and continuity, hyperactivity and inertia, and between impulsiveness and indecisiveness. Dissonance between *Liver-Lung* foments a struggle between expressiveness and self-restraint, fervor and indifference, spontaneity and reserve, chaos and order.

Because she's a *Wood* type, Sally is predisposed to unbridled *Liver Qi*, which generates excess pressure and tension to produce hyperactivity, heat, spasm, and volatility. Eventually overwork, lack of proper nutrition, and prolonged emotional intensity deplete *Blood* and *Moisture*, leaving Sally reactive, dry, fatigued, restless, sullen, and depressed, especially before her period.

The therapeutic strategy needed to assist Sally in recovering her equilibrium includes relieving pressure, dispelling *Heat*, relaxing spasm, and replenishing *Blood* and *Moisture*. Exercise that includes stretching and softening muscles will relieve pressure and spasm and equalize circulation between her extremities, chest, and abdomen. This cools her head while warming her hands and feet. Appropriate herbs and foods will nourish *Blood*, restore *Mois-*

ture, encourage circulation, and dispel *Heat* and *Wind*. Acupuncture will foster the efficient function of her internal organs by modulating the movement of *Qi* and *Blood*, quieting her mind, and tempering her mercurial moods.

Sally tends to use up all her available energy and to rest only when she is exhausted, rather than sustain adequate reserves. Her pacing and timing are critical—activity and work need to be balanced by adequate leisure, and she must learn to be comfortable with the feeling of energy without experiencing a compulsion to expend it immediately.

WOOD: Liver Patterns

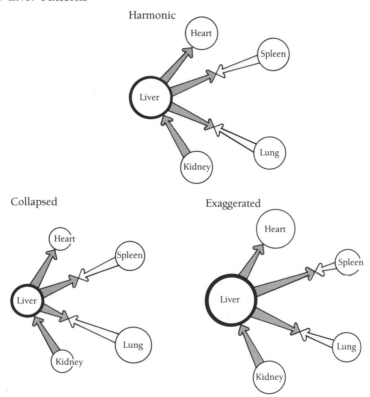

Harmonic and Dissonant Patterns

In the *harmonic Liver* pattern, the *Kidney* and *Heart* maintain stability while the *Spleen* and *Lung* provide the tension necessary for movement and adaptation. In the *exaggerated Liver* pattern, the *Kidney* and *Heart* become hyperactive, and the *Spleen* and *Lung* become hypersensitive and erratic. In the *collapsed* pattern, the *Kidney* and *Heart* become drained and weakened while the *Spleen* and *Lung* become overbearing and congested.

Whereas Sally is a composite sketch of a *Wood* type, acting out *exaggerated* and *collapsed* scenarios, Dan is a real patient who sought help for a very particular problem. Dan fits the *Wood* pattern because his talents and style of operating as well as the problems he experiences under duress correspond to the mode of action and the character of the *Liver Network*. Like Sally, he has the strengths and weaknesses of *Wood*.

DAN: HOW COME I'M NOT BETTER YESTERDAY?

Dan marches into the clinic as if he owns the place. Dropping his coat and briefcase on a chair, he spreads out onto the couch. By bellowing that he's arrived, he commands immediate and total attention.

Dan complains of needing to eat every few hours to avoid feeling weak, dizzy, and congested in his chest and throat. This congestion obstructs his free access to air, provoking anxiety, which then triggers rapid breathing and feeling faint, hot, and nauseated. His physician has told him that he has hypoglycemia and food allergies. Dan declares, "I've been all over the place and done all the tests. I'm fed up with not getting results. I hear you're good, and I want you to cure me. Which room do you want me in? I have another appointment in an hour."

As Dan lies down on the treatment table, he says, "I'm thirty-five, I've lived in numerous cities, and started many businesses. Six years ago I could run all day, go without a meal until dinner, and work all night. Now I not only have to sleep, but I have to get up in the middle of the night for a snack. If I wait too long, I wake up with a headache pounding in my temples. This thing is interfering with my freedom. I can't just go to any restaurant because if I eat the wrong foods, my chest tightens up and my head gets stuffy. I've had to forgo even an occasional drink over business. Fix me. By the way, there's one other little problem. Sometimes I can't get it up, and when I do, boom it's over. I never used to have any trouble in that department."

Dan's body is well proportioned and muscular. He points to a midriff bulge that is another recent acquisition, which he attributes to his craving for the abundant carbohydrates that keep him going. He has been told to eat a lot of protein, but beef often causes allergic reactions.

TREATMENT

Dan's tongue is enlarged and pale with greasy yellowish-white fur and a red line that goes from the tip along both edges. His face and neck are slightly flushed. His pulse is quick and taut, as well as weak and soft in the positions that correspond to the *Spleen* and *Kidney*. Dan begins to look anxious and fearful of the acupuncture needles and wants to know how long this treatment will take. In response to his temerity, I choose three points: between the thumb and forefinger on the *Large Intestine* meridian; between the first and second toe on the *Liver* meridian; and above the inside ankle on the *Spleen* meridian. Dan feels every needle strongly, even with mild stimulation. Slight perspiration forms on his upper lip, palms, and feet.

Within ten minutes after the needles are in place, Dan falls into a deep sleep with slow, regular breathing and a serene expression on his face. After twenty minutes the needles are removed, and Dan comments that he feels mellow but a bit uneasy being so relaxed since he's accustomed to operating at a fast pace.

He gets back into his tie, jacket, and shoes without rushing, announcing, "I feel great. So is this it, or do I need more treatment?"

I let Dan know this is the beginning of an ongoing process that requires more acupuncture, herbs, and a modification of his diet. Total reliance on convenient carbohydrates like bread and pasta for quick energy must be replaced by more complex carbohydrates like rice, protein-rich legumes, and fat-free animal foods that will generate and sustain energy without creating stagnation. High-fiber foods, both raw and cooked, will help to disperse *Qi* by stimulating intestinal activity; steamed and boiled foods will help to disperse phlegm and at the same time moisturize and eliminate *Heat*. Dan needs to avoid greasy, spicy, and creamy foods, which tend to create congestion of *Qi* and *Moisture* and accumulation of *Heat* and phlegm.

Since he has lost the ability to regulate his own metabolism, his body requires reeducation. Success will depend on modifying his diet, work style, and sleep pattern, as well as receiving acupuncture and herbal treatments. Acupuncture enables Dan to experience how it feels to function effectively without always being in "overdrive." He agrees to try this approach for a while and leaves the clinic with herbs that disperse *Qi* and *Moisture* and tonify the *Spleen*. He takes these herbs before eating to improve his assimilation, help him last longer between meals, and lessen his allergic reactions. In the morning and evening he takes a constitutional formula that harmonizes the *Liver* and *Spleen*. This relaxes the *Liver*, activates the *Spleen*, eliminates *Heat* and *Wind*, and both nurtures and distributes *Qi* and *Blood*.

INTERPRETATION AND STRATEGY

Erratic intensity and hyperfunction characterize Dan. He has been in overdrive for so long that he cannot slow down without feeling unnatural, even threatened. He becomes bound up and volatile without the constant opportunity for discharging his nervousness. This *exaggerated Liver* pattern oppresses the *Spleen*, resulting in an inability to accumulate reserves, demonstrated by his major complaint—the inability to endure too long without eating.

The dynamic of the *Liver* dominating and overstimulating the *Stomach*   169 and *Spleen* causes *Nutritive Qi* to be utilized immediately without the appropriate diversion of some of this into stored reserves. The *Liver* should be able to store resources in the form of *Blood*, but when it becomes hyperactive it drains its own resevoir and the *Kidney*'s as well. Since *Water* nurtures *Wood*, this is a case of the rebellious child (*Liver*) making inordinate demands upon its mother (*Kidney*). That's why impotence and premature ejaculation have become a problem.

The words *quick* and *short-lived* characterize a lot of Dan's history. He has pursued many life-styles and careers without sustaining any vocation long enough to build a secure base that would provide continuity and foundation. Dan has become unbounded and ungrounded by his insatiable appetite for change and challenge.

It is important to gain Dan's trust and cooperation so that he can direct some of his drive into reorganizing his existence, throwing himself into the project of healing himself with the enthusiasm he has for starting a new business. The *Wood* type recoils at the prospect of following orders or adopting someone else's agenda. Dan needs to know that he is in charge and that there are choices. He doesn't want to be pushed.

He'd like to rely on the acupuncture to do his work for him, but as he begins to feel better, he is willing to be more aware of the consequences of his own behavior. He then has the choice to use himself differently. Dan must come to this realization through his own experience rather than on the faith of another's authority. Acupuncture softens Dan's temperament so that he can experience a more serene self.

The dynamic between *Earth* and *Wood*, *Spleen* and *Liver*, organizes the production and distribution of *Nutritive Qi* and *Blood*, the buildup and breakdown of energy and tissue. Dispersing the stagnant *Qi* and *Heat* from the *Liver* while dispersing the stagnant *Moisture* and *Qi* from the *Spleen* will improve the interaction between the *Liver* and *Spleen*. Treatments lessen Dan's excessive hunger, steady his erratic energy and moods, and begin to generate a surplus of *Qi*, which will strengthen the *Kidney* and restore his flagging reserves.

The dynamic between *Metal* and *Wood*, *Lung* and *Liver*, organizes rhythm and flow. Dispersing the stagnant *Qi* (phlegm) of the *Lung* while moisturizing the *Lung* and *Liver* will restore their proper relationship. Treatment relieves Dan's symptoms of difficult breathing and mucus congestion and helps him to become comfortable with limits by stabilizing his energy so that he is less anxious about having too much or too little. He can be full of energy without being full of tension or agitation. The main differences between the *Liver-Spleen* and *Liver-Lung* patterns are the predominance of digestive disturbance in the former and dysfunctional elimination or discharge in the latter. In either, *exaggerated Liver Qi* interferes with the smooth functioning of peri-

stalsis and respiration, both of which depend on the harmonious interaction of contraction *(Metal)* and expansion *(Wood)*. Dan's case typifies a primary *Wood-Earth* conflict and a secondary *Wood-Metal* conflict.

Resolving the conflicts between *Liver-Spleen* and *Liver-Lung* helps Dan with his problems. Within four months of his first visit, Dan has regained control of his eating problem—he has three regular meals a day and sleeps through the night. Although he needs a snack if he has been working hard, he no longer has the same desperation about it. Some congestion persists, but without the former anxiety about or difficulty in breathing. Because he feels more in control of his life, he is more patient, less nervous, and more optimistic. With more consistent energy throughout the day and the return of his sexual stamina, Dan feels that treatment is working for him.

Summary of Dan's Patterns		
Signs and Symptoms	Interpretation	Interpretation
	According to *Qi, Moisture, Blood*	According to *Organ Networks*
Unsustained energy Impotence Premature ejaculation Pale tongue Weak pulse	Depletion of *Qi, Blood*	Weakness of *Kidney*
Headache at night Excessive hunger Agitation Redness on tongue Yellow tongue fur Rapid pulse	Accumulation of *Heat*	Disharmony of *Liver-Spleen*
Greasy tongue Mucus congestion	Accumulation of *Moisture*	Disharmony of *Liver-Spleen*
Erratic emotions Impulsive behavior Irregular breathing	Stasis of *Qi*	Disharmony of *Liver-Lung*

Prescriptions for Therapy

Harmonize *Liver-Spleen*
Disperse *Qi*
Disperse *Moisture*
Cool interior

Harmonize *Liver-Lung*
Tonify *Qi*
Tonify *Blood*
Consolidate *Moisture*
Disperse *Qi*

WOOD		
PIONEER		*LIVER*
Mental Faculties	**Biological Functions**	**Organs—Tissues—Fluid**
Clarity Judgment Foresight Decision	Filling Arousal Expansion Acceleration	*Liver* and *Gallbladder* Eyes and eyebrows Tendons and nerves Nails, bile, tears

WOOD

Exaggerated patterns arise from:	**Collapsed patterns arise from:**	**Aggravations occur with:**
Congestion of *Qi* and *Blood* Accumulation of *Heat* and *Dampness* Generation of *internal Wind* Disharmony of *Liver-Spleen* *Liver-Lung*	Depletion of *Blood* and *Moisture* Accumulation of *Heat*, *Wind*, and *Dryness* Weakness of *Spleen*, *Kidney*, *Liver*	Spring and summer *Wind* and *Heat* Sour and greasy and spicy food Alcohol, opiates, amphetamines 11 P.M.–3 A.M. and 11 A.M.–3 P.M.

Characteristic Features of Psyche

Undistorted	**Exaggerated**	**Collapsed**	**Difficulty With**
Confident Assertive Bold Ambitious Competitive Powerful Direct Committed Decisive	Arrogant Aggressive Reckless Driven Antagonistic Tyrannical Confrontational Compulsive Impulsive	Pretentious Peevish Erratic Premature Contrary Ineffectual Devious Fickle Ambivalent	Intensity Restraint Equality Sharing Cooperation Ambiguity Obstacles Anger

Characteristic Features of Soma			
Undistorted	**Exaggerated**	**Collapsed**	**Difficulty With**
Supple, muscular, square physique Thick, coarse skin and swarthy complexion Strong, slim, sinewy hands and feet	High blood pressure Oily skin/hair Boils Cramps of long muscles, hands, feet Vertigo Ringing in ears Constipation with cramps/ spasms Sciatica Pain in ribs Heartburn Difficult swallowing Eye/ear pain Shingles Awkward and accident-prone Hard, thick nails Breast pain Tendon injuries	Labile blood pressure Hypoglycemia Blurry vision Sensitivity to light or sound Cystitis, urethritis Itchy eyes, urethra, anus Tendonitis Dry, brittle nails Lax joints and tense muscles Irritable colon Chronic tension in neck and across shoulders	Occipital/lateral headaches Migraine TMJ syndrome Facial neuralgias Peripheral nerve dysfunction Hypertension Sexual dysfunction Painful menses PMS Substance abuse

SO, YOU THINK YOU'RE A WOOD TYPE

KEYS TO UNDERSTANDING WOOD

- seeks challenge and pushes to the limit
- enjoys and does well under pressure
- admires speed, novelty, and skill
- loves action, movement, and adventure
- likes to be first, best, and only

TYPICAL PROBLEMS

- intolerance and impatience
- volatile emotions
- extremism: impulsive or overdisciplined self-indulgent or self-punishing
- vascular headaches, muscle spasms, high blood pressure, nerve inflammations, migratory pain
- abuse of stimulants and sedatives

CRITICAL TIMES

- *exaggerated Wood—Liver* congestion: spring and late summer, 11 P.M.–3 A.M. and 7 A.M.–11 A.M.
- *collapsed Wood—Liver* depletion: summer and fall, 11 A.M.–3 P.M. and 3 A.M.–7 A.M.

A FRIENDLY REMINDER

The power of *Wood* comes from the capacity to rapidly expand and build up pressure. *Wood* types need to modulate their intensity and stay flexible, to be able to retreat and yield as well as surge forward and be undaunted.

CHAPTER NINE
FIRE

Do you not see
That you and I
Are as the branches of one tree?
With your rejoicing
Comes my laughter;
With your sadness
Start my tears
Love,
Could life be otherwise
With you and me?
Tsu Yeh
Tsin dynasty, A.D. 265–316

FIRE IS DAZZLING, EVANESCENT, TREMBLING, EXCITING, AND ALL-embracing. Summer, the time when plants and creatures develop to their fullest potential, marks the ascendance of the power of *Fire*. Summer conjures up a sense of splendor and fulfillment as we stretch to the limits of our capacity. A brilliant sun climbs to its zenith over full-bloom magnolias amidst the hum of bees buzzing. In summer, *Yang* is dominant—light, warmth, activity, and interaction are at a peak. *Fire*, like summer, is expansive, radiant, outgoing, and warm. As the sun accelerates the life streams of the earth, the *Heart* squeezes the living juices of the blood through the vessels, imbuing the body with mindfulness.

The *Heart* and *Kidney* are like two ends of a rainbow, distinct and unfathomable, drawing between them the multicolored luminous ribbon of our being, a dimension bounded on one end by *Water* and on the other by *Fire*. *Fire* represents the universal and enveloping space into which we grow and expand. As *Water* determines our longevity, *Fire* determines our breadth and scope. *Water* is seed and root, *Fire* is flower and fruit. Like Dionysus, *Water* is associated with the subconscious, primal forces of nature, whereas like Apollo, Greek god of the sun, *Fire* symbolizes wakefulness and the development of wisdom and compassion. This relationship between *Water* and *Fire* is expressed by Jill Purce in *The Mystic Spiral*:

Situated between the poles, on our journey through the spherical vortex, we see at either end our source and goal. We are pulled in

176

both directions, since the longing for the womb . . . has its counterpart in the passionate longing of the mystic for union with God.

THE ARCHETYPE FOR FIRE: THE WIZARD

Fusion is the organizing principle for the *Wizard*, who seeks to imbue the mundane with the extraordinary, merging human aspirations with divine purpose. Just as the *Fire* of love unites male and female to form new life, so the *Wizard* wields a miraculous power to overcome separation by welding divergent elements into one. His excitement and enthusiasm generate the heat required for the reaction of fusion to occur. With this tremendous catalytic energy, he brings the transforming power of light, love, and awareness into the world.

Enchanting and persuasive, the *Wizard* is a natural salesman, selling not so much the product itself as the experience of possessing an instrument of magic, a veritable talisman, that endows us with the power to transcend our ordinary existence. The magic, however, is in the *Wizard*, not in the merchandise. So when this awesome barker of dreams vanishes, and the remarkable can opener that would open up a whole new world becomes merely a practical device, we are not dissatisfied or disappointed: the very experience of astonishment and joy that the *Wizard* inspires makes us glad.

Using personal magnetism and the gift of expression, he can assemble a group of individuals into one body. Whether as a team, chorus, classroom, audience, congregation, or political party, the *Wizard* gathers us up into a shared expanse of vision and feeling. Through this marriage with the hearts and minds of others, we realize a virtue of our humanness.

HECTOR: EXEMPLAR OF FIRE

Affectionate and expressive, Hector possesses a lively sense of humor, a jovial, optimistic attitude, and a generosity of spirit. He is genuinely concerned about the happiness of those around him, and because of his openness, it's easy for him to involve himself with the needs and desires of friends, family, and even strangers.

Hector is both imaginative and articulate and has a passion for contact through touch and conversation. He is a good orator and teacher because of his love of speech. Through his capacity for communication, he reaches out to people and makes friends easily.

Hector lives just below the surface. His thoughts and feelings are readily exposed: he wears his heart on his sleeve and has a rich inner life that is easily affected by other people. He has ready access to his intuition and is often considered by his friends to be a mind reader because he knows what's happening without being told. He scans his world with antennalike intelligence, receiving and integrating a plethora of information and impressions.

Constantly responding to stimuli, he may appear to quiver like a hummingbird, simultaneously motionless and vibrating. He has a rosy, almost flushed complexion and shining, darting eyes. Glowing with warmth and energy, Hector easily attracts the attention of others around him. Imbued with the hot, bright, magnetic quality of *Fire*, he can be awesome and seductive as a performer or leader. Like the power of *Fire* to inflame and transform, through his charisma Hector stirs our yearning for transcendence.

Playful and demonstrative, Hector showers his family with feelings and attention when he is around them. However, he is often not at home when there is something more engaging going on elsewhere. Hector needs plenty of interaction to satisfy his requirements for recognition, stimulation, and contact. Since Hector thrives on intimacy and pleasure, and relishes the gamut of experiences and sensations, he may seem like an insatiable hedonist. But Hector is not selfish with his pleasure; in freely exhibiting his own delight, he shares it with others.

Because Hector has trouble insulating himself from the constant barrage of external influences, his powers of discrimination and discernment can be overloaded, resulting in anxiety and confusion. Sometimes he cannot separate his own thoughts and feelings from those around him. His confusion can develop into a sense of dread if he feels bombarded by unwanted and unpredictable events. He may come to loathe surprises, which frighten rather than please him. Under stress, Hector can become hyperactive, nervous, and have difficulty focusing his attention. His hands become warm and moist, and he perspires freely when he is excited or busy. Hector likes things hot: spicy food, warm weather, and emotional fervor feed his naturally heightened awareness, and he can "burn" with unbridled intensity.

But when *Fire* is blazing too fiercely, it can burn out its own source, turning into cold ashes. Overexcited or overextended, he is unable to slow himself down or pull himself together. This can result in an inability to rest, sleep, and replenish his resources. When he reaches the limit of his capacity, his heart could suffer arrhythmia, cramps, and enlargement due to the exhausting demands made upon it. Should his *Fire* burn itself out, Hector's glow will turn to pallor, and his warmth and intimacy will turn to isolation and melancholy. In order for *Fire* to generate joy and fulfillment, it must remain within bounds. The fire in a furnace warms a house, whereas in the forest, out of control, it wastes and destroys the land. Hector must contain his power or be consumed by it.

Hector gives and demands a lot. His friends, family, and associates may feel that they become fuel for his needs and desires. Because of his charm, it is easy for people to become caught up in Hector's exhilarating world—

they are attracted to his brightness like moths to a flame. And when Hector "burns out," he may leave a trail of empty and exhausted people who have given him their all.

Peacefulness of spirit and tranquillity of mind are the hallmarks of the harmonious working of the *Heart*. When the *Heart* is disturbed by confusion and sudden shifts of reality, it becomes unable to maintain calmness and clarity. Anxiety, agitation, and fearfulness ensue. Lucidity and security become turbidity and dread. Compassion becomes sentimentality, and speech and expression become exaggerated, losing meaning and relevance. Senseless babbling and disjointed thoughts are the outcome of this disorientation and homelessness of the *Spirit*.

Whereas the dissembling of the *Water* type takes the form of a shrinking of the self through isolation and diminution, the dissembling of the *Fire* type takes the form of dissolution of the self through merging between the inner and outer world. There is a loss of identity and the faculty to discriminate between self and other. When *Fire* is vigorous and contained, Hector is able to weather the stress of success or failure, gains or loss, with relative equanimity, maintaining individuality and relationship.

HOW WE RECOGNIZE HECTOR AS A FIRE TYPE

Hector reveals the true nature as well as the *exaggerated* and *collapsed* features of the *Fire* type. He is affectionate, open, expansive, generous, intuitive, warm, and bright. When Hector is overdriven by his own tendencies, he is disposed toward heat, fervor, dryness, redness, and excitability.

Unrestrained *Heart Qi* generates *Heat* and agitation, which can produce mania, delusional behavior, and bizarre experiences like hallucinations, nightmares, and rushes of physical sensation. Hector's whole body becomes flushed and feverish as he tries to rid himself of excess metabolic heat through profuse sweating and intense thermal radiation from the head, hands, and feet.

Impassioned by the thrill of imagined pleasures, Hector feeds on fantasy, sometimes generating unrealistic expectations of fulfillment. The momentum created by unanchored exhilaration results in disappointment when actual life does not match dreams. When this happens, it can be difficult for Hector to recover his buoyancy—he feels as if his spirit has been lost, like a high-flying kite that a swift wind has ripped away. Hector's emotional pendulum swings between the inflation of euphoria and the deflation of anguished discouragement—he can be alternately frenzied or melancholic, gregarious or isolated, talkative or passive, seductive or timid.

When his *Qi* is exhausted, Hector becomes pale, subject to cold, easily frightened and confused. Sensitivity turns to vulnerability, and intuition becomes veiled with darkness and doubt. Withdrawn and morose, he dwells on tales of unrequited longing and vivid morbid images of suffering. Hector is an incurable romantic whose life can assume the maudlin qualities of a television melodrama.

Whether *exaggerated* or *collapsed*, Hector's boundaries—his sense of himself—are soft. They easily expand or shrink under emotional stress; Hector merges, becoming everyone, or dissipates, becoming no one. He is undone by his penchant for relinquishing his self-possession, his own self-sense. His challenge is to maintain his mooring, a clear, discrete identity without sacrificing his sensitivity and openness. His virtue is his compassion, the capacity to know, feel, and understand what others experience.

THE EVOLUTION OF DISTORTED PATTERNS OF FIRE

For the *Fire* type the key relationships are between the *Heart* and *Lung* (*Fire* restrains *Metal*) and between the *Heart* and *Kidney* (*Water* inhibits *Fire*).

FIRE: Heart

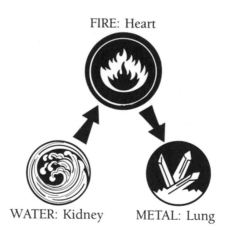

WATER: Kidney   METAL: Lung

When excessively strong, the *Qi* of the *Heart* can attack the *Lung*. The *Qi* becomes too dispersed, leaving the envelope of the skin open and loose, unable to guard the body and contain the *Essence* and *Spirit*. When *Fire* overcomes *Metal* there is an *excess* of *Dryness* and *Heat*, which leads to problems such as dry cough, thirst, night sweats, and sores in the nose and throat. Emotionally this person becomes restless and sensitive—easily moved from laughter to tears and prone toward melancholy and anxiety. Conflict heightens between the desire for expression and effusion (*Heart*) and the need to preserve boundaries, set limits, and maintain defenses (*Lung*). It then becomes difficult for the *Fire* type to make distinctions, besieged by a fugue of intense feelings of pleasure and pain, grief and happiness, which may overwhelm him and over which he has little control.

Dominated by the *Heart*, the *Lung* cannot adequately nurture the *Kidney*. The *Kidney* becomes weak, and *Water* cannot properly restrain *Fire*. When this happens, the *Heat* generated by the *Heart Yang* can damage the *Yin* of the *Kidney*, resulting in painful scanty urine, soreness of the back, and disturbances of libido and potency. Uninhibited *Fire* disturbs attention, expression, and sensation. Weak *Water* (depleted *Kidney Essence* and *Moisture*) disposes a person to be easily distracted and doubtful. Stuttering occurs when the tempo of thoughts and speech lose their synchrony. Accentuated and magnified, impressions conveyed by the five senses may become unreliable and overwhelming. These altered states of perception in which reality becomes plastic and fluctuating may be familiar to those who have used psychedelic substances, involved themselves in intense spiritual practices, or suffered sudden emotional or physical shock. This kind of experience represents a stress on the integrity of the *Heart-Kidney* relationship, the interaction between *Shen* and *Jing*, *Spirit* and *Essence*.

When *Heart Qi* is *exaggerated*, the *Liver* overheats and becomes brittle like dry wood, and the *Spleen* becomes scorched like parched, sun-baked earth. The body and character lose their resiliency and become stiff, dry, and easily inflamed. The muscle and joints may be feverish and painful, eyes irritated, tongue sore, vision and hearing distorted. This can devolve into a *collapse* of *Heart Qi*, at which time a person becomes hypersensitive, fragile, and close to the edge of hysteria.

The key problems for *Fire* are dehydration, perturbed circulation of blood, and instability of mental function. The *Heart* is the home of the *Spirit* (*Shen*), and the *Blood* houses the mind. By perfusing the body with *Blood*, consciousness pervades all realms of soma and psyche. *Heat* generated by *exaggerated Fire* consumes the body's *Moisture* and dries the *Blood*. *Yang* destroys *Yin*. Metabolic activity as well as the pace of thoughts and impressions in the mind become unpredictable with surges of energy and emotion alternating with periods of vapid dullness. Not knowing how he will feel from one moment to the next causes Hector apprehension and insecurity.

In order to maintain fluidity and steadiness, the *Fire* type requires continual moisturization of the body and gentle inhibition of the tendency toward extreme dissipation and excitation. When the living sap of the body withers, life loses its softness, luster, and juiciness. Hector needs to drink sufficient liquids and avoid overindulging in heating and drying foods such as curry, sugar, alcohol, coffee, tea, chili, and salt. He requires the time and space for solitude and restitution, to regain inner calm and clarity. Developing powers of discipline and discrimination, his *Metal* aspect, and culti-vating the rootedness of *Water* through identification with family, ancestry, and history will help him with the steadiness that enables him to thrive.

MARIA: IS IT WARM IN HERE OR IS IT JUST ME?

Wearing an anxious smile, Maria flops onto a chair. Her eyes dart around the room like a camera, registering every detail. She appears both nervous

FIRE: Heart Patterns

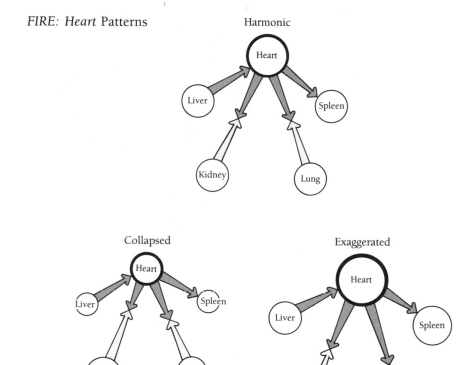

Harmonic and Dissonant Patterns

In the *harmonic Heart* pattern, the *Liver* and *Spleen* maintain stability while the *Lung* and *Kidney* provide the tension necessary for movement and ad-aptation. In the *exaggerated Heart* pattern, the *Liver* and *Spleen* become hy-peractive and the *Lung* and *Kidney* become hypersensitive and erratic. In the *collapsed* pattern, the *Liver* and *Spleen* become drained and weakened while the *Lung* and *Kidney* become overbearing and congested.

and excited about her visit. As she removes her jacket she comments, "Is it warm in here or is it just me?"

Maria says, "I have a part in a film right now, and I have itchy red welts on my neck and face like hives. Can you do anything for that? I've been controlling it with Benadryl, but it's not working so well and it makes me feel jittery."

Asked about her health and what sorts of problems she's had in the past, Maria replies, "I've had a recurring problem with cystitis, for which I've taken a lot of antibiotics. I get canker sores in my mouth, and around my period I become sensitive, have hot flashes, my hands and feet swell up so I can't wear my ring or my good shoes, and I have bad dreams. It's also the time I'm most likely to get a bladder infection."

Maria comments that she has a weakness for stimulants like coffee and chocolate, especially before a performance. She uses them to feel "on" and likes being high. She comments that she's particularly thirsty while she's working, craving ice water or other cold drinks. I ask if she ever feels cold, and she says that after a hot flash she may feel a chill.

<h3>TREATMENT</h3>

Maria lies on her stomach and loosens her collar since the first acupuncture point is along the spine at the base of the neck. The needle is inserted about three-eighths of an inch deep and is twirled in place for about fifteen seconds. Maria reports when she feels a sensation of fullness or heat at the point, after which the needle is gently withdrawn.

She turns over so that points above each wrist on the *Pericardium* channel can be treated. This time she reports a sensation of warmth and tingling, after which the needles are removed. Points are used along the *Large Intestine* channel on the hand, the *Lung* channel above the wrist, and the *Kidney* channel below the ankle, and a special point is used above the bridge of the nose between the eyebrows. These needles remain in place for twenty minutes.

Maria volunteers that she felt more sensations than I asked her about, not only tingling and heat, but also waves of vibrations going up and down her back and legs. For a while she felt very hot and her heart beat quickly; now she feels cool and her heart calm. She wants to know if everyone has this experience and what these feelings mean. Asked whether her sensations are pleasant or unpleasant, she replies that as long as it's not abnormal, she likes it. I reassure her that it is not abnormal since acupuncture is experienced idiosyncratically by everyone. Although Maria wants to keep talking as she lies on the table, I suggest that she close her eyes and rest quietly.

<h3>INTERPRETATION AND STRATEGY</h3>

Maria's tongue is red at the tip, and her pulse is soft, weak, and rapid. Arising   183 from hyperactivity of the *Heart*, the hives represent *Heat* in the *Blood* that is trying to escape through the skin, governed by the *Lung*. This is an example of the *Qi* of the *Heart* invading the *Lung*, of *Fire* burning *Metal*. Red tongue, mouth sores, thirst, and hot flashes are mounting evidence that there is too much *Heat (Yang)* and not enough *Moisture (Yin)*. The fact that her pulse is also weak and that she seeks stimulants to keep herself going indicate the beginning *collapse* of *Qi*.

Normally the *Fire* from the *Heart* descends to warm the lower region of the body, including the *Kidney*. In Maria's case, the excess *Heat* causes irritation and inflammation of the delicate mucous membrane lining the bladder and urethra, causing cystitis. The *Heat* causes *Moisture* to evaporate and be held in suspension under the surface of the skin, manifesting as puffiness of the hands and feet.

Maria's troubles reflect the disturbed interaction between the *Heart-Lung* and *Heart-Kidney*. The dynamic of *Fire* and *Metal*, *Heart* and *Lung*, organizes our boundaries. The secretion of the *Heart*, which is perspiration, appears on the outer surface of the body, while mucus, the secretion of the *Lung*, softens and lubricates the skin and its underside.

The dynamic of *Fire* and *Water*, *Heart* and *Kidney*, organizes the continuum of our reality. The *Heart* evokes our communication and contact with the world, while the *Kidney* processes our inner impressions and establishes the root and substance of our individual and ancestral identity. When the *Heart* is dominant, the hot nature of its *Qi* can damage the *Yin* of the *Kidney* and *Lung*. It is necessary to clear the excessive *Heat* and nurture *Yin* by generating *Moisture—Yin* can be used to balance *Yang*.

The acupuncture point on the spine clears *Heat* in general, and the points on the *Pericardium* clear *Heat* from the *Heart Network* and calm the *Spirit*. The point on the *Large Intestine* channel is specific for red, itching skin and promotes elimination of *Heat* via the bowels. The points on the *Kidney* and *Lung* channels tonify those *Organ Networks* and distribute *Moisture* upward toward the chest and head. An herbal prescription to harmonize the relationship between the *Heart* and *Kidney* will disperse *Heat*, tonify *Moisture*, tranquilize the mind, and stabilize the will.

Maria delights in the immediate transformation that occurs when she connects with an audience, changing everyday reality into a charged and intimate drama. She gravitates toward such peak experiences. She is quick to share her feelings and give feedback about her sensations. Eager to communicate and establish close contact, she is open to forming a friendship in addition to receiving help.

When Maria says, "Is it warm in here or is it just me?" she is articulating a conflict between *Fire* and *Metal*. She feels a confusion about boundaries, merges with her surroundings, and has difficulty knowing who she is as distinct from those around her. This dilemma between fusion and separation characterizes the distortion of the *Heart-Lung* relationship. Maria may sometimes have a hard time distinguishing herself from the role she is playing. She can't tell whether her subjective feelings are her own or a shared experience.

Maria's rapid pulse and red tongue also reveal *Heat*, which evolves into an antagonism between *Yin* and *Yang*. As the *Essence (Yin)* of the *Kidney* degenerates under the overbearing influence of the *Heart Fire (Yang)*, more symptoms of *Heat* and weakness appear. Maria's penchant for stimulants aggravates this.

Maria's *exaggerated* condition has begun to devolve into *collapse*. The strategy at this stage is to disperse *excess* and supplement *deficiency*, to clear *Heat* and generate *Moisture*. For Maria it's important to appreciate the power of *Fire* to suddenly consume internal resources. When *Fire* gets out of control, the *Yin* of the *Kidney* and *Lung* can be quickly depleted.

The *Fire* type easily becomes unstable, requiring a secure, peaceful environment with a regular routine to balance overly expansive tendencies. Squandering reserves for the sake of heightening experience betrays a predisposition to distort the relationship of *Heart* and *Kidney*. *Fire* types need to be wary of melting the candle by basking too long in the limelight without having a quiet sanctuary in which to replenish the *Yin* necessary to keep their *Yang* in check. With *Yin* restored and *Yang* steadied, the *Spirit* is calm and the root is secure.

Maria needs to eat foods that moisturize and cool without creating *Cold* or weakness. She is attracted to fasting and cleansing because it makes her temporarily feel calm and comfortable. More important than cleaning out, Maria will benefit from juicy fruits and vegetables, warm soups, and adequate liquid intake. She should also have denser root vegetables, sea vegetables, and legume or fish protein, which will strengthen her *Kidney Qi*. Raw and cooked foods can be used to balance her changing states of hyper- and hypoactivity: warm, cooked foods will stimulate her metabolism when she is tired, and cool or raw foods will slow down her metabolism when she is overexcited. Minimal use of hot, spicy condiments, ice cream, frozen yogurt, or iced drinks will preserve stability and guard against extremism.

With treatment twice a week for six weeks, the red, itchy welts disappear and the hot flashes before her period also diminish. Cutting back on stimulants and reordering her life to include cooling-off periods hastens Maria's rate of recovery. Her tendency toward chronic cystitis improves, though it requires more treatment.

After six months of intermittent treatment, Maria continues to have periodic episodes of mild itching and cystitis, especially after strenuous performances or long tours away from home. She learns to manage her occasional symptoms by regularly using an herbal formula that harmonizes the *Kidney* and *Heart* and one that disperses *Moisture* and dispels *Damp Heat*. Every few months Maria comes in for what she calls a "tune-up" or maintenance visit to reevaluate what herbs to take and readjust her diet and habits.

Summary of Maria's Patterns		
Signs and Symptoms	**Interpretation**	**Interpretation**
	According to *Qi, Moisture, Blood*	According to *Organ Networks*
Cystitis Hot flashes Canker sores Hives Red-tipped tongue Rapid pulse	Accumulation of *Heat*	Disharmony of *Heart-Lung* and *Heart-Kidney*
Thirst Swollen hands and feet	Depletion of *Moisture*	Weakness of *Kidney* and *Lung*
Bad dreams Excitable and sensitive Craves stimulants Weak pulse	Depletion of *Qi* and disturbed *Spirit*	Weak *Kidney* Unstable *Heart*

Prescriptions for Therapy

Harmonize *Heart-Kidney*
Cool interior
Disperse *Moisture*

Harmonize *Heart-Lung*
Tonify *Moisture*
Consolidate *Moisture*

FIRE		
WIZARD		*HEART*
Mental Faculties	**Biological Functions**	**Organs—Tissues—Fluid**
Impression Communication	Dilation Sensation	*Heart/Small Intestine* Tongue and external ear
Intuition Comprehension	Perfusion Extension	Arteries and arterioles *Blood* and perspiration

FIRE

Exaggerated patterns arise from:	**Collapsed patterns arise from:**	**Aggravations occur with:**
Congestion of *Blood* Accumulation of *Heat* Depletion of *Moisture* Disharmony of *Heart-Lung* *Heart-Kidney*	Depletion of *Blood* Loss of *Heat* Weakness of *Liver*, *Heart*, and *Spleen*	Hot weather and summer Hot, spicy, and sweet food Alcohol and psychedelics 11 A.M.–3 P.M. and 11 P.M.–3 A.M.

Characteristic Features of Psyche			
Undistorted	**Exaggerated**	**Collapsed**	**Difficulty With**
Lively	Excitable	Startled	Boundaries
Communicative	Garrulous	Mute	Space
Charismatic	Seductive	Flirtatious	Separation
Optimistic	Grandiose	Credulous	Stimulation
Sanguine	Pollyanna	Giddy	Future
Aware	Hypersensitive	Confused	Unknown
Tender	Sentimental	Sensitive	Dreaming
Empathetic	Merging	Lost	Expression
Devoted	Adoring	Infatuated	Sleep
Enthusiastic	Avid	Selfish	Thinking
Alert	Anxious	Panicky	Pleasure and Pain

Characteristic Features of Soma			
Undistorted	**Exaggerated**	**Collapsed**	**Difficulty With**
Soft, willowy physique	Enlarged *Heart*	Slow, irregular pulse	Disturbed sleep
Graceful hands and feet	Profuse/ frequent perspiration	Weak *Heart*	Disorders of *Heart*/arteries
Soft, warm, moist, stretchy skin	Flushed face	Chills or over-heats easily	Disturbances of heart rate and rhythm
Long neck, arms, and legs	Irregular/rapid heartbeat	Low blood pressure	Disturbances of speech and sensation
	Chest pain	Faints or gets dizzy easily	Disorders of blood pressure and circulation
	Painful urination	Anemic	
	Strong, erratic pulse	Pale with flushed cheeks	
	Overheats easily	Tires easily from excitement	
	Sores of mouth, tongue, lips	Cannot sustain sexual excitement	
	Pulmonary hypertension	Premature orgasm	
	Dry, painful eczema		
	Easy sexual excitement but difficult to please		

So, You Think You're a Fire Type

Keys to Understanding Fire

- relishes excitement and delights in intimacy
- keenly intuitive and passionately empathetic
- believes in the power of charisma and desire
- loves sensation, drama, and sentiment
- likes to be hot, bright, and vibrant

Typical Problems

- anxiety, agitation, and frenzy
- bizarre perceptions and sensations
- nervous exhaustion and insomnia
- palpitations, sweating, hypoglycemia, rashes, palsy
- abuse of mind-altering substances

Critical Times

- *exaggerated Fire—Heart* congestion: summer and fall, 11 A.M.–3 P.M. and 3 A.M.–7 A.M.
- *collapsed Fire—Heart* depletion: late summer and winter, 11 P.M.–3 A.M. and 3 P.M.–7 P.M.

A Friendly Reminder

The power of *Fire* comes from the capacity to liberate heat and light and realize joy and fulfillment. *Fire* types need to temper their chemistry and contain their fervor, conserving as well as sharing their resources, withdrawing and separating as well as embracing and merging.

CHAPTER TEN

EARTH

There is nothing which heaven does not cover,
and nothing which earth does not sustain.

Chuang Tzu
369–286 B.C.

EARTH IS AS MASSIVE AS A CRAGGY MOUNTAIN RANGE, AS GENTLE AS A rolling grassy hill, as inviting as a verdant meadow, as absorbing as a rich alluvial valley receiving rivers of sediment and rain. Parading across boundaries, the Rockies, Appalachians, Andes, Himalayas, Alps, and Caucasus encircle and unite territories and villages, tribes and nations. In the sheltering hollows and crevices of the earth's body, creatures sculpt terraces, fields, and paddies and graze in marshes, forests, and open plains. *Earth* cradles and nurtures the life that depends upon it.

As summer wanes and fall approaches, there is a hiatus, a period in which time seems to stop and the glory of summer hangs suspended. Late summer marks the ascendance of the power of *Earth*, the time of ripening, when all that has grown and matured throughout spring and summer lies ready for harvest. Momentarily free of the cycle of birth, growth, decay, and death, this is a secure time of peace and plenty during which we appreciate the flowering of our labor. The *Spleen*, like Indian summer, corresponds with the *Phase* of *Earth*. Receiving and sharing solid and liquid, perceptions and ideas, the *Spleen* incorporates food and experience into the substance of who we are.

Earth—the soil that feeds us and the ground that locates us in time and space—imparts stability. A tree is as sturdy as the soil in which it is rooted. A sapling that grows out of gravel or sand is easily uprooted, whereas one that wraps its roots around granite stands sturdy, almost impossible to dislodge. When *Earth* is too porous, the structure that holds us securely in place erodes, whereas if too dense, we can become stuck in one spot, unable to move in any direction. *Earth*'s density and mass sustain our momentum, keeping us aligned in the direction of our desired goal.

Just as a gyroscope spinning in place keeps an aircraft flying steadily along a prescribed path, *Earth* generates the capacity for changing direction without losing balance. *Earth* represents our center of gravity, the point of reference around which all other aspects of character and structure orient themselves, the axis around which they revolve.

THE ARCHETYPE FOR EARTH: THE PEACEMAKER

Unification is the guiding principle of the *Peacemaker*. Through her power to establish and sustain relationships, she nurtures and promotes our connectedness with each other and our world. Focusing on what is mutually shared, she synthesizes what is divided and antagonistic into what is unified and interdependent. The *Peacemaker* values serenity and stability, mediating conflict with her gift for converting discord into harmony. She is the master of positioning and leverage, able to alter her perspective, grasping what is central to achieving the most cooperation with the least sacrifice. Chameleonlike, she can assume and enhance the attributes of those around her, putting people at ease in an environment of trust.

The *Peacemaker* embodies sympathy and caring, a ready advocate for those in greatest need—of friendship, sustenance, and recognition. Negotiating peace for its own sake, she tirelessly serves humanity as the great balancer and equalizer, the preserver of families and societies.

DOROTHY: EXEMPLAR OF EARTH

Dorothy holds her world up and together with practical, down-to-earth intelligence, anticipating and meeting the needs of her family, friends, and co-workers. As the nucleus of her network she constructs the matrix and context for the life that thrives around her.

Although Dorothy can be readily diverted to help another, she keeps her own quandaries to herself, hiding worry behind a congenial, cheerful front. Dorothy is sweet; she has an amiable disposition, an engaging smile, and a sweet tooth. She respects one maxim in particular:

> Kind hearts are the garden
> Kind thoughts are the roots
> Kind words are the blossoms
> Kind deeds are the fruits

Popular, accommodating, and grounded in herself, Dorothy can afford to give and take with ease. Contributing her advice with diplomatic craft, she eagerly organizes other people's lives with a facility for resolving their personal or social dilemmas.

Dorothy is fleshy and strong rather than sinewy or tight. Her power is in her mass, carried in a round body with solid hips and thighs planted firmly on the ground. Although Dorothy does not move quickly, she is efficient, accomplishing tasks with deliberation and focus. A patient listener, she draws people out in conversation so that even a stranger feels comfortable.

Dorothy's home functions as her center of operations, the place where she contentedly mixes work, recreation, and domestic life. She has a territorial attachment to her household as a locus and extension of herself. Protective and loyal, her identity is tied in the knot of her family. As a spider spins a web, Dorothy builds familial relationships, mothering and incorporating friends into an extended social network. Dorothy is the glue that binds groups together. Being indispensable fulfills her need to be useful and stay connected. In a busy, indifferent world, she creates an oasis of caring, risking the loss of herself if she becomes completely immersed in others.

Dorothy has difficulty saying no, often compelled to take on more than her share of other people's projects or predicaments. This extra weight increases her own mass, and she becomes prone toward languidity and sluggishness. Like oversaturated soil, Dorothy can feel thick and heavy, as if caught in a muddy quagmire. When this happens immobility engulfs her, and even rising from a chair becomes an arduous task. Caught in the labyrinth of her own commitments, inertia and a loss of perspective defeat her attempts to find a way out of her entanglements.

Just as silos full of harvested grain engender a feeling of abundant prosperity, Dorothy feels enriched and complete when she is filled to her limit. Similarly, her impulse is to be generous—her deepest wish is that everyone have as much as they need and want. She resists change that she anticipates might jeopardize security and stability. Attached to plenty and threatened by scarcity, she is willing to add to but reluctant to relinquish or replace relationships, positions, locations, resources. As a squirrel collects acorns in his nest, she stores away surplus to assure that needs are met.

The inherent capacity to absorb makes Dorothy vulnerable to becoming overburdened and overweight. Just as the *Spleen* incorporates and then distributes *Nutritive Essence* in order to diminish or augment body mass, Dorothy's physical form fluctuates, reflecting the constant reorganization of her social and material life. Dorothy uses her body by pulling herself together, gathering herself up, and then spreading herself out.

Pleasing other people, something utterly important to Dorothy, can leave little room for fulfilling her own desires, creating an empty feeling in the midst of a life that seems replete. Because she sometimes confuses her hunger for satisfaction with a craving for food, eating becomes a means of filling up. Being continually full slows her metabolism and assimilation of nutrients. Food sits undigested in her stomach, uncomfortably inflating her abdomen with stagnant fluid and gases. Lacking sufficient energy from the food she ingests, she eats more and profits less.

Retarded digestion engenders an urge for the quick fix of sugar and starch. Unable to benefit from the longer-lasting nourishment derived from complex carbohydrates, vegetables, and proteins, she seeks the support of easily digested vitamins and other concentrated food supplements. She see-

saws between the urge to fill up and the discomfort of being overfull. Rarely feeling right, she opts for strenuous weight-loss regimens in hopes of attaining the natural balance of eating only when truly hungry. She tries both fasting and the lavish consumption of raw vegetables and fruits. Raw foods and juices have a cold, wet nature that contribute to greater attrition of her digestive power, which eventually makes a strategy of dieting ineffectual.

If Dorothy's environment is constant and generous, she functions optimally. With social, emotional, and physical nourishment unsteady and unpredictable, like feast and famine, she can be greedy and acquisitive in the face of opulence, fearful of deprivation and impoverishment in sparse times. When Dorothy loses her stability, she oscillates between being empty and full, indulgent and renunciatory, self-centered and self-deprecating, grandiose and defeated, meddling and apathetic, bingeing and starving. If she can restrain herself from overcompensating, Dorothy's instinctive proclivity for poise and balance return.

Just as the *Spleen* forms and reconstitutes the *internal* milieu, Dorothy generates our social medium—she designs the space, casts the players, and sets the mood so that everyone can do their part. It is not always clear exactly what it is that Dorothy does—her role is amorphous and undefined, soft like her body, curved without edges, spilling over into the sometimes unrecognized work of mothering the world. Dorothy may feel herself unformed or underdeveloped, inseparable from her project, her family, her environment, shaped by it as much as the sculptor of it. Her work is to serve, to connect, to raise awareness, and to facilitate action. Without her instinct for arrangement and harmony and her zeal for togetherness, the human arena would be considerably more lonely, desolate, and austere.

HOW WE RECOGNIZE DOROTHY AS AN EARTH TYPE

Dorothy has a sociable, sunny disposition and is supportive, pliant, reliable, and politic, infusing balance, consistency, and focus into her extended network of relationships. She has a way of deliberately insinuating herself in other people's affairs that gains people's trust and appreciation. Like *Earth*, she is always there, permeating and infiltrating her social environment, serving and providing.

Obsessed, Dorothy becomes entangled in a web of details and complexity. She overperforms her role as intermediary and caretaker so that what was moderating becomes overbearing and inhibiting and what was nurturing becomes intrusive and overprotective. When the influence of the *Spleen* is too pervasive, there is more absorption than transformation, more density than activity, more mass than energy. Thoughts, feelings, fluids, and food are amassed, settle, and congeal rather than amble freely.

When concern and involvement become worrisome burdens, she loses her ability to hold herself up and together. Collapsing into a lugubrious inertia, she is engulfed by self-pity and dissatisfaction. Dramatic fluctuations in appetite, weight, and self-esteem are a consequence of her loss of poise. Dorothy's easy, relaxed manner takes on an nebulous quality, and she vacillates, scattered and wishy-washy without self-confidence or clarity. She can be so consumed with wondering what she should do that she does nothing. This overwhelming ambivalence defeats her attempts to rescue her self or even ask for help.

Being called upon to bring people together rouses Dorothy to action and rescues her the way an incoming tide frees a beached whale from the sand, returning her to a buoyant and fluent milieu. Just like the mammals of the sea, Dorothy is a tribal, social animal. As important as it is for Dorothy to maintain her network for herself, it is essential to the group's survival that she be there for them.

THE EVOLUTION OF DISTORTED PATTERNS OF EARTH

For an *Earth* type, conflict tends to develop between *Earth* and *Water (Spleen-Kidney)* and *Earth* and *Wood (Spleen-Liver)*. *Earth* restrains *Water*, and *Wood* restrains *Earth*. Together the *Spleen* and *Kidney* organize the distribution and storage of *Moisture*, whereas the *Spleen* and *Liver* govern the allocation and supply of *Nutritive Essence* and *Blood*. Disturbance of these relationships creates stagnation of *Qi*, *Moisture*, and *Blood*.

EARTH: Spleen

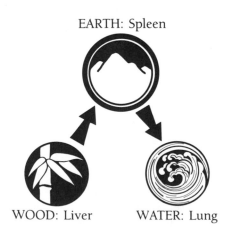

WOOD: Liver   WATER: Lung

When an overbearing *Spleen* restricts the *Kidney* too harshly, the *Kidney's* function of discharging unnecessary fluids and metabolic wastes diminishes, causing *Dampness* to accumulate in the lower half of the body. Edema and swelling occur in the abdomen, hips, legs, and ankles, and urination is scanty or inadequate. The joints of the ankles, knees, and hips suffer because of the added weight, and the back becomes weak. Swelling of the intestines and cysts of the ovaries may develop because of this stagnation of fluids. Too much *Moisture* trapped in the body produces spongy, tender flesh and muscles. The *Qi* and *Blood* do not circulate freely, and other organs, deprived of *Moisture* and nourishment, get dry, irritated, and weak. When tissue is saturated with fluids, secretions become gelatinous and sticky. A paradox emerges: *Dryness* and *Wetness* coexist because water is present but not accessible. Dorothy feels dry but not thirsty. Her membranes and joints are swollen, while her abdomen, back, and limbs stay cold and damp.

There is an intrinsic tension between *Earth* and *Water*. *Earth* wants to share (distribute) and accommodate (absorb), and *Water* wants to withhold (store up) and harden (consolidate). When *Earth* is *exaggerated* this manifests behaviorally as meddling interference, too much arranging and enveloping, and not enough distance and relinquishment—letting things be. With *collapsed Earth* there is too much softness, receptivity, and being enveloped and not enough firmness, resoluteness, and confinement—"staying in your own space."

Tension between the *Spleen* and *Liver* becomes a problem when stagnation of *Spleen Qi* generates congestion of *Blood* and *Qi* in the *Liver*. Stagnation of *Blood* can manifest as heavy menstrual flow with viscous clotted blood and the growth of fibroid tumors in the uterus. Lack of circulation of *Spleen* and *Liver Qi* also causes poor digestion in the form of intestinal gas, distension, constipation and diarrhea, and abnormal appetites.

Earth-Wood conflict revolves around the polarity between continuity, security, and predictability on the one hand and change, risk taking, and spontaneity on the other. The need to ease social and emotional discomfort is pitted against the urge toward freedom and arousal. Dorothy's emotions become heavy and intense when her *Liver* is too weak to stimulate and disperse the muddy energy of *Earth*. She then falls prey to soppy sentimentality and irascible sensitivity—everything feels so weighty and earthshaking that her reactions are disproportionate to the situation.

Like tropical air laden with humidity, things get sticky and turbid. Dorothy's complexion and eyes turn murky and her thinking muddled as a generalized stasis makes it impossible for her to take action on her own behalf. When the *Spleen* accumulates excessive *Moisture*, the *Heart* becomes congested: the heart enlarges, blood pressure rises from excess fluids, and awareness becomes hazy. Edema results from fluid oozing into the intercellular spaces of the limbs and leaking into the cavities of the abdomen and chest. Obesity due to this overaccumulation further undermines the physiologic capacity to bear the burden and cope.

The therapeutic goals for Dorothy are to redistribute *Moisture*, mobilize stagnant *Qi*, and improve digestion. Learning to recognize whether she is too "dense" (static and congested) or too "porous" (scattered and dissipated) will prompt her to rearrange her commitments, activity, and appetites according to her inner state. She requires a routine that activates her physically and diverts her mentally. Regular and appropriate nourishment, emotional and intellectual, is a means of avoiding "feast and famine" cycles that promote stagnation—which leads to deprivation—which eventually leads to diminished metabolic efficiency and emotional despondency and discouragement.

EARTH: Spleen Patterns

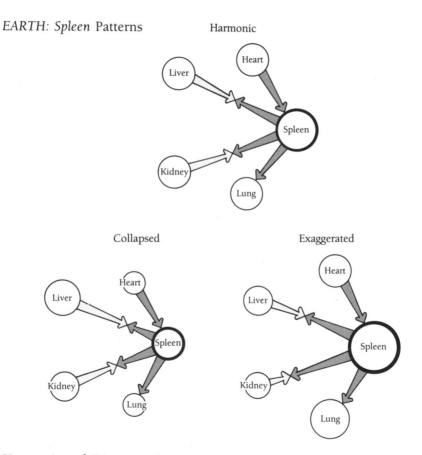

Harmonic and Dissonant Patterns

In the *harmonic Spleen* pattern, the *Heart* and *Lung* maintain stability while the *Kidney* and *Liver* provide the tension necessary for movement and adaptation. In the *exaggerated Spleen* pattern, the *Heart* and *Lung* become hyperactive and the *Kidney* and *Liver* become hypersensitive and erratic. In the *collapsed* pattern, the *Heart* and *Lung* become drained and weakened while the *Kidney* and *Liver* become overbearing and congested.

Fluids, starches, sugars, fats, and sticky glutinous foods are Dorothy's undoing, particularly in the form of confections and pastries, pastas, milk, cheeses, and rich sauces made with butter or oil. Dorothy needs ample roughage and fiber to move the more glutinous foods that she likes through her system. Warm, dry condiments (ginger, pepper, parsley, and cardamom) help her eliminate excess gas and moisture. She should also avoid refrigerated or iced foods because the *Cold* engenders *Dampness* and depresses the "digestive fire" of *Stomach* and *Spleen*. Relieving stagnation through mobilization of *Qi* and *Moisture* can be accomplished through exercise that requires muscular effort coupled with movement. Herbal and acupuncture treatment is helpful because it activates *Qi*, eliminates *Dampness*, and regulates digestion.

Being the consummate arranger that she is, Dorothy needs to organize patterns of continuous, predictable changes in activity and attention, protecting herself against becoming stuck due to a lack of options or scattered because of a lack of structure. Dorothy must stay grounded yet maintain her ability to move and change—focused yet free to detach and reorient herself so that she may juggle poise and mobility.

RICHARD: JOIN MY TEAM

Richard saunters leisurely into the clinic, even though he is late. He explains casually, "I took a wrong turn and got lost on the way here; I hope you can still make room for me. I'm looking forward to having you join my health team." He makes himself comfortable and with a winning smile agrees to wait until I am free.

Richard engages me in his story in the waiting room. Pointing under his ribs on the right side, he says, "I've been having pains here, and they won't let up. My doctors says it's not hepatitis, though I've had that before, and he doesn't know what to do. I'm a fund-raiser; my work is helping people give their money away, so I spend a lot of time socializing. That doesn't bother me, but two or three times a year my back goes out and I get laid up in bed. My doctor says my prostate might need surgery, but I don't fancy the knife, not yet, at least. Besides bad gums and some loose teeth, I'm in fine fettle."

"What about the hepatitis?" I ask.

Richard says, "The first time I got it I was in the navy. Second time I was on vacation in Mexico and ate at a bad street stand. It took six months before I pulled myself together. Ever since then I seem to react poorly to more than a couple of drinks or too many French fries. If I overdo it, I wake up with a foggy, heavy feeling in my head, like I can't see straight, and a dull, swollen pain under my ribs. Then my prostate kicks in. Fact is, even too much coffee can make that worse. It's ironic that only the things I love   197 are a problem: good food, good liquor, and strong coffee with plenty of cream and sugar."

Richard's abdomen is soft, distended, and cool below the navel. His tissue is not firm but yielding, with a layer of fat where there used to be muscle. His tongue is pale and flabby with a thick, sticky fur, and his pulse is weak, full, and spongy like his tissue. All this suggests too much fluid and congestion: the *Spleen* is not doing the job of transforming and distributing food or liquid.

"Do you get cold easily?" I inquire.

Richard replies that cold, rainy weather makes his back hurt and that he relies on hot coffee to warm him up in the morning. Treatment will be aimed at dispersing stagnation by activating circulation and elimination.

Because Richard's belly is cool, moxa is burned on a site below the navel called the *Sea of Qi*. This region is the reservoir of life force, of inherited and acquired *Essence*, and the origin of all the channels. Moxa here warms and arouses the *Qi* of the entire body, especially of the *Kidneys* and *Intestines*.

A point on the *Liver* channel below the ribs, at the site of Richard's discomfort, relieves stagnation in the *Liver* and *Spleen*. A point on the *Spleen* channel above the ankle harmonizes the interaction between the *Liver*, *Spleen*, and *Kidney*, dispersing accumulated *Dampness* and congestion, relieving the swelling in the prostate for that reason. It also has the general effect of tonifying the *Spleen* and improves its ability to transform and distribute *Moisture*.

Another point just above the ankle on the *Kidney* channel strengthens the *Kidney* and promotes diuresis, eliminating excess fluid from the tissue. On the top of the foot, between the first and second toe, a point on the *Liver* channel mobilizes *Qi*, stimulating and regulating the *Spleen* and *Stomach*. Altogether this treatment harmonizes the *Liver* and *Spleen*, strengthens the *Kidney*, and invigorates metabolic heat (the *Yang* of the *Spleen* and *Kidney*). Richard luxuriates in the freedom that nothing is required of him, and he thoroughly enjoys the treatment process.

Richard distinguishes himself by his sympathetic, easygoing manner, a talent for organizing people, his pleasure at savoring food, and the soft, comfortable form of his body. He uses himself to create and maintain contacts within an extensive circle. He becomes a medium through which people share their economic harvest.

The flaccid quality of his flesh, tongue, and pulse all indicate the collapse of *Spleen Qi*. The feeling of heaviness and distension in his head, abdomen, and prostate results from chronic stagnation of *Moisture*. Soreness and swelling in the hepatic region reflects obstruction of the *Liver Network*, while deterioration of the teeth and aching in the lumbar region reflect debility of the *Kidney*.

Earth transforms, and *Wood* mobilizes. The *Spleen* generates *Blood* and *Qi*, and the *Liver* stores *Blood* and regulates *Qi*. Together the *Spleen* and *Liver* organize the production and distribution of the nutritive substance that becomes blood and tissue. *Earth* absorbs, and *Water* consolidates. Surplus *Nutritive Qi* created by the *Spleen* is collected and preserved as acquired *Essence* by the *Kidney* for lubrication, reproduction, and regeneration. Together the *Spleen* and *Kidney* govern the perfusion and storage of *Yin* substance, *Moisture*, and *Essence*.

The first issue to deal with for Richard is the stagnation of *Qi* and *Moisture* that results in congestion and weakness of the *Liver* and *Kidney*. Digestion and assimilation are less the issue than the excess accumulation that arises from inadequate circulation and elimination. Therapy will also emphasize correcting *Kidney* and *Liver deficiency* by tonifying *Qi* and *Blood* while maintaining circulation of *Qi* and *Moisture*. As *Liver* and *Kidney* function improve, the prostate problem will resolve itself since it will no longer be needed by the body as an overflow depository of fluid wastes. As *Qi* and *Yang* grow, Richard's metabolism will function more efficiently, and he will lose weight. His decreased mass will relieve some of the stress on his lower back and circulatory system. A healthier *Liver* will circulate the *Blood* and *Qi* throughout the body, and a stronger *Kidney* will eliminate unnecessary *Moisture*.

Richard reluctantly agrees to reducing his consumption of coffee, alcohol, pastry, and bread, all of which generate *Dampness* and promote swelling of the liver and prostate. Warm, cooked foods will minimize his need for the quick energy provided by stimulants and refined carbohydrates.

The pain under Richard's ribs is gone after the second treatment, and the swelling of his liver subsides after the fourth visit. His prostate and urinary function improve enough to obviate his present concern about surgery. Although Richard's symptoms have cleared, he is advised to remain on herbal supplements for a year because of the chronic weakness of his *Liver* and *Kidney*. Pleased that his condition is so amenable to this form of therapy, Richard begins to spread the word about his success and encourages many others to try Chinese medicine.

Summary of Richard's Patterns		
Signs and Symptoms	**Interpretation**	**Interpretation**
	According to *Qi, Moisture, Blood*	According to *Organ Networks*
Swollen *Liver* Prostatitis Foggy, heavy head Thick, sticky tongue fur Full, spongy pulse	Stagnation of *Qi* and *Moisture*	Disharmony of *Liver-Spleen* and weakness of *Spleen*
Soft, cold abdomen Weak gums Loose teeth Weak, sore back Pale, flabby tongue Weak pulse	Depletion of *Qi* and vital *Heat*	Disharmony of *Spleen-Kidney* and weakness of *Kidney*

Prescriptions for Therapy

Harmonize *Spleen-Liver*
Disperse *Qi*
Disperse *Moisture*
Warm interior

Harmonize *Spleen-Kidney*
Tonify *Qi*
Consolidate *Moisture*
Warm interior

EARTH		
PEACEMAKER		SPLEEN
Mental Faculties	**Biological Functions**	**Organs—Tissues—Fluid**
Remembering Intention Ideation Attention	Balancing Transforming Absorbing Distributing	*Spleen* and *Stomach* Lips, mouth, eyelids Muscles, Saliva, lymph, chyle

EARTH

Exaggerated patterns arise from:	**Collapsed patterns arise from:**	**Aggravations occur with:**
Congestion of *Qi* and *Moisture* Accumulation of *Heat* and *Dampness* Generation of *internal Wind* Disharmony of *Spleen-Liver Spleen-Kidney*	Depletion of *Qi* and *Blood* Accumulation of *Damp* and *Cold* Weakness of *Liver, Spleen, Kidney*	Late summer and change of season Humidity, *Heat*, and *Cold* Sweet, sticky, and cold food 7 A.M.–11 A.M. and 7 P.M.–11 P.M.

Characteristic Features of Psyche

Undistorted	**Exaggerated**	**Collapsed**	**Difficulty With**
Nurturing Supportive Relaxed Oriented Sociable Sympathetic Considerate Agreeable Poised Attentive	Overprotective Meddlesome Inert Stuck Crowding Involved Worried Conforming Lugubrious Overbearing	Spoiling Clinging Amorphous Vacillating Ingratiating Attached Scattered Wishy-Washy Precarious Fawning	Change Disorientation Self-sacrifice Efficiency Ambivalence Identity Independence Concentration

Characteristic Features of Soma			
Undistorted	**Exaggerated**	**Collapsed**	**Difficulty With**
Round, firm physique Large, thick musculature Soft, smooth, peachy skin Hands and feet seem small Broad hips and shoulders	Conjunctivitis Excess appetite Water retention Irregular bowels and urination Swollen prostate Tender gums PMS with lethargy, aching, hunger, and swelling Sores on scalp Heavy, aching head and eyes Sticky, puffy eyelids Sticky mucus in nose and throat Sticky saliva and perspiration Swollen, sensitive *Spleen* or *Liver*	Tends to form soft lumps and swollen glands Sore, weak lumbar region Weak ankles and wrist Hunger but can't decide what to eat Prolapse of *Stomach*, *Intestine*, *Uterus* Varicose veins Slow healing of cuts Bruises easily Spongy, tender muscles Bleeding gums Tooth decay Hard to lose weight Bloats easily Poor muscle tone	Metabolic, muscle, and lymphatic dysfunction Venous disorders Digestive disorders Weight management Fluid balance

So, You Think You're an Earth Type

Keys to Understanding Earth

- wants to be involved and needed
- likes to be in charge but not in the limelight
- agreeable and accommodating: wants to be all things to all people
- seeks harmony and togetherness
- insists upon loyalty, security, and predictability

Typical Problems

- worry, obsession, and self-doubt
- meddling and overprotective
- overextended and inert
- lethargy, indigestion, unruly appetites, water retention, muscle tenderness
- unrealistic expectations and disappointment

Critical Times

- *exaggerated Earth—Spleen* congestion: late summer and winter, 7 A.M.–11 A.M. and 3 P.M.–7 P.M.
- *collapsed Earth—Spleen* depletion: fall and spring, 7 P.M.–11 P.M. and 11 P.M.–3 A.M.

A Friendly Reminder

The power of *Earth* comes from the capacity to link, nurture, and sustain. *Earth* types need to balance their devotion to relationship with solitude and self-expression, developing self-reliance as well as building community.

CHAPTER ELEVEN
METAL

Autumn

Wind passes over the lake.
The swelling waves stretch away
Without limit. Autumn comes with the twilight,
And boats grow rare on the river.
Flickering waters and fading mountains
Always touch the heart of man.
I never grow tired of singing
Of their boundless beauty.
The lotus pods are already formed,
And the water lilies have grown old.
The dew has brightened the blossoms
Of the arrowroot along the riverbank.
The herons and seagulls sleep
on the sand with their
Heads tucked away, as though
They did not wish to see
The men who pass by on the river.

Li Ch'ing Chao
A.D. 1081–1143

METAL IS AS AUSTERE AS A VAST ARID PLAIN BEFORE WINTER RAINS, AS sharp as a high mountain peak slicing through mist into a clear empty sky. This *Phase* embodies the power of restraint, separation, and refinement.

Autumn is a time of withering and decay. Fallen leaves decompose, returning to the soil as the remains of crops are plowed under. Expired blossoms and fallen fruit fertilize the soil for next year's growth. The sap of trees settles into the interior, sinking down toward the roots. It is time for eliminating what is unnecessary, storing up only what is needed for winter. As the trees shed foliage, creatures prepare their shelters for the stark hibernation of winter as life slows down, collapsing inward. Corresponding to the temperament of this season, the *Lung*, the organ of *Metal*, sucks in and refines the *Qi*, sending it downward to nourish our roots with pure *Essence*. Ruling the skin, the outer limit of the human body, the *Lung* protects against external invasion and safeguards internal resources.

Metal, derived from the earth, is a pure substance generated by a process of reduction. Derived from the concept in alchemy of turning base metals into gold, this *Phase* represents the transformation of the gross materials of nature into pure "essence." Fall is a time for evolution through reduction. Matter returns to its source in preparation for its later re-creation—the rotting fruit leaves behind its seeds, and this corroding matter nourishes the kernels that multiply in spring.

With fall comes a sense of gathering in, stocking up, mingled with a sense of loss as the light begins to fade and the air chills. *Yin* waxes as *Yang* wanes. This is another season of change, but as spring was an expansive time of breaking through and proliferation, fall is a contractive time of pulling in and dying back. The life cycle completes itself in autumn. The *Nei Jing* says that the energy of fall is the "killing energy"—sharp, retracting, and finishing.

THE ARCHETYPE FOR METAL: THE ALCHEMIST

Transmutation is the guiding principle for the *Alchemist*, who seeks the perfection of form and function. Through his power of discernment, he distills what is good and pure from what is coarse and primitive. In his striving to extract order from chaos, he molds situations so that people perform their tasks with elegant precision.

Defining and refining, the *Alchemist* is the keeper of standards and measures, the source of aesthetic and moral values, the defender of virtue, principle, and beauty. He is the master of ceremony and discipline. Like an abbot ensconced in his sanctuary, serene, detached, unflappable, he instructs us in the meaning of ritual and doctrine, providing the structure that enables people to apply the metaphysical to the mundane.

LOUIS: EXEMPLAR OF METAL

Immaculate, impeccable, and well organized, Louis has a place for everything and keeps everything in its place. Methodical, efficient, and disciplined, he is a man who lives according to principle. Applying his analytic and critical mind, Louis derives satisfaction from taking things apart and putting them back together. It suits his sense of order and control. His gift is in designing systems. By pruning concepts, protocols, and objectives, he insures that a family affair, political campaign, factory, or corporation runs according to schedule. Although Louis may not inspire passionate devotion, he is well appreciated for his integrity and commitment to reason.

With smooth skin draped over a slim frame, Louis has fine, angular features. Sensitive to all aspects of his internal and external environment, he has a particularly keen sense of smell. His self-awareness is bounded by a well-developed talent for detachment and discrimination: he is adept at separating his own ideas and desires from those around him. Skilled at carving distinctions, Louis cuts through ambiguity.

Everyone knows exactly where they stand with Louis. Neither gullible nor easily ruffled, Louis remains aloof, difficult to know intimately. He prefers not to take work home with him and doesn't mix business with pleasure. Louis maintains some emotional distance from his spouse and children yet is always correct and fair, providing equal time and favor in meeting his family's needs. He dislikes conflict and disorder, preferring conformity over strangeness, composure over excitement. Pleased when others are satisfied with their role and obligations, he expects his life to be agreeable and sensible. His patience persists as long as people do their share and follow established practices, insuring that events transpire according to plan.

Louis judges right and wrong, success or failure, according to how closely actions match principles. He sometimes overidentifies with standards, methods, and schedules and covets his own authority and expertise, disinclined to relinquish any part of it. When the execution of his carefully rendered schemes is derailed, he can fall back on a rigid adherence to rules and regulations in an effort to reassert control over disturbingly fluctuating circumstances. His striving for perfection can be a source of disappointment, since no one may be able to meet his standards, including himself. Emotionally this translates into his reluctance to share himself with others. Disillusioned with his efforts to make the world flawless and good, Louis sometimes resorts to reinstating order by means of punishment and prohibition. In the face of having the righteous and reasonable denied him, he is willing to sacrifice the pleasures of spontaneity and intimacy for the sake of safety and control.

This pattern of constant inhibition interferes with rhythmic activity. When the cadence of respiration and elimination is interrupted in his lungs, skin, and intestines, this may lead to problems such as asthma, constipation, lack of perspiration, and dryness of skin or mucous membranes. Louis can also develop increased sensitivity to odors and changes in temperature and humidity, which trigger sneezing, sinus congestion, and headaches. Increased skin sensitivity predisposes him to dryness or itching from irritants like poison oak or exposure to wind and sunlight.

Asthma and constipation are somatic expressions of his inability to exhale, release, and go with the undulating flow. Louis resists tumult by tightening down, so that his chest may become overdeveloped, swollen with stagnant air that he cannot expel, reducing his capacity to inhale fully. He could become like the caricature of a Prussian officer with stiff neck and spine, barrel chest, tight pelvis, and a fundamental unyielding rigidity.

This stiffening also appears as suppressed emotional expression and fixed mental attitudes. When insecure, Louis becomes flat and mechanical in his responses in order to protect against the influence of intangibles such as feelings or personal tastes. His penchant for correctness can easily slip into self-righteousness and a subservient reliance on experts, leaving no room for innovation and independent thought. In this way Louis armors himself against irrationality and change, disappointment and disillusionment. Faced with an insoluble conflict practically or morally, he breaks down like the intelligent machine that can no longer compute, having lost touch with his own internal standards and principles. His self-reliance shattered, the resulting insecurity leads to meekness and a desire to be ruled and molded by those whom he fears and admires. He mimics his superiors, those more powerful than he, alternating between snobbish arrogance and obsequious deference.

Because of his yearning for and admiration of the human potential for conscience, reason, and virtue, he is often able to rise above the apparent corruption and disarray of mundane life, to appreciate the symmetry and beauty of all forms and the goodness of all souls.

HOW WE RECOGNIZE LOUIS AS A METAL TYPE

Louis's true nature expresses itself through his sense of symmetry, self-discipline, purity of ideals, and logical mind. It is important to him that people fulfill their obligations and act equitably. Louis prefers that things have shape, sequence, and definition, and he is most comfortable in a setting in which he can determine how events should unfold.

As the *Wood* type was expansive and potentially chaotic, like a "bull in a china shop," the *Metal* type is contractive and potentially overstructured, like a puffed-up military officer. When Louis's tendencies become *exaggerated*, perfectionism, authoritarianism, and dogmatism replace flexibility, self-discipline, and critical thinking. The single-minded focus on control causes inhibition of peristalsis, restricted breathing, a flattening of affect, and a blunting of sensation and perception.

Persistence of this internal stiffening can also trigger a *collapse* into internal disorder: a decay of personal values and self-definition. Inner resolve is replaced by reliance upon outer constraints. Unable to adapt to changing circumstances, plagued by disappointment and sorrow, Louis vacillates between credulousness and morbid cynicism as he searches for external answers for internal doubts and grief. It is an irony that the *Metal* type, ordinarily a paragon of rationality and self-control, can become rudderless, without substantial definition, bewildered by internal forces and grasping at external rules to anchor his reason. What was a fixation upon an inflexible   207 set of standards and values becomes a morass of moral confusion and doubt. The tendency toward personal cleanliness, household order, and careful expression can stand on its head as Louis collapses and surrenders to sloppy dress, domestic disarray, and a cacophony of impulses that elude his control.

When the stability of *Metal* is undermined, the need to differentiate and order things intensifies. Devotion to correct behavior and thinking, and adherence to fixed distinctions between good and bad, right and wrong, arise from the need to be in control. Peace becomes dullness, openness is stultified, and order becomes ritualized routine. Critical, judgmental, and perfectionistic behavior compensates for inner feelings of ambivalence, ambiguity, self-doubt, and the lack of moral conviction.

Having "the courage of your convictions" describes the harmonious synthesis or resolution of the opposition between *Metal* and *Wood*. *Metal* provides the standard or measure, the moral values, and *Wood* gives the impulse and power to realize these values in action—in other words, ethical behavior. *Metal* and *Wood* represent a complementary set of relations: contraction and expansion, inhibition and excitation, reduction and proliferation, restraint and striving. Whereas the *Wood* type can explode like a volatile time bomb with a short fuse, the *Metal* personality can shrink inward, like old Jell-O, stiff on the surface and gooey at the core.

Between *Metal* and *Fire* exist the polarities of tight and loose, analytic and intuitive, sensitive and sensual, and distinct and merged. As *Fire* reveres passion and empathy, *Metal* esteems mindfulness and right action. When these are joined together, a kind mind prevails. Wedding virtue with love describes the harmonious synthesis between *Metal* and *Fire*. Whereas the *Fire* type becomes dispersed through excitement and euphoria, the *Metal* type becomes stuffy through suppression and tedium.

Yet when Louis is at his best, he interacts easily with other people, secure within, easily distinguishing his own thoughts, feelings, and values from those around him. He feels neither vulnerable to outside influences and opinions nor compelled to impose his standards or sensibilities on others. True to himself, he feels protected and receptive, articulate and inspired, righteous and sure.

THE EVOLUTION OF DISTORTED PATTERNS OF METAL

The polarities between *Metal* and *Wood* (*Lung* and *Liver*), and *Metal* and *Fire* (*Lung* and *Heart*), characterize the *Metal* type. The *Lung* and *Liver* govern the upward and downward, inward and outward, circulation of *Qi*. The *Lung* and *Heart* affect the perimeter of the body, opening and closing, tightening and loosening, pores, sweat glands, and vessels.

When the *Lung* is overly strong, the *Liver* and *Heart* are relatively weak.

METAL: Lung

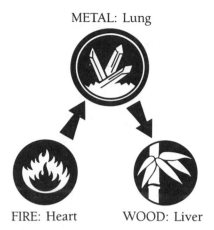

FIRE: Heart   WOOD: Liver

Since the *Lung* commands the *Qi*, it is easy for it to inhibit the function of other *Organs*. In particular the *Liver* becomes too subdued, with a consequent suppression of feeling and expressiveness. By comparison, *Wood* or *Fire* types have less command over their impulses, whereas a *Metal* type is capable of exerting such complete self-control that he becomes reserved and remote.

When the *Lung* excessively restricts the *Heart*, *Fire* diminishes, causing the person to become chilly and emotionally closed. Through contraction of the skin and depression of peripheral circulation, the *Lung* confines warmth and *Moisture*, *Qi* and *Blood*, to the body's core. This suppression of *Qi* can cause lack of motility, and the confinement of *Heat* can cause *Dryness* from the evaporation of fluids, both of which may contribute to constipation or asthma. Entrapped *Heat* might also cause inflammation or irritation as in laryngitis, sinusitis, dermatitis, ileitis, colitis, and urethritis. A *Fire* type, in whom *Qi* is always at the surface, is flushed, warm, and perspires readily. The *Metal* type is the opposite. His energy is contained beneath the surface, his complexion wan, his skin cool, tight, dry, and he rarely perspires. It is difficult for someone like Louis to discharge and rid himself of toxicity or negativity. Retention of physical or mental wastes can accumulate on the one hand, congealing into tumors, or constrict the emotional field on the other, resulting in a diminished capacity for feeling and responsiveness.

The *Spleen*, mother of the *Lung*, becomes depleted after prolonged constriction of *Qi*, which interferes with the digestive and assimilative activities of the stomach and intestines. Consequent *deficiencies* of *Moisture* and *Nutritive Essence* escalate into a condition of severe *Dryness*, the signs of which may be a lack of secretions, emaciation, anemia, poor appetite, and a ghostly, ethereal appearance.

As the succulent moisture of life shrivels, the body becomes fixed, cal-   209 lused, and inanimate. Because his skin is tight and his perspiration is as scarce as rain in the desert, Louis rarely catches colds. But if his defenses are overwhelmed, an infection may penetrate quickly to the interior of the body, giving rise to high fevers without the evaporation of perspiration to cool the intense heat. Under such circumstances, what would otherwise be an ordinary flu could develop into a severe bronchitis or pneumonia.

When the *Lung* is exhausted, the rhythmic functions of the body lose their regularity and synchronicity. This is manifested by alternating heat and

METAL: Lung Patterns

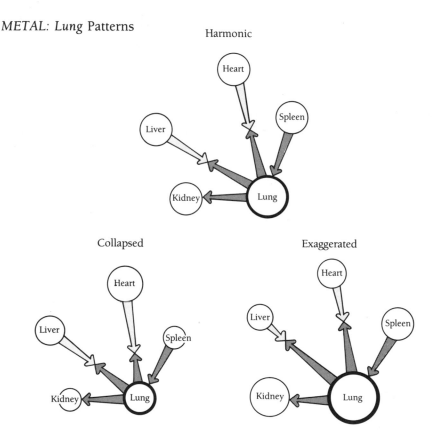

Harmonic and Dissonant Patterns

In the *harmonic Lung* pattern, the *Spleen* and *Kidney* maintain stability while the *Liver* and *Heart* provide the tension necessary for movement and adaptation. In the *exaggerated Lung* pattern, the *Spleen* and *Kidney* become hyperactive and the *Liver* and *Heart* become hypersensitive and erratic. In the *collapsed* pattern, the *Spleen* and *Kidney* become drained and weakened while the *Liver* and *Heart* become overbearing and congested.

chill, dryness of mucous membranes and clamminess of the skin, itching and numbness, constipation and diarrhea, shortness of breath and hyperventilation, intermittent and rapid heartbeat, sadness and giddiness, indifference and sensitivity, blandness and frenzy. Vascular congestion in the legs and bladder weakness result when the *Lung* no longer draws the *Qi* from the extremities to the core or from the pelvis to the chest. The skin as the envelope of the body becomes easily penetrable and unable to defend against assault by pernicious influences, whether emotional, climatic, or microbial.

The key issues for Louis are stiffness, dryness, and inhibition. The *exaggerated* tendency toward inner restraint of bodily sensation and emotional expression retards the circulation of *Qi*, the pulsatory activity of the viscera, and impedes the distribution of bodily juices that lubricate and soften the skin, muscles, and mucous membrane. To preserve his self-sufficiency and openness, Louis needs to cultivate a buoyancy of spirit and a resiliency of structure. Keeping his skin elastic with massage or brushing helps him to avoid becoming callused and indifferent to sensation and emotion. Aerobic exercise, a high-fiber diet, and a moderate fluid intake are especially important for Louis. Opening his bowels, relaxing his chest, and stimulating his skin will help him remain pliant and keep his mind receptive to new ideas and inspiration. Socially, Louis can use his talent for design to insure that involvement with other people becomes a ceremonial if not a celebrated part of his daily life. It is important for him to place himself in situations that demand spontaneity as well as discipline: faith and instinct as well as knowledge and reason. Herbs and diet would help him to regulate and supplement *Qi* and *Moisture*. Acupuncture would be directed toward regulating *Blood* and *Moisture* in the skin, relaxing the chest, and activating the *Liver*, thereby preventing patterns of stiffness and dryness from crystallizing into stasis and rigidity.

STELLA: I LIVE BY THE BOOK

Stella is a trim, crisply dressed woman with fine, curly dark hair. Calm and composed, prepared with a list of her symptoms and questions written out on a note card, she waits courteously for an invitation to speak. Stella asks, "Could you tell me your fee and whether this session will include treatment as well as consultation?" I explain the fee structure and the services that I offer.

She continues, "The reason I've come is that my breasts are continuously hard and fibrous, and over the last six months, my periods have become spotty and infrequent. My skin and hair are dry, and my hands and feet get icy cold for no apparent reason. I do regular exercise, eat with care, never drink, smoke, or overindulge. I don't understand these problems. I've always   211 lived by the book. My energy is good, digestion is fine, I sleep well, and am rarely sick. I don't mind not having the period, but I'm concerned that it may be related to my breast problem. I won't take drugs or hormones, so I wanted to try acupuncture. I'll consider the herbs, but I don't like the idea of taking medicine."

TREATMENT

Stella's pulse is thin, tight, and buoyant; her tongue is pale pink with dry fur, and there is a hint of redness at the front edges and tip. Stella comments that her mouth and throat often feel dry. She's not really thirsty, but she drinks four glasses of water a day because she thinks she should. Her ovaries are tender. Even though her hands and feet are cold, her chest and abdomen feel warm. In the past Stella says she has had pain in her ovaries with spotting during ovulation.

The warmth of her abdomen and the coldness of her extremities indicate that her circulation is obstructed, which confines the *Heat* in the interior. A disorder of the *Liver* is often responsible for this problem, so the treatment will use points that help the *Liver* move the *Blood* and *Qi* from the center of the body to the extremities.

A point on the top of the foot between the third and fourth toe on the *Gallbladder* meridian will help liberate the *Qi* and *Blood* from the interior by activating the *Liver* and *Gallbladder* and drawing the *Qi* down from the chest. Above the wrist on top of the forearm, a point on the *Triple-Burner* meridian will draw the energy from the chest into the arms. In the middle of the chest, a point on the sternum will disperse the stagnant *Qi* and circulate the *Blood* in the breasts. Between the navel and the pubis bone is a point called *Gate of the Source*, which circulates the *Qi* and *Blood* in the lower abdomen and benefits the uterus and ovaries.

As Stella lies stiffly quiet, she begins to quiver as if she were shivering. She says she is not cold and that she doesn't understand why she is shaking. I explain that this is a manifestation of the release of *Qi* and that she will feel warm and relaxed when this activity subsides and not to worry about it. A tear spills from each eye as she relates that she doesn't feel upset but she seems to be crying. I comment that this too is a sign of the release of bound-up energy taking an emotional form. She comments that now her mouth feels moist as well. Both the secretion of tears and saliva is literally a sign that the juices are flowing. Stella is surprised and impressed by the changes that she is feeling and apologizes for being emotional.

INTERPRETATION AND STRATEGY

Everything about Stella is well defined, from the clothes she wears to the clarity of her self-expression. She is fastidious, careful, and pleased with the rhythm and method of her life. Stella does not like displaying her emotions—

she is both private and well managed—so her response to treatment makes an impact on her. She is not easily moved, especially in the company of strangers.

As a *Metal* type, part of what upsets Stella is that the smooth-running system of her life is being disturbed. She is reluctant to alter her habits by taking herbs since she does not take kindly to disruptions of her regular routine. But she is willing to consider the idea if she can justify the use of herbs and incorporate them into her life-style.

A central relationship for the *Metal* type is between the *Lung* and *Liver*, between the circulation of *Qi* and the distribution of *Blood*. When *Metal* dominates *Wood*, the *Qi* and *Blood* can become confined and suppressed. The prolonged stagnation of *Qi* and *Blood* in a localized region such as the breasts or ovaries engenders the formation of congealed masses such as tumors.

Stella shows signs of both *deficiency* and *excess*, but neither is preeminent or extreme. Her tongue is pale, her pulse is thin, her skin is dry, and her periods are scanty. These are all signs of a *deficiency* of *Blood*. The redness around the edges of her tongue, tightness of her pulse, hardening of the breasts, and warmth of her chest and abdomen are signs of stagnation of *Qi* and *Blood* as well as confined *Heat* in the interior. Overall, Stella has a strong constitution as evidenced by her infrequent sickness, high energy, healthy appearance, and well-integrated life-style.

The strategy for Stella is to disperse the *Qi* and tonify the *Blood*. This will alleviate the conflict that has developed between the *Liver* and the *Lung* and reverse the process of stagnation, guarding her against the formation of masses. When the *Qi* in her chest loosens, the *Heart* will be able to perform its function of circulating *Blood* to the hands and feet, and the *Liver* will be able to distribute *Blood* throughout the chest, breasts, and abdomen.

Since Stella has some hesitancy about taking herbal medicine and because she is already committed to eating wholesome food, for the time being I suggest an herbal food recipe to be cooked with grains, vegetables, and protein. I advise her to avoid eating hot, spicy foods that increase internal *Heat* and *Dryness*. The edible herbs include the roots of white peony, ligusticum, and polygonatum, combined with lycii berries, red dates, and safflower. Together with the seasonings of turmeric and fresh ginger and a few more ordinary ingredients like eggplant, leeks, shiitake mushrooms, and carrots, this recipe will improve circulation, build *Blood*, tonify *Qi*, and generate *Moisture*.

The moistening, softening, and nurturing effects of these supplementing herbs and foods will restore the smoothness and elasticity of Stella's skin, the luster and texture of her hair, and the circulation within her breasts and reproductive organs. Later, when she is comfortable with the herbs in her diet, she can begin using medicinal formulas. Acupuncture and herbs to- 213 gether will harmonize the *Lung* and *Liver*, *Qi* and *Blood*, and strengthen the *Heart* and *Kidney*.

Over the subsequent three months, Stella's midcycle bleeding ceases, her breasts soften following each period, and her circulation improves to better warm her hands and feet. She savors her herbal meals and is amenable to taking herbal medicine until the hardness in her breasts is completely gone. She is relieved that she doesn't have to continue acupuncture for too long but agrees to return for a follow-up in a few months to monitor her continuing improvement.

Summary of Stella's Patterns		
Signs and Symptoms	Interpretation	Interpretation
	According to *Qi, Moisture, Blood*	According to *Organ Networks*
Hard breasts Tender ovaries Midcycle bleeding Tight pulse Cold extremities	Stagnation of *Qi* and *Blood*	Disharmony of *Liver-Lung*
Warm chest and abdomen Dry mouth Reddened tongue	Accumulation of Heat	Disharmony of *Lung-Heart*
Scanty, infrequent periods Dry skin and hair Thin pulse Dry tongue	Depletion of *Blood* and *Moisture*	Weakness of *Kidney* and *Liver*

Prescriptions for Therapy

Harmonize *Lung-Liver*
Disperse *Qi*
Disperse *Blood*
Cool interior

Harmonize *Lung-Heart*
Tonify *Blood*
Tonify *Moisture*
Consolidate *Moisture*

METAL		
ALCHEMIST		*LUNG*
Mental Faculties	**Biological Functions**	**Organs—Tissues—Fluid**
Analysis	Emptying	*Lung/Large Intestine*
Definition	Inhibiting	Nose/skin/membranes
Discrimination	Contracting	Body hair
Synthesis	Descending	Mucus secretions

METAL

Exaggerated patterns arise from:	**Collapsed patterns arise from:**	**Aggravations occur with:**
Congestion of *Qi* and *Moisture*	Patterns arise from: Depletion of *Qi* and *Moisture*	Fall and spring *Wind* and *Heat-Cold*
Depletion of *Moisture*	Accumulation of *Damp* and *Cold*	Cold, dry, spicy, and bitter food
Accumulation of *Heat*	Invasion of *Wind*	Sweet, sticky, and cold food
Disharmony of *Lung-Liver* *Lung-Heart*	Weakness of *Spleen, Lung, Kidney*	3 A.M.–7 A.M. and 3 P.M.–7 P.M.

Characteristic Features of Psyche			
Undistorted	**Exaggerated**	**Collapsed**	**Difficulty With**
Methodical	Ritualistic	Ceremonious	Control
Discerning	Prejudiced	Dilletante	Disappointment
Scrupulous	Perfectionistic	Petty	Emotional
Accepting	Stoical	Resigned	expression
Neat	Austere	Sloppy	Intimacy
Calm	Indifferent	Numb	Authority
Disciplined	Strict	Compliant	Relativity
Honorable	Self-Righteous	Hypocritical	Disorder
Precise	Dogmatic	Lacks	Spontaneity
Reserved	Cool	conviction	
		Elusive	

Characteristic Features of Soma			
Undistorted	**Exaggerated**	**Collapsed**	**Difficulty With**
Erect, trim symmetrical physique Light, clear, dry, smooth skin Delicate features with small bones and compact muscles	Overexpanded chest Dry cough with tight chest Sinus headache Nasal polyps Dry hair, skin, and mucous membranes No perspiration Stiff spine, neck, and posture Coarse skin with large pores Constipation with tense intestine Inhibited peristalsis Dry, cracked nails and lips Scanty urine Dry nose-throat Tight muscles Intermittent pulse	Narrow chest Frail physique Delicate skin Short of breath Stress incontinence Congested nose, throat, sinus Moles and warts Headaches from sadness and disappointment Loss of body hair Clammy hands-feet Easy perspiration Varicose veins Cracked, dry, or soft nails Soft, enlarged lymph nodes Sneeze or cough with changes in temperature and humidity	Respiratory disorders Skin ailments Dehydration Elimination Lubrication Venous circulation Lymphatic circulation

SO, YOU THINK YOU'RE A METAL TYPE

KEYS TO UNDERSTANDING METAL

- likes definition, structure, and discipline
- respects virtue, discretion, and authority
- seeks to live according to reason and principle
- holds self and others to the highest standards
- reveres beauty, ceremony, and refinement

TYPICAL PROBLEMS

- indifference and inhibition
- autocratic, strict, and persnickety
- formal, distant, and unnatural
- stiff joints and muscles, dry skin and hair, shallow breathing, sensitive to climate, poor circulation
- self-righteousness and disillusionment

CRITICAL TIMES

- *exaggerated Metal—Lung* congestion: fall and spring, 3 A.M.–7 A.M. and 11 P.M.–3 A.M.
- *collapsed Metal—Lung* depletion: winter and summer, 3 P.M.–7 P.M. and 11 A.M.–3 P.M.

A FRIENDLY REMINDER

The power of *Metal* comes from the capacity to shape and refine. *Metal* types need to compensate for their rationality, self-control, and meticulousness with passion, spontaneity, and social involvement.

CHAPTER TWELVE
WATER

Of all the elements, the Sage should take water as his preceptor.
Water is yielding but all-conquering. Water extinguishes Fire,
Or finding itself likely to be defeated, escapes as steam and
     re-forms.
Water washes away Soft Earth, or, when confronted by rocks, seeks
     a way round.
Water corrodes Iron till it crumbles to dust; it saturates the
     atmosphere
So that Wind dies. Water gives way to obstacles with deceptive
     humility,
For no power can prevent it following its destined course to the
     sea.
Water conquers by yielding; it never attacks but always wins the
     last battle.
The Sage who makes himself as Water is distinguished for his
     humility,
He embraces passivity, acts from nonaction and conquers the world.

Tao Cheng
Eleventh century A.D.

WATER IS AS SUBTERRANEAN AS AN UNDERGROUND STREAM, AS DARK AND fertile as the womb, as enduring as the jade-colored sea. *Water* ascends to fullness in the frost of winter as plants submerge their energy into their roots, animals thicken their hides, and ponds harden into ice. Movement slackens as matter and energy concentrate. This is a time of apparent quiescence and stasis, yet beneath the surface is the hidden activity of gestation and germination that will bring forth renewal in spring. Before seeds and bulbs germinate, they demand a spell of chilly slumber. During this period of hibernation the essence of life persists in its most primitive state. The bear huddled in the corner of a darkened cave may be mistaken for dead except for his subtle warmth and slow, shallow breath. During winter he lives from accumulated reserves, resting until aroused by the hunger that swells as spring signals the intense activity of a new cycle. The *Kidney* abides within us like the bear in its cave, harboring the germ of being, the *Essence*, that feeds and renews our life force.

Like Dionysus, Greek god of nature, *Water* represents the primal incho-

218

ate forces of human nature, the realm of the collective and personal unconscious. *Water* is the primeval ooze out of which form materializes as life. It
links past and future, ancestor and descendant, and is the source of our
inherited intelligence.

THE ARCHETYPE FOR WATER: THE PHILOSOPHER

Revelation propels the *Philosopher* in her relentless quest for truth. She brings
to light that which is hidden, uncovering new knowledge, dispelling mystery,
eroding ignorance. Scrutinizing life until the meaning and significance of her
impressions coalesce into the germ of understanding, she is like an old-time
prospector with a nose for nuggets, sifting through the gravel of notions and
beliefs, tireless in her effort to apprehend the nature of reality. Just as the
miner digs through tons of ore before unearthing a single gem, the *Philosopher* searches doggedly for truth, which, like a diamond, is esteemed not
only for its radiant sparkle, but for its abiding hardness as a tool to advance
civilization. It takes millennia to crystallize the residual mineral essence of
fossils into this precious stone. Time is the pick and shovel of the *Philosopher*, who exhumes the bones of culture that endure. The *Philosopher* yearns
for meaning that transcends the rudderless meandering of human affairs.

As she offers insight to the world, she relies on her hope that knowledge
will be married with wisdom, power with compassion, aware that destiny is
the final authority. Able to envision what can be, she is critical of what is
by comparison. She discerns the inevitable disparity between apparent and
ultimate reality. As the custodian of our memories and dreams, she articu-
lates our aspirations, our ends, but does not define for us the machinery of
their realization, our means.

KATE: EXEMPLAR OF WATER

Kate is a visionary. Her keen imaginative intellect has great scope. She has
a sense of where things begin and where they're going. Insatiably curious
and willing to play with ideas, Kate wins respect for her thoughtfulness and
originality. She does well when inspired by the enthusiasm and motivation
of others. Left to her own devices, she is a thinker rather than a doer. Kate
so savors the life of the mind that it is easy for her to just sit and cogitate
while the world goes on around her.

Lean or fleshy, Kate's sturdy frame, sculpted features, and soft, graceful
hands define her appearance. Encircling her high forehead and lucent eyes,
her silky hair remains lustrous even as it becomes gray with age. Like an
owl with its furrowed, piercing gaze, she has acute perceptions and a quietly 219

pensive, serious demeanor. Hidden by the veil of night, the owl perches silently, listening and waiting. Kate is at home in the dark and secluded spaces of her inner life, where her attention extends beyond the pedestrian details of daily life. Alive in the world of ideas, she is relatively indifferent to the world of the mundane.

A paragon of integrity, she is unwilling to compromise principles for the sake of peace or pleasure. Bordering on eccentricity, even heresy, she resolutely holds on to her views, regardless of the fact that they may be outside of or in opposition to the mainstream. With candor she voices her truth, emanating a scrupulous toughness of spirit, accepting the consequences of her unswerving commitment to a path, belief, or cause. Hovering on the edge of stubborn adherence, she is willing to withstand self-sacrifice.

Kate experiences herself as resilient and self-sufficient, preferring the rest of her family to be the same. Relishing the accessibility of warmth and intimacy, she also requires the freedom to withdraw emotionally into a protective shell of solitude. Devotedly loyal and committed, she regards the continuity of her family as more important than harmonious daily happiness.

Solitary by nature, she runs the risk of being isolated socially, relying on other people to push through her armor, captivate her, draw her out. Because Kate inhabits a deep interior world, it's hard to know what she's thinking or feeling from the outside. Taciturn and removed, she is not always aware of how the distance she maintains limits her relationships. She periodically seals herself off from external affairs, seeming not to require the society of others because she is cloistered within her own mind, divining from the source, the well of her being. Yet at a certain point she emerges from her cocoon to reconnect with society so the seeds of understanding germinating within may flower in the world.

Under conditions of prolonged estrangement, Kate can become so physically inactive and reclusive that, as if in suspended animation, she becomes unresponsive and inaccessible. This hard, deadened expression leads to apathy and depression. Negativity and a cynical attitude begin to color her perceptions, sabotaging her desire for and expectation of fulfillment. Suspicious of people using her for their own ends, she loses faith easily. She sees others as merely living in the moment, wasting time and resources, while she plans prudently for the next hundred years. Enjoyment of the ordinary pleasure of contact with friends and co-workers eludes her grasp as she observes the world turn false and unreal juxtaposed to the vivid profundity of her inner life. Her private thoughts and dialogues become her most precious possessions, her secret refuge from the clamor and clutter of life outside her mind.

Entrapped in a pattern of retreat, Kate dreads her life becoming an endless winter of hibernation without the promise of spring. She resists rising out of bed in the morning, her back sore, her limbs stiff and chilly. Her libido and gusto for life and love fade. Moaning and groaning, she feels grouchy, muttering complaints about minor aches and pains. Kate engages in minute self-scrutiny of the way her body feels and functions. Fascination with the workings of her physical processes verges on a hypochondriacal concern with all manner of discomforts. She focuses a clinical gaze on all of her anomalies and eccentricities, noting a protruding vein or bone here, a mole or bump there.

Kate's intense inward focus builds upon itself, reinforcing the insular, self-protective cave within which she dwells. Her ideas and desires, unable to find expression, are like seeds that sprout in darkness but cannot grow without light. Kate is aware of her grim self-exile but is powerless to engage her will and overcome her paralysis of life-affirming impulses. Like a dark star, she sucks life energy into herself but does not radiate luminous warmth.

Yet in the depths of her despondency and loneliness, Kate harbors the potential spark for self-renewal. At the extreme of her inward regression and contraction, *Yin* turns to *Yang* as nighttime yields to dawn, and her stored reserve of vitality is enough to feed her recuperation, restore her strength, and rekindle her fervor for life. Kate is patient. Holding tenaciously to a durable sense of herself, she knows that the spirit within can be reanimated by harnessing her will and creativity. Time is her healer, permitting the well that has been drained to refill itself. Kate endures; she is a survivor.

How We Recognize Kate As a Water Type

Firmly rooted in herself, Kate is tough, self-possessed, and idiosyncratic to the point of unconventional. Like an underground spring, she has reserves of strength that can be tapped if you dig deeply enough.

If Kate's tenacity, prudence, introspection, and solitary independence become *exaggerated*, she hardens, appearing crusty and cynical, arthritic, cold, and deadened, as if fossilized. Once frozen, Kate cracks, like a sheet of ice. Her dissembling takes the form of fear, a constant premonition of extinction through a loss of substance and will. She becomes suspicious and stingy, worried that everyone wishes to appropriate her thoughts and feelings, her secrets and her warmth. Without a live connection with other people, her grasp upon a reality outside of herself becomes tenuous. And when her vitality is attenuated through prolonged isolation, the integral structure of Kate's identity collapses. Her native sense of self, of continuity and future, that "I was born, I exist, I will survive," melts into a terror of invasion and absorption, of drowning in a vast, undifferentiated sea. What was tough and hard becomes porous and fragile: faith, desire, and motivation collapse. She succumbs to her asocial tendencies and escapes into a self-   221 imposed Siberian tundra. What was defined and emergent in her becomes as inchoate and primitive as formless protoplasm. *Water* takes the form of the vessel that contains it—Kate cannot take shape without developing the expansive, actualizing aspects of her being. As a *Water* type, Kate has a propensity either to harden and compact herself into stone or to lose form, becoming undefined and amoebalike and, in a sense, anonymous.

As with all the types, Kate's strengths in *Water* need to be balanced by the connectedness of *Earth*, the warmth and expressiveness of *Fire*, the arousal to action of *Wood*, and the structure of *Metal*. Development of these aspects will enable Kate to enjoy the independence and creative gifts of her temperament.

THE EVOLUTION OF DISTORTED PATTERNS OF WATER

Domination by the *Kidney* particularly stirs conflict with the *Heart* and *Spleen*. The *Yin* nature of the *Kidney* is characterized by *Coldness* and *Moisture*. *Excess* of *Yin* dampens the *Fire* of the *Heart* and the digestive *Fire* of the *Stomach* and *Spleen*. The *Kidney* rules the lower body as the *Heart* and *Lung* rule the upper region. Kate's energy is concentrated in the lower back, legs, hips, and lower abdomen.

WATER: Kidney

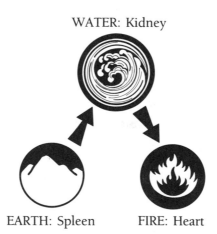

EARTH: Spleen   FIRE: Heart

The *Yin* of the *Kidney* manifests as *Moisture*, internal secretions, and other essential substances like bone marrow, cerebrospinal fluid, reproductive hormones, semen, and urine. A *Water* type tends to be large-headed and large-boned, well developed in the hips, pelvis, and legs. Her arms and upper torso may appear small and relatively underdeveloped by comparison, giving her a pear shape.

When *Water* suppresses *Fire*, a person becomes sensitive to cold and has difficulty both in making contact with people and maintaining a positive and optimistic attitude. It is difficult to light a fire when the wood is soggy from being drenched with rain. *Fire*'s expansive, comforting warmth is overcome by *Water*'s wetness and cold. Unbalanced by *Fire*, which reaches out, communicates, and generates warmth and excitement through commingling, Kate is at risk of being withdrawn, isolated, and insecure.

WATER: Kidney Patterns

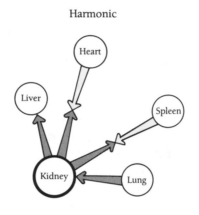

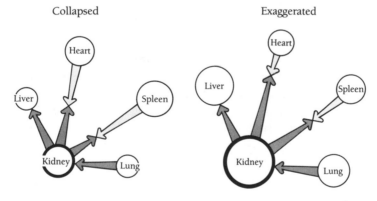

Harmonic and Dissonant Patterns

In the *harmonic Kidney* pattern, the *Lung* and *Liver* maintain stability while the *Heart* and *Spleen* provide the tension necessary for movement and adaptation. In the *exaggerated Kidney* pattern, the *Lung* and *Liver* become hyperactive and the *Heart* and *Spleen* become hypersensitive and erratic. In the *collapsed* pattern, the *Lung* and *Liver* become drained and weakened while the *Heart* and *Spleen* become overbearing and congested.

As a result of this overpowering of *Yang* by *Yin*, a progressive retardation of metabolism, activity, and expression occurs. Enlargement of the heart, due to an excessive volume of circulating fluids, and edema, an overflow of fluids, occurs as the *Yang* declines and the watery aspect of *Yin* grows. *Coldness* increases, causing the core energy of the body to become congealed and hardened, which can lead to the formation of tumors, nodules, and lumps, especially in the lower abdomen, reproductive organs, spinal cord, or brain. This may also take the form of hardening of the arteries, particularly in the brain, leading to early senility or stroke. Increased blood volume strains the heart and elevates blood pressure by forcing the heart to pump greater volumes of blood than it can easily handle. In Western medicine the strategy is to administer a diuretic to dispel water, easing the demands on the heart.

Outwardly, a *Water* type would appear impervious and fixed, like a statue sculpted out of moist clay. Inwardly, she is emotionally inaccessible, and because the warmth of the *Heart* is muted, she appears cold-hearted.

The effect of this upon the *Spleen* shows as flabby musculature, a pot belly, a tendency toward edema, loose bowel movements, and a lack of interest in food. When the *Lung* becomes drained by the *Kidney*, shallow breathing and dryness of the nose and throat may develop, along with emphysema and urinary retention. Because of the concentration of fluid in the hips and pelvis, strain on the lumbar region may result in chronic discomfort and instability of the lumbosacral spine and arthritis of the hips and knees. However, in spite of all their infirmities and immobility, people dominated by *Water* maintain a sharp, perceptive mind and intellectual inquisitiveness. Their struggle is to keep creative ability and mental acuity from being submerged by currents of cynicism, pessimism, or stoic resignation.

The therapeutic objectives for the *Water* type are to circulate *Moisture*, maintain warmth, and promote physical activity, social interaction, and emotional expression. Foods that are salty and astringent cause retention of fluids and should be carefully consumed. Bitter and spicy foods that promote excessive loss of heat and secretions can lead to dissipation of *Kidney Essence*. Regular exercise is essential to preserve muscle tone, blood circulation, and the even distribution of warmth and fluids. Strong social bonds keep the *Water* type involved and motivated to communicate her creative visions and put her knowledge into practice.

HOMER: BETWEEN A ROCK AND A HARD PLACE

Homer enters the clinic limping. Taking careful and deliberate steps, he approaches a chair and with a barely audible sigh eases himself down. He holds himself stiffly in place, reluctant to relax in case he needs to carry himself into the treatment room.

Homer says with a wry grin, "Doc, it's like I'm between a rock and a hard place. When I'm sitting down, I can't stand up, and when I'm standing, I can't sit down. I've been a welder for twenty-five years. When I was a young guy, I could scale bridges and skyscrapers in any kind of weather. Now as soon as there's a chill in the air, I get stiff and it's hard for me to shift around to do my work. I'm not outdoors anymore—I have my own shop where I do jobs and metal sculpture. Lately I can't hold my tools or maintain one position without an aching pain in my back, hands, and hips. I'm only fifty, with lots more metal to bend. I need some grease on these bones so they won't squeak so bad.

"I've tried aspirin, but it doesn't help much and bothers my stomach. At night I take a nip of whiskey to warm up, relax, and dull the pain enough for sleep. My spirits get low, and I start to lose hope—especially if I'm cold and numb. The whiskey helps free me up. I don't want to become an alcoholic, and that's why I'm here. I'm willing to try acupuncture and herbs if it gets me back to work. The pain I can live with; it's not having my hands that really gets to me."

I ask Homer whether anything else bothers him. Homer remarks that food tastes lousy, his appetite is poor, and he has been losing weight. Whiskey before dinner and bed stimulates his appetite, makes the food go down better, and minimizes the gas and belching after he eats.

TREATMENT

Acupuncture will increase Homer's circulation, improve his digestion, and alleviate the pain and stiffness in his joints. The needles are inserted into points that correspond to the *Kidney*, *Stomach*, *Spleen*, and *Pericardium*, located on the low back, ankle, knee, and wrist. The points in the low back correspond to the site of Homer's pain and stiffness. They will invigorate the *Kidney* and strengthen the spine and lumbar region.

Homer doesn't feel the needles go in, but he can feel a full, drawing sensation around them. After a few minutes he reports a warm current running down the back of his legs to his heels, a feeling neither familiar nor painful. He heaves a sigh, and his mouth wrinkles into a bemused grin.

Homer likes the warmth of my hand on his cold back. Since he needs to be warmed up, I wrap the handle of the needles with a tight ball of the herb called moxa. These wool-like leaves are ignited, penetrating the acupuncture site with a nourishing heat. Warmth is conducted through the needle into the deeper tissue. With mild surprise Homer comments, "I don't know if I'm imagining this, but my feet are warming up." Homer lies on the treatment table for twenty minutes before the needles are removed.

Expecting to feel his usual stiffness and pain, he rises cautiously—to find himself moving and bending more freely. He has responded well to treatment, and even if his symptoms slyly creep back over the next few days, 225 he will make steady progress, with relief lasting longer after each treatment.

To enhance his recovery, Homer soaks his feet in a hot ginger foot bath in the evening. This activates circulation of *Blood*, *Qi*, and *Moisture* in his lower back and legs, assisting the *Kidney* and supporting the *Heart*, relaxing his muscles and easing his sleep.

INTERPRETATION AND STRATEGY

For Homer, *Water* is overcoming *Fire* and invading *Earth*. His stiff joints and back are associated with the *Kidney*, his digestive disturbance with the *Spleen*, and his melancholy, poor circulation, and troubled sleep with the *Heart*. *Earth* should control *Water*, but because of the weakening of *Fire*, *Earth* is inadequately nourished and loses its ability to restrain *Water*. Homer loses his interest in food, which ultimately results in the depletion of *Qi* and *Kidney Essence*.

Steady and constant work, anxiety about his capacity to continue, and his willingness to endure the pain but not the limitations of his illness are attitudes associated with a *Water* type. Homer is pleased to be rooted in one place, chipping away at the same thing, year after year. Homer undertook a lifetime commitment, progressing from a skilled laborer to his own business. He had the imagination to transform his trade knowledge into a creative, aesthetic medium. His gratification stems from building structures out of iron and steel, things that last.

Homer can put aside physical discomfort in order to stick with the work at hand with a stoic acceptance. He takes responsibility for his woe, seeking help when his own solutions are not working. Even though Homer works with other people, within that environment he remains set apart, maintaining a realm in which he follows his own creative path. It is characteristic of the *Water* type to resolutely maintain a self-sufficient, inviolable sphere even when surrounded by others.

Homer is also a good illustration of what can happen to the expression of the creative impulse when the inner fire begins to collapse. The *Heart Network* is the vehicle through which we come to the fullest expression of our being. *Water* needs *Fire* to fulfill its ends. When *Yang* deteriorates, *Yin* hardens, unable to flow, and someone like Homer ossifies.

Homer's "rock" is his persevering determination, and the "hard place" is the physical rigidity and petrification of his body. In Homer's younger life he could work hard all day and night under any conditions. The result of this unrelenting use of his inner resources defeated him by undermining *Fire* and *Earth*. When Homer's excessive *Water* quenches *Fire* and overcomes *Earth*, his *exaggerated* tendencies *collapse*.

Homer's instinct to use whiskey to warm and activate his *Blood* resembles the use of alcohol infused in medicinal herbal wines to augment the warming and activating properties of herbs, especially for the treatment of arthritic conditions. Alcohol stimulates the *Heart* and dilates the blood vessels, temporarily improving circulation and relaxing the mind. Homer should avoid cold and raw foods because they have a chilling, dampening effect on the *Kidney*, *Spleen*, and *Heart*.

The strategy for Homer will be to strengthen and harmonize the areas of weakness that exist in *Water*, *Fire*, and *Earth*. The *Kidney* depends upon the *Spleen* and *Stomach* for replenishment of *Essence* and upon the *Heart* for the circulation of *Essence* and the "spreading of joy." An herbal formula disperses stagnation, strengthens the *Kidney*, and warms his body. This also helps to revive his appetite, improve his digestion, free his joints, and raise his spirits.

After three treatments Homer's pain and stiffness were ameliorated. He returned to his usual level of work with an increased tolerance for the cold environment of his shop. After three months of herbs and acupuncture with sustained improvement, Homer prepared a strong brew of ginseng root to warm and consolidate the *Qi* of his whole body, especially the *Kidney*. He gave up whiskey and for six months had no complaints. Then he experienced a return of stiffness in his hips and hands. Another dose of ginseng reversed this relapse, and a year later he remained free of pain.

Summary of Homer's Patterns		
Signs and Symptoms	**Interpretation**	**Interpretation**
	According to *Qi, Moisture, Blood*	According to *Organ Networks*
Stiff, sore joints and back	Stagnation of *Qi, Moisture, Blood*	Weakness of *Kidney, Heart,* and *Spleen*
Poor appetite Weight loss Coldness	Depletion of *Qi, Blood,* and *Vital Heat*	Disharmony of *Kidney-Spleen* and weakness of *Kidney*
Poor sleep Melancholy	Depletion of *Blood* and *Vital Heat*	Disharmony of *Kidney-Heart* and weakness of *Kidney*

Prescriptions for Therapy

Harmonize *Kidney-Spleen*
Disperse *Qi*
Disperse *Moisture*
Disperse *Blood*
Warm interior

Harmonize *Kidney-Heart*
Tonify *Qi*
Tonify *Blood*
Warm interior

WATER		
PHILOSOPHER		*KIDNEY*
Mental Faculties	**Biological Functions**	**Organs—Tissues—Fluid**
Imagination	Consolidation	*Kidney* and *Bladder*
Perception	Retention	Brain and bones
Retention	Germination	Spinal cord and fluid
Reflection	Regeneration	Ovaries and testes
		Sexual secretions
		Urethra, anus, inner ear, head-pubic hair

WATER

Exaggerated patterns arise from:	Collapsed patterns arise from:	Aggravations occur with:
Congestion of *Moisture* and *Blood*	Depletion of *Moisture, Blood, Essence*	Winter and summer
Accumulation of *Heat* and *Cold*	Congestion of *Moisture* and *Blood*	*Cold, Dampness,* dryness
Disharmony of *Kidney-Heart*	Accumulation of *Cold*	Cold, sweet, raw, salty foods and beverages
Kidney-Spleen	Weakness of *Spleen, Lung, Kidney*	3 P.M.–7 P.M. and 3 A.M.–7 A.M.

Characteristic Features of Psyche

Undistorted	Exaggerated	Collapsed	Difficulty With
Candid	Blunt	Sarcastic	Sociability
Introspective	Withdrawn	Catatonic	Introversion
Modest	Reticent	Anonymous	Conformity
Watchful	Penetrating	Voyeuristic	Generosity
Objective	Detached	Cut off	Hypochondria
Curious	Scrutinizing	Critical	Isolation
Ingenious	Eccentric	Fanciful	Communication
Careful	Suspicious	Phobic	Exposure
Particular	Demanding	Fussy	Trust
Thrifty	Covetous	Miserly	Confidence
Sensible	Cynical	Pessimistic	
Lucid	Preoccupied	Absentminded	

Characteristic Features of Soma			
Undistorted	**Exaggerated**	**Collápsed**	**Difficulty With**
Strong, dense, lean physique	Hypersensitive vision-hearing	Dulled vision-hearing	Memory and alertness
Long, large bones	Headaches above eyes and vertex	Ringing in ears	Disturbances of sensory and motor function
Sculptured face	Lack of sweat and urine	Weak and stiff spine, lower body, joints	Distorted shape of bones/ joints/teeth
Long, narrow head and face	Hardening of blood vessels and cartilage	Degeneration of disks-cartilage	Disturbed growth and reproduction
Deep-set eyes	Rigidity of joints-muscles	Cold buttocks, legs, feet	Inefficient excretion or conservation of fluids
Narrow shoulders, wider hips	kidney and bladder stones	Frequent urination	Cysts, swellings, sclerosis of reproductive and urinary organs
Long fingers and toes	Bony tumors	Osteoporosis	Disrupted cycles of sleeping and waking
	Precocious sexuality	Prematurely gray, thin hair, wrinkled skin	
	Weak digestion	Infertility, frigidity, impotence	
	Shrinking gums	Lacks stamina	
	Needs little sleep	Hard to wake up	
	Atonic constipation	Loss of appetite	
	Dark or bronze complexion	Weak abdominal muscles	
	Hypertension	Dark, pasty skin	

So, You Think You're a Water Type

Keys To Understanding Water

- articulate, clever, and introspective
- self-contained and self-sufficient
- penetrating, critical, and scrutinizing
- seeks knowledge and understanding
- likes to remain hidden, enigmatic, and anonymous

Typical Problems

- emotionally inaccessible and undemonstrative
- isolation and loneliness
- tactless, unforgiving, and suspicious
- hardening of the arteries, deterioration of teeth and gums, backache, chilliness, loss of libido

Critical Times

- *exaggerated Water—Kidney* congestion: winter and summer, 3 P.M.– 7 P.M. and 11 A.M.–3 P.M.
- *collapsed Water—Kidney* depletion: spring and late summer, 3 A.M.– 7 A.M. and 7 A.M.–11 A.M.

A Friendly Reminder

The power of *Water* comes from the capacity to conceive, concentrate, and conserve. *Water* types need to offset their toughness, bluntness, and detachment with tenderness, sensitivity, and openness, risking softness and contact, exposure and attachment.

III

THERAPY

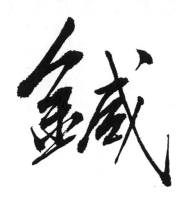

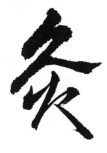

Acupuncture and Moxibustion

CHAPTER THIRTEEN

ACUPUNCTURE: A UNIFIED FIELD OF INVISIBLE CHANNELS

Beginnings and Endings (for Efrem)

The Acupuncturist
Told me how Chinese medicine
Connects the Grief emotion
To the intestines
As he treated me
For a painful
Somewhat mysterious malady

Beginnings and Endings
Separations
How to say good-bye
Holding the sadness in,
Or as he said once before
Some Deep Holding
Holding in the grieving
For a long time—yes said I
At least 21 years
Since my mother's death
And also Elsa, and he said
The recent separation
Yes I agreed, and he said

Beginnings and Endings
That's really all he needed
To say that day
Because with his treatment
I cried and cried
My body shaking, quaking,
Tears filling up my ears
The needles sticking out all over me

Today was a healing feeling experience
Some part of what is trapped inside
Could no longer be repressed, denied,
Had to be expressed, so may
My future life be blessed
With an ability to calmly flow
To let it go—to tell it on the mountain
To tell my story
In all of its intricate
Weavings and blendings
Beginnings and Endings

Lincoln Bergman

WHEN I RETURNED TO MY FAMILY AFTER ACQUIRING ACUPUNCTURE skills, it appeared as wizardry that a few needles placed strategically could perform instant wonder. I was able to help my aunt open jars that had remained sealed to her arthritically crippled grasp and aid a sculptor strengthen his limp arm so that he could again carve wood. My father had been unable to help either of them. I felt as if I had found a secret key to knowledge buried within the folds of a foreign culture. To my father's Western mind, it is suspiciously curious that a throbbing between the temples vanishes when a needle is inserted in the foot, or that melancholy lifts after stimulating a point above the wrist, or that an improperly positioned fetus turns itself around after burning herbs on the little toe. Seeing the body as permeated by streams of vital force makes these events more comprehensible, even reasonable.

GATES OPEN INTO A MATRIX OF CHANNELS

Organ Networks communicate with each other via an invisible web of channels transporting *Qi* and *Blood*. The *Qi* courses through the body in perpetual motion similar to water in a riverbed. Like the matrix of waterways that cover the surface of the earth, these channels empty into one another, intersect, and have underground as well as surface streams, connecting the interior with the exterior of the body.

Acupuncture points are located in small depressions in the skin called "men" or "gates." Access can be gained to the internal circulation of *Qi* and *Blood* through acupuncture points. In ancient times, when Chinese cities were fortified by walls, gates were opened to receive sustenance and closed to keep harm away. Acupuncture points are gateways, subtle portals of the body that are opened and closed to adjust its dynamic.

Thin, solid, sterile stainless-steel needles enter the channels, activating or inhibiting the flow of *Qi* and *Blood*. Fourteen major pathways traverse the body from the top of the head to the tips of the fingers and toes. Many principal acupuncture points are located below the elbow and knee—where the *Qi* changes its polarity from *Yin* to *Yang* and gathers force as it moves from the extremities toward the core. Stimulation of these points exerts profound influence upon the equilibrium of the organism as a whole.

Depending on our assumptions about how the body works, different possibilities arise for solutions to its problems. While doing clinical study in Shanghai, Efrem treated a three-year-old boy who, since the age of eight weeks, was retarded because of meningitis. Western medicine was able to save his life but could not help him to speak, walk, feed himself, or dispel his dull and passive demeanor. After ten weeks of acupuncture, the boy was vocalizing, standing, eating by himself, and interacting with animation and cheer. He began to walk, and his manual dexterity improved, enabling him to explore and manipulate his environment. In this short period he went through a metamorphosis from a listless infant to a bright and responsive child. In Chinese terms, the illness had shut down the capacity of his *Kidney* to sustain his growth and development, severing the cohesion of *Spirit* and *Essence*. By supplementing *Kidney Qi* and activating all the channels with acupuncture, psyche and soma were reunited, and his family felt that their child had come home to them.

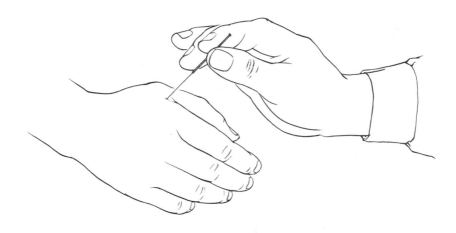

Acupuncture Needle Insertion

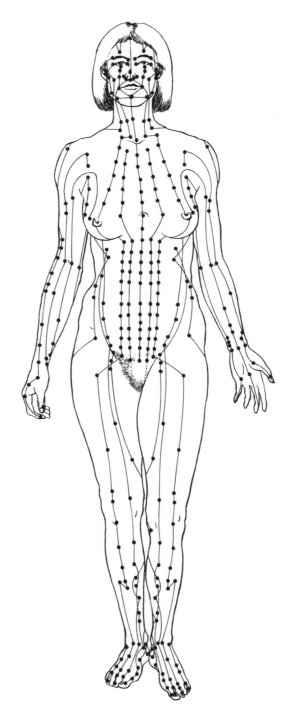

Acupuncture Points upon Channels of *Qi*

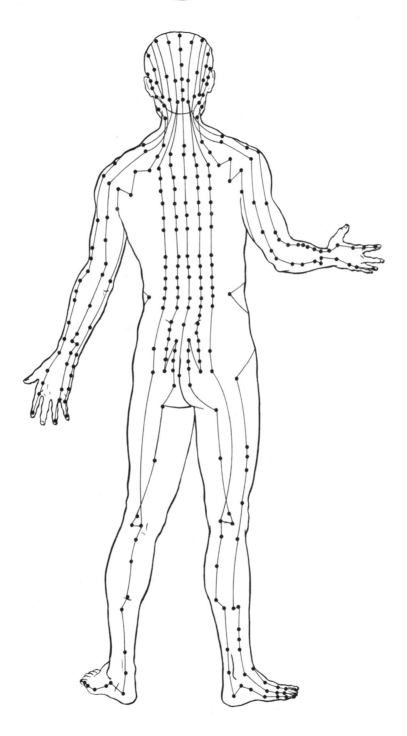

Acupuncture Points upon Channels of *Qi* 239

CORRESPONDENCE THEORY AND REORGANIZING PATTERNS OF ILLNESS

Legends abound about the origins of acupuncture. One story is that acupuncture was discovered by observing that soldiers wounded by arrows and spears recovered from ailments in other parts of their bodies. Trial and error over many centuries evolved into a refined and detailed clinical methodology based on this system of correspondences. Another tale holds that semidivine sages mapped the pathways of *Qi* and chronicled the effects of ingesting herbs. What was invisible to the ordinary eye was visible to their enlightened perception.

By eliminating congestion and activating circulation of *Qi*, acupuncture interrupts and disorganizes patterns of illness. For example, a throbbing, hot, full feeling in the head accompanied by coldness in the hands and feet suggests an *excess* of *Qi* in the head and a *deficiency* in the extremities. By stimulating points on the hands and feet, congested *Qi* and *Blood* are dislodged from the head and redistributed throughout the body. The headache retreats, and a comfortable sense of warmth and connectedness pervades the body.

Acupuncture is most effective when functional disturbances have not yet developed into organic or structural impairments. Migraine headaches are more responsive to treatment than pain due to a brain tumor. However, even in degenerative disorders like the joint deformities of arthritis or the chronic inflammation of nerves and muscles, frequent long-term treatment can bring about relief of pain and sometimes impressive recovery of function.

HOW DOES ACUPUNCTURE WORK, ANYWAY?

The metaphor of the mechanic and the gardener helps us to differentiate between Western and Chinese explanations of the phenomenon of acupuncture. Conventional Western wisdom perceives acupuncture as limited to the amelioration of pain. For example, neurophysiological experiments have demonstrated that acupuncture modifies the transmission of neural impulses between the spinal cord and the brain, forming the basis of what is known as the "gate control" theory. This theory postulates that the action of pain fibers in the spinal cord is blocked by acupuncture. Acupuncture is also known to stimulate the release of endogenous morphinelike substances called endorphins, brain hormones produced by the body as a response to stress. Their release during the exertion of running or swimming accounts for what is referred to as "jogger's or swimmer's high." Endorphins induce a euphoric sense of well-being, serving as an adaptive and regenerative resource for coping with pain, one form stress takes.

While neurological and hormonal hypotheses describe how acupuncture alleviates pain, they do not adequately explain its diverse therapeutic effects. Other experiments, including the study of acupuncture-assisted surgery, have shown that acupuncture not only inhibits pain, but also directly affects peripheral microcirculation, rhythm and stroke volume of the heart, blood pressure, levels of circulating immunoglobulins, gastrointestinal peristalsis, secretion of hydrochloric acid, and the production of red and white blood cells. Acupuncture seems to adjust all the physiological processes of the organism, possibly through activation of the homeostatic function of the autonomic nervous system. Recent clinical research using acupuncture in the treatment of alcohol, tobacco, drug, and food addiction suggests that stimulating points along the vagal branch of the autonomic nervous system in the external ear decreases cravings and withdrawal reactions. These clinical and experimental findings reflect the state of our understanding from the perspective of Western medical science.

The central issue from the classical Chinese medical point of view is not why acupuncture works, but rather how and when to use it. The dynamic balance that Chinese medicine equates with health manifests as smooth and constant movement. When *Qi* and *Blood* stagnate, the processes of elimination and regeneration deteriorate, constituting the basic condition underlying many forms of illness.

Pain is also considered to be the result of congested *Qi*, *Blood*, or *Moisture*. If poor circulation persists, tissues (muscle, tendons, nerves, blood vessels, internal organs) become swollen, fibrous, and hardened, which further impedes adequate circulation, undermining the functional capacity of the organism. Because pain is associated with observable phenomena like swellings, nodules, and tumors, pain that exists without observable cause is assumed to be the product of hidden or invisible stagnation. This echoes the circular logic of correspondence thinking. Acupuncture is a process of stirring up the *Qi* so that stasis is overcome, thereby restoring circulation, reducing swelling, alleviating pain, and promoting healing.

THE MECHANIC AND GARDENER REVISITED

The mechanistic approach of Western science supposes that acupuncture works by jamming pain signals in a complex neurological circuit much like computer engineers reprogram sophisticated information systems. The body becomes an electronic and biochemical network of transmitting and receiving stations with messages flowing back and forth along specific single-function pathways. So we have a picture of acupuncture blocking and unblocking valves, opening and closing switches, latching and unlatching gates. Because of such a narrow focus, the possibility of multiple and simultaneous interactions is overlooked.

Within the Chinese medical zeitgeist the acupuncturist is a practical ecologist who never loses sight of the whole while attending to any of the parts. Since this model assumes the synchronicity of response throughout the organism, it's reasonable that stimulation of a local site will have global impact and that stimulation of an array of sites can have specific outcomes. Treating the surface of the extremities with needles affects the deep organs of the chest and abdomen, and at the same time, points of the abdomen will affect the head, arms, and legs. It is not acceptable in Chinese medicine for pain to be erased while the patient's emotional state declines, for the mobility of the knee to improve while the digestion and circulation deteriorate.

Acupuncture is not like a drug that is supposed to produce a discrete and limited result. In Western medicine a given drug or procedure results in a limited, desired effect, plus so-called side effects, which are adverse changes in the organism as a whole. In Chinese medicine, this logic is reversed, so that global changes in the whole organism result in the disappearance of specific symptoms. In acupuncture "secondary" effects are intended, all part of one continuous process of change.

Conceptualizing acupuncture as limited to the treatment of pain, or as a disease-specific therapy, contradicts the very heart of Chinese medicine, which takes multifarious effects for granted. The acupuncturist operates much like a shepherd herding goats into a corral or a farmer diverting river water into terraced fields in an attempt to orchestrate a fortuitous convergence of natural forces.

BIOELECTRIC OSCILLATING FIELDS

Some Western scientists and doctors have become interested in acupuncture; they provide a nexus where ancient theories of Qi and modern theories of biology and physics converge. Several biological theorists assert that electromagnetic fields organize and shape living organisms but are so subtle they are imperceptible. They suggest that the flux of these fields determines health and growth. Robert Becker, M.D., a researcher in electrophysiology, has demonstrated that certain electrical fields and currents are essential for tissue regeneration, and he has used microcurrent to heal nonunion bone fractures. In *The Body Electric*, Becker comments:

> Although neuro-physiologists had studied pain . . . for decades, there was still no coherent theory of it. . . . The prevailing view in the West was that if acupuncture worked at all, it acted through the placebo effect. . . . I proposed a more elegant hypothesis. The acu-

puncture meridians, I suggested, were electrical conductors that carried an injury message to the brain. . . . For currents measured in nanoamperes and microvolts, the amplifiers would have to be . . . a few inches apart—just like the acupuncture points! . . . like dark stars sending their electricity along the meridians, an interior galaxy that the Chinese had somehow found and explored. . . . If the integrity of health really was maintained by a balanced circulation of invisible energy through this constellation . . . then various patterns of needle placement might indeed bring the currents into harmony. . . . Our readings indicated that the meridians were conducting current. . . . Each point . . . had [an electrical] field surrounding it, with its own characteristic shape. It was obvious . . . that at least the major parts of the acupuncture charts had, as the jargon goes, "an objective basis in reality."

The contemporary practice of acupuncture has begun to synthesize classical with modern concepts and methods. Acupuncture can now be conceptualized as a bioelectric information-modulating system. In ancient China the metaphors for the body reflected the development of irrigation systems and waterways for commerce that were unifying society during the Han dynasty. Today the overarching concern of societies is the use and acquisition of energy resources. Society used to be powered by water; now it is fueled by electricity. In ancient times fields grew golden grain; in the modern world fields have become the playground in which electromagnetic pulses oscillate. The ancient metaphor of currents of *Wind* and *Water* now coexists with metaphors of currents of information in worldwide photoelectronic systems and networks. As in ancient times, the body continues to be perceived as a miniature projection of its social context, with microprocessing systems and electromagnetic fields and conductors. These metaphors are complementary—the universe of *Qi*, "the web that has no weaver," and the fields and forces of the quantum physicist are only a half step apart.

ACUPUNCTURE TREATMENT: WHAT TO EXPECT

AN UNUSUAL INTERVIEW

The practitioner makes a diagnostic assessment that takes into account the patient's present and past symptoms and complaints (medical history), inherited constitution (family history), environment (social and natural), life-style (work and habits), and psychology (thoughts, emotions, and relationships) and involves observation of facial and tongue color and physical palpation of the body and pulse.

243

HOW THE NEEDLES FEEL

Needles penetrate anywhere from a fraction of an inch to several inches, depending on the thickness of flesh and muscle at a given location. Since the needles are extremely fine, minimal pain accompanies insertion. Sensations such as tingling, heaviness, soreness, and pressure are not only common but desirable because this indicates that the *Qi* is present and being summoned. Sensations may occur around the acupuncture point as well as along the channel of which it is a part. Sometimes people feel the *Qi* moving in areas far from the point of insertion.

Response to treatment is highly individual. A drifting, dreamy sense of well-being and relaxation is usual, as is an elevation of spirits. The needle itself goes unnoticed or feels like a small pinch followed by a sensation of numbness, ache, traveling warmth, tingling, or heaviness around the area. Following acupuncture it is as normal to experience the desire to continue resting as it is to feel immediately animated, though sometimes this sense of invigoration is delayed until the days following treatment. Most people are relieved to find that treatments are not especially uncomfortable and, in fact, look forward to the experience.

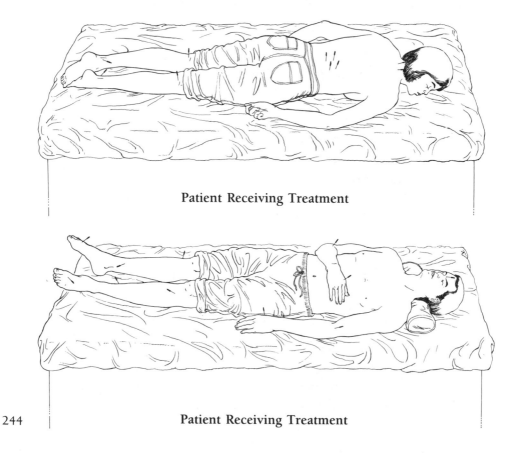

Patient Receiving Treatment

Patient Receiving Treatment

HOW ACUPUNCTURE POINTS ARE CHOSEN—PRINCIPLES OF TREATMENT

An acupuncturist considers many factors in selecting appropriate points for treatment. Some of these include

1. the channel nearest the site of the problem
2. points known to benefit particular conditions
3. points that affect specific *Organ Network* function
4. points that harmonize the *Five Phases*

The first guiding principle is the topographical relationship between the channels and the site of the symptoms. According to this, it would make sense to treat nasal congestion using a local point outside the nostril, *Large Intestine 20* (called *Welcome Fragrance*), assisted by *Large Intestine 4* (known as the upper *Gate of Qi*), a distal point located between the index finger and the thumb. This latter point is chosen for assistance because it exerts a strong influence upon the upper body, especially the face and neck, and because it governs movement upward from the chest and downward to the abdomen. Because of this, it is used for dental pain, thyroid surgery, sinus headaches, and coughs as well as for constipation and facilitating childbirth.

This leads to the second principle, which relies on the effectiveness of classic sites for treating certain problems. Several examples: heating *Bladder 67* on the little toe can correct malposition of the fetus; bleeding *Lung 11* along the thumbnail can relieve swelling of the throat; needling *Pericardium 6* above the wrist can alleviate angina pectoris; and needling *Small Intestine 3* on the side of the hand can relieve acute spasm of the neck.

Another principle is the selection of points based on their power to promote unique functions of the *Organ Networks*. For example, since the *Spleen* transforms *Moisture*, and edema and phlegm appear when this function is depressed. *Stomach 40* and *Spleen 9* have the property of invigorating the *Spleen* and dispelling *Dampness*. Since the *Liver* stores and nurtures the *Blood*, when this function is impaired, anemia and apathy develop. Needling *Liver 3* harmonizes the *Liver*, enabling it to revitalize the *Blood* and arouse the mind. Selecting points according to the dynamics of *Qi*, *Blood*, and *Moisture* is called treating the "root," and selection based upon symptoms is called treating the "branch."

The last principle dealt with here, though many more exist in theory and practice, concerns *Five-Phase* correspondence thinking. The lattice of channels and streams that organize and govern the processes of the human organism act as a semipermeable membrane, a filter and interface between the organism and its environment. Five points on each channel corresponding to each of the *Five Phases* are the links and passages in this web, connecting interior rhythms of *Qi* with macrocosmic cycles of activity. These powerful nodal points of change, located below the elbow and knee, can   245 affect all conditions solely on the basis of *Five-Phase* interrelationships. Allergies or depression that occur in the spring and fall are a manifestation of a transitional conflict between the *Liver* and *Lung* within the body and the *Phases* of *Wood* and *Metal* in nature. Using the points that correspond to *Wood* and *Metal* on the *Liver* and *Lung* channels serves to harmonize the interaction of these two *Organ Networks* and to place the organism in sync with the seasonal cycle. The body as hologram embodies the whole within each part—embedded within each *Organ* channel are points of resonance akin to each of the five *Organ Networks*. Each channel has a point of *Wood, Fire, Earth, Metal,* and *Water*.

Within this framework, symptoms and signs of illness are used to reveal the fundamental conflicts between the *Organ Networks* using the language of the *Five Phases*—these are the basic relationships from which symptoms emerge. For example, a restless, frightened, confused, exhausted person, unable to sleep and experiencing sharp pains in the chest and back, feels on the verge of mental and physical collapse. This array represents the breakdown between *Water* and *Fire,* between the *Kidney* and the *Heart*. The crucial objective is to reestablish a viable relationship between the *Kidney* and *Heart* by using points that harmonize *Water* and *Fire*. With this kind of treatment, process is reorganized, which brings about the relief of symptoms as a byproduct.

How Long Will It Take?

Duration and frequency of treatment vary since each person is a unique riddle to be solved. Some need only a few sessions, while others need the accumulated benefit of weeks or months of attention. This depends on factors such as the severity of the complaint, how long the person has had it, and the extent to which living patterns exacerbate the condition. A session lasts about an hour and is scheduled as often as every day or as little as twice a month. As symptoms improve, fewer visits are required, individual progress being the yardstick.

Angus had fallen off a roof and suffered contusions that left him unable to walk without severe pain. He was told he would have chronic arthritis for the rest of his life and would never be able to return to his occupation as a roofer. After the third visit he experienced whole days without pain for the first time in six months. By the fifth visit he was able to walk normally without discomfort, and within a few weeks he returned to work at his trade. Shirley had uterine fibroids that were growing monthly. She wanted to avoid surgery until she reached menopause, at which time the fibroids might shrink on their own. After eight months of weekly treatment her fibroids diminished markedly, and her periods became regular with a cessation of heavy bleeding, debilitating pain, and weakness.

Generally, after six to twelve sessions there will be some subjective response to treatment: recovery from the main complaint or a more generalized sense of improvement, including increased alertness and tranquillity, more restful sleep, or better circulation. These positive signs suggest improvement, offering promise that the specific symptom may be alleviated with continued treatment. For chronic problems the process is often extended, and progress may be recognized more by hindsight, when people look back and remember how they felt before treatment.

Changes that can be recognized by the doctor include improvement of the pulse and appearance of the tongue, vitality and tone of the skin and muscles, clarity and brightness of the eyes, lucidity of thinking and expression, evenness of temperament, and buoyancy of spirit. Often the pulse will respond quite favorably immediately following a treatment, even though the patient does not note a change. Conversely, symptoms may improve dramatically without comparably significant alterations in the pulse.

In China today, where health care is inexpensive and readily accessible, acupuncture is usually administered in a series of ten to twenty treatments and as often as twice a day in serious or acute conditions. The potential of acupuncture is maximized by frequency, continuity, and perseverance. Serious, chronic illness requires persistent and long-term treatment in order to achieve results. Many factors influence the outcome of treatment. Based on animal research it appears that the placebo effect or suggestibility is not the determining factor. In other words, acupuncture works in spite of the patient's expectations or beliefs.

Simple ailments such as the common cold, tension headaches, strains, and sprains, when treated in their early stages, can be resolved in one to five treatments. Rheumatoid arthritis, cystic ovaries, or asthma may require treatment over six months to two years. There are miraculous cures of apparently intractable problems and times when recovery is beyond the scope of acupuncture in spite of dedication, persistence, and faith. Acupuncture can also be helpful for people who can't be cured but whose pain can be ameliorated in an advanced terminal disease or whose immunity, appetite, digestion, sleep, and energy can be improved.

Acupuncture is a subtle and potent technique for initiating change that may engender strong reactions as well as gradual transformations. There is often a struggle between the need for change and the desire to maintain that which is stable and familiar. Everyone wishes for cure without change, for recovery without effort.

Aggravations that occur during the process of treatment are referred to as "healing crises" if, after their resolution, a person feels better than before. The doctor and the patient need to work together to intelligently evaluate the effects of treatment and mutually determine its course.

Both response and responsibility involve the capacity to react and interact. It is the patient's responsibility to respond as fully and freely as possible.   247

It is the doctor's responsibility to interpret progress and guide the patient, being responsive to his or her desires, expectations, needs, and limitations. It is the doctor's responsibility to both teach and learn from the patient and the obligation of the patient to explore the new perspectives and suggestions offered by the doctor.

ACUPUNCTURE IN A SHANGHAI CLINIC

When Efrem was an intern in Shanghai at the Shu Guan Hospital Acupuncture Clinic, he was particularly excited by the enthusiasm generated by many doctors and patients working together. Rather than patients being isolated in private rooms, ten people at once were treated communally in a room crowded with tables and chairs. The atmosphere was neither frenetic nor chaotic, but friendly, vocal, and intimate. Some people had traveled long distances to be seen at this clinic renowned for resolving difficult cases. It felt thrilling to be in an environment in which helping was what everyone was doing. Patients were helping each other by sharing both their individual stories and their common intention to make the most of this opportunity for treatment. Doctors were supporting each other with continual exchanges of advice and assistance. There was no competition between doctors, no motive for personal profit or gain, and among patients there was no expectation of privilege or ownership of a doctor's time or attention. This atmosphere, charged with a spirit of mutual support and intense commitment, seemed to accelerate recovery time. People who had languished for years under other medical regimens changed dramatically in a matter of weeks.

Acupuncture practiced in this way seemed to incorporate several principles that maximized its benefits. These were to focus the treatment on the patient's concerns, to make treatment as frequent as necessary, to keep it affordable, and to tailor it to a person's physical and emotional capacity. The future of acupuncture in North America will in part depend on access to hospital settings, outpatient clinics, and the economic support of private and public insurers.

WHAT ACUPUNCTURE CAN TREAT

Acupuncture can treat disorders of *Qi*, *Blood*, and *Moisture* and problems of *Organ Networks* and their associated channels—but this obviously does not correspond to the Western vocabulary of named diseases and conditions. Acupuncture may be helpful for withdrawal from addictions such as sugar, coffee, cigarettes, cocaine, and alcohol; stress reduction; postsurgical recovery; signs of aging; and decreased immunity. The World Health Organization of the United Nations has listed conditions for which it considers acupuncture appropriate:

Infections
  colds and flu
  bronchitis
  hepatitis

Musculoskeletal
and Neurologic
  arthritis
  neuralgia
  sciatica
  back pain
  bursitis
  tendonitis
  stiff neck
  Bell's palsy
  trigeminal neuralgia
  headache
  stroke
  cerebral palsy
  polio
  sprains

Internal
  asthma
  high blood pressure
  ulcers
  colitis
  indigestion
  hemmorrhoids
  diarrhea
  constipation
  diabetes
  hypoglycemia

Mental-Emotional
  anxiety
  depression
  stress
  insomnia

Dermatologic
  eczema
  acne
  herpes

Eyes-Ears-Nose-Throat
  deafness
  ringing in the ears
  earaches
  poor eyesight
  dizziness
  sinus infection
  sore throat
  hay fever

Genitourinary and Reproductive
  impotence
  infertility
  premenstrual syndrome (PMS)
  pelvic inflammatory disease (PID)
  vaginitis
  irregular period or cramps
  morning sickness

"My arthritis had it so I couldn't use my fingers much. After my first treatment, I could open a jar again. I hadn't done that in a long time."
                                        Jeanne Forsmith, age 74

"It wasn't really cramps that bothered me, but two weeks before my period I would get bloated, stop sleeping well, feel irritable, depressed, angry, and my breasts would swell up and hurt. If I stood too long, my lower legs would ache,

and I got real tired no matter how much I slept. The worst thing was the ex-haustion and being a grouch with my family. All those things got better real gradually with acupuncture. I had to take herbs, too. It's been almost two years, and I still go for treatment once a month before my period."

Cynthia Fields, age 38

"My rash was red and itchy all over both legs. In the night I'd scratch and have scabs by morning. I tried regular doctors and homeopathy for two years. I tried everything. After my first acupuncture treatment it started getting better. After six visits it was pretty much clear. Then I tried to quit smoking. It's been a year and a half since my last treatment and the rash hasn't come back, and I haven't smoked, either."

Helena Muscal, age 22

"I have osteoporosis and kidney problems. I slipped and fell and was in a brace from my neck to my tailbone in constant pain from compression fractures in my upper back. The pain didn't stop for ten months, keeping me awake nights. I began acupuncture, and the pain began to ease up. The first thing to happen was that I started sleeping at night. Within two months the pain went away. After four months I shed my brace. I had more energy. For the many months before treatment I never went through a day without pain—now I go for days, and I can take care of myself and function."

Tom Bylar, age 44

"I broke my ankle so badly, I needed one steel plate and four pins. The stiffness and throbbing was awful. I noticed enough improvement to discontinue after five acupuncture sessions. My range of motion increased, and the stiffness decreased. The most remarkable thing was how the muscle spasm and pain diminished and stayed gone after treatments. I know it hastened my recovery period since I could stretch and use my ankle more."

Joanna Rinaldi, age 37

"For months my blood pressure was so high that I was dizzy all the time and couldn't stand up. I was frightened because it was barely under control with medication. Within forty-eight hours after one of my acupuncture treatments the pressure dropped so low that my doctor had to take me off medication. It re-mained normal, and I can walk around now without feeling dizzy."

Esther Zipin, age 88

"For three years I had no energy, no stamina. I had been diagnosed as having both the AIDS and Epstein-Barr viruses. I also had yeast throughout my digestive tract, which made it difficult for me to eat. With physical effort like walking, I got short of breath and felt pain in my chest. In the beginning, acupuncture made

me feel spaced out and tired. After about two months I felt more energetic, my digestion improved, and I stopped having shortness of breath. After eight months of treatment twice a week combined with taking herbal tonics daily, I regained my strength and felt as if I could return to work and a normal life-style. It's been six months since my last treatment, but I won't hesitate to get more acupuncture if I start feeling sick again."

Frank Bell, age 31

"I was on a seesaw of antidepressant and antianxiety drugs for years until I began to use acupuncture to stabilize my dosage levels. It occurred to me that maybe I could use acupuncture to get off drugs altogether. I got three treatments a week for five months, and I'm now free of two very addictive medicines, both of which were prescribed by psychiatrists. I'm relieved to feel back in control of my life again."

Stephanie Mills, age 35

"I had been diagnosed as having chronic prostatitis and urethritis, which anti-biotics hadn't helped long-term. After ten acupuncture treatments my difficult urination and painful ejaculations disappeared."

Emilio Perez, age 51

"Since my childhood I'd been dependent on inhalers and antiasthma medicines. Along with acupuncture treatments for six months, I eliminated spicy and cold foods from my diet. Now I can play basketball without needing bronchodilators, and I only take medicine occasionally if I get a bad case of hay fever."

Robbie Johnson, age 33

"My doctors said I would recover on my own, but after a year I hadn't improved. I had facial paralysis and numbness from Bell's palsy, and I couldn't close my eye at night. After six treatments I was able to sleep with both eyes closed, and after nine treatments my mouth stopped drooping and the numbness was gone."

Sylvia Black, age 47

METHODS OF TREATMENT

Methods of manipulating the needle affect treatment, depending on whether the objective is to consolidate or disperse the *Qi*, to accelerate or retard it. Other methods stimulate acupuncture points without the insertion of needles. One technique, called moxibustion, uses the focused heat generated by burning "moxa," the compressed dried leaves of Chinese mugwort. This has a potent invigorating effect on the body and is particularly suitable for conditions of extreme *deficiency* or *Cold*. Moxibustion is a method of augmenting *Qi*, exploited in emergencies to prevent escape of the life force, reviving   251 consciousness and averting *collapse*. Points can also be activated by acupressure and *tui na* ("twee nah"), a traditional system of massage, mobilizing *Qi* and promoting blood circulation by manual contact with skin, muscle, nerve, and bone. This method is often used to treat infants, children, and the elderly, who may be too sensitive to tolerate acupuncture. Cupping, which employs vacuum suction with glass globes or bamboo jars, is a technique that quickens the *Blood*, dispersing *Wind*, *Heat*, and *Dampness*. Muscle injury, acute bronchial congestion, joint pain, and headache may be helped with this method.

CONTEMPORARY TECHNIQUES

Modern technology has made possible the use of electrical stimulation without acupuncture needles. Muscle training, facial toning, and the control of intractable pain are some of the uses of this noninvasive microeletric stimulation. Electroacupuncture devices help improve athletic performance and the recovery time following injuries. Microcurrent is being used to heal muscle and nerve impairments associated with neurosurgery, spinal cord injury, stroke, and palsy and to speed recuperation from surgery by reducing swelling and inflammation. These instruments can also revive facial tone, shape, texture, and color, counteracting the effects of aging by improving the metabolism of muscle and skin.

A variety of approaches to acupuncture therapy were developed on different continents. Differences in technique among Asia, Europe, and North America do not suggest one approach is superior to another. Some acupuncturists use deeper insertion and stronger manipulation, others employ more needles with shallow insertion and minimal manipulation. Some techniques are more traditional and others more modern. There is both dialogue and experimentation amongst practitioners in pursuit of relevant models and methods for Westerners.

ACUPUNCTURE FIRST AID: ACUPRESSURE MASSAGE

The stimulation of acupuncture points by applying pressure with the fingertips can sometimes be effective for relieving acute symptoms. The guideline is to apply enough pressure to get results without causing unnecessary discomfort.

Subjective feedback is useful in locating the acupuncture point and in finding the proper level of stimulation. Since the most reactive points are tender or sensitive when pressed, this can help to determine their location. Massage of these points should feel strong but not intolerably painful. If it hurts, it should "hurt good." If some soreness cannot be felt, the pressure is probably not strong enough.

Generally, use a finger that does not have a long nail, or the knuckle of the index finger, and press firmly while rotating in a tight circle. Where there is very little flesh, such as on the fingers or toes, it is acceptable to use the edge of a fingernail. Duration of the massage is determined by the tolerance of the subject or the diminution of symptoms. Stimulation of a single point can last thirty seconds, five minutes, or be continued for twenty minutes in one-minute sequences with rests in between. Points may be massaged sequentially in the order listed.

FIFTY ACUPUNCTURE POINTS FOR SELF-CARE

Point Combinations According to Body Areas

Head and Neck—*G.B. 39 + S.I. 3*
Cheeks and Jaw—*S.I. 3 + S.I. 19*
Nose, Mouth, and Throat—*St. 44 + L.I. 4*
Chest and Ribs—*G.B. 40 + Pe. 6*
Upper Abdomen—*St. 36 + Pe. 6*
Lower Abdomen—*St. 43 + Li. 3*
Groin and Pubis—*Li. 3 + Ki. 8*
Sides and Waist—*G.B. 40 + U.B. 40*
Lower Back,
Sacrum, and Hips—*U.B. 60 + G.B. 34*
Upper Back,
Scapula, and Nape of Neck—*U.B. 58 + S.I. 3*
Upper Arms
and Shoulders—*T.B. 5 + L.I. 11*
Forearms and Hands—*L.I. 10 + L.I. 4*
Outer Knee, Calf,
and Ankle—*G.B. 34 + G.B. 39 + U.B. 60*
Inner Knee, Calf,
and Ankle—*Sp. 9 + Sp. 6 + Ki. 3*
Feet—*G.B. 40 + Sp. 4 + Ki. 1*

Point Combinations According to Specific Ailments

Common Cold and Flu: *L.I. 4 + Lu. 7 + Ki. 7 + G.V. 14*
Fever—*L.I. 11*
Chills—*T.B. 5*
Sinus congestion—*U.B. 2*
Nasal congestion—*L.I. 20*
Cough—*Lu. 5–6*
Wheezing or chest pain—*C.V. 17*
Earache—*T.B. 17*
Headaches: *G.B. 39 + L.I. 4 + U.B. 58*

Frontal pain—*E.P. Yin Tang*
Temple pain—*E.P. Tai Yang*
Eye pain—*G.B. 14*
Occipital pain—*G.B. 20*
Parietal pain—*G.B. 8*
Vertex (top) pain—*Li. 3*
Neck pain—*G.V. 14*
TMJ pain—*S.I. 3 + S.I. 19 + St. 44*
Indigestion: *St. 36 + L.I. 4 + Sp. 4*
Nausea—*Pe. 6*
Stomach cramps or pain—*C.V. 12*
Distension—*Sp. 9*
Belching or hiccups—*Pe. 6*
Intestinal flatulence or cramps—*St. 25*
Constipation—*L.I. 11*
Diarrhea—*St. 43*
Genitourinary Disorders: *Li. 3 + Ki. 8 + Sp. 6*
Bladder or urethral pain—*Li. 8*
Female Reproductive Disorders: *Sp. 6 + Sp. 9 + Li. 3*
Premenstrual anxiety/sensitivity—*Ht. 7*
Breast pain/swelling—*C.V. 17*
Delayed menstruation—*Pe. 6*
Excessive bleeding—*Sp. 10*
Uterine pain—*C.V. 4*
Ovarian pain—*Ki. 5*
Male Reproductive Disorders: *Sp. 6 + Ki. 7 + Li. 3*
Testes pain—*Ki. 5*
Prostate pain—*Ki. 8*
Ejaculation pain—*Li. 8*
General Irritability and Tension: *L.I. 4 + Li. 3 + G.B. 21*
Anxiety and Insomnia: *E.P. Yin Tang + Ht. 7 + Sp. 6*
Weakness and Fatigue: *Ki. 7 + St. 36*
Itching: *L.I. 11 + Li. 3*
Leg Cramps: *Li. 3 + U.B. 58 + G.B. 34*

Emergency First Aid

Fainting, seizure: *G.V. 26* and *St. 36*
Cessation of breathing: *Ki. 1* and *C.V. 17*
Shock: *Pe. 6* and *St. 36*
Heat exhaustion: *G.V. 14* and *L.I. 11*
Difficult or prolonged labor: *Sp. 6* and *G.B. 21*
Postpartum bleeding: *Sp. 10* and *Li. 3*
Severe diarrhea: *C.V. 4 + St. 43*

Harmonizing Organ Networks

These pairs of points can be massaged simultaneously or sequentially in the order given. Apply slightly greater pressure to the second point in the sequence.

Kidney and Heart:
    Kidney symptoms more prominent—*S.I. 4 + Ki. 3*
    Heart symptoms more prominent—*U.B. 58 + Ht. 7*
Heart and Lung:
    Heart symptoms more prominent—*L.I. 4 + Ht. 7*
    Lung symptoms more prominent—*S.I. 4 + Lu. 9*
Lung and Liver:
    Lung symptoms more prominent—*G.B. 40 + Lu. 7*
    Liver symptoms more prominent—*L.I. 4 + Li. 3*
Liver and Spleen:
    Liver symptoms more prominent—*St. 36 + Li. 3*
    Spleen symptoms more prominent—*G.B. 34 + Sp. 4*
Spleen and Kidney:
    Spleen symptoms more prominent—*U.B. 58 + Sp. 6*
    Kidney symptoms more prominent—*St. 36 + Ki. 3*

HOW TO LOCATE THE POINTS

Acupuncture points are located according to anatomical landmarks. Distance between landmarks is determined by a relative measurement, different for each individual, called "body units." One body unit is equivalent to the width of the second joint of the thumb. Three body units are equivalent to the width of the other four fingers when they are held together. In addition, large areas of the body, including the limbs, abdomen, chest, and head, are measured according to specified numbers of body units between anatomical landmarks. The distance between the crease of the elbow and the crease of the wrist is twelve body units; between the crease of the knee and the external ankle bone is sixteen body units; between the crease of the knee and the internal ankle bone is fifteen body units; between the pubis and the navel is five body units; and between the navel and the lower border of the sternum is eight body units. All the first-aid points can be located by referring both to the diagrams and the written descriptions.

Lung Channel (Lu.):
    1. *Lu. 5*—in the hollow of the elbow on the thumb side next to the large biceps tendon.
    2. *Lu. 6*—on the inner aspect of the forearm, on the thumb side, ap-   255

Abbreviation Key

Lu. = Lung

L.I. = Large Intestine

St. = Stomach

Sp. = Spleen

Ht. = Heart

S.I. = Small Intestine

U.B. = Urinary Bladder

Ki. = Kidney

Pe. = Pericardium

T.B. = Triple-Burner

G.B. = Gallbladder

Li. = Liver

G.V. = Governing Vessel

C.V. = Conception Vessel

E.P. = Extra Points

1. *Lu. 5*
2. *Lu. 6*
3. *Lu. 7*
4. *Lu. 9*
5. *L.I. 4*
6. *L.I. 10*
7. *L.I. 11*
8. *L.I. 20*
9. *St. 25*
10. *St. 36*
11. *St. 43*
12. *St. 44*
13. *Sp. 4*
14. *Sp. 6*
15. *Sp. 9*
16. *Sp. 10*
17. *Ht. 7*
18. *S.I. 3*
19. *S.I. 4*
20. *S.I. 19*
21. *U.B. 2*
22. *U.B. 40*
23. *U.B. 58*
24. *U.B. 60*
25. *Ki. 1*

26. *Ki. 3*
27. *Ki. 5*
28. *Ki. 7*
29. *Ki. 8*
30. *Pe. 6*
31. *T.B. 3*
32. *T.B. 5*
33. *T.B. 17*
34. *G.B. 8*
35. *G.B. 14*
36. *G.B. 20*
37. *G.B. 21*
38. *G.B. 34*
39. *G.B. 39*
40. *G.B. 40*
41. *Li. 3*
42. *Li. 8*
43. *G.V. 14*
44. *G.V. 20*
45. *G.V. 26*
46. *C.V. 4*
47. *C.V. 12*
48. *C.V. 17*
49. *E.P. Yin Tang*
50. *E.P. Tai Yang*

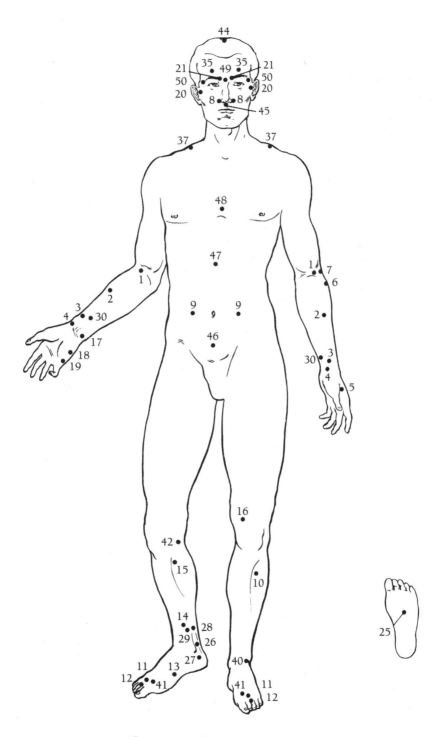

Fifty First Aid Acupressure Points

Abbreviation Key

Lu. = Lung

L.I. = Large Intestine

St. = Stomach

Sp. = Spleen

Ht. = Heart

S.I. = Small Intestine

U.B. = Urinary Bladder

Ki. = Kidney

Pe. = Pericardium

T.B. = Triple-Burner

G.B. = Gallbladder

Li. = Liver

G.V. = Governing Vessel

C.V. = Conception Vessel

E.P. = Extra Points

1. Lu. 5
2. Lu. 6
3. Lu. 7
4. Lu. 9
5. L.I. 4
6. L.I. 10
7. L.I. 11
8. L.I. 20
9. St. 25
10. St. 36
11. St. 43
12. St. 44
13. Sp. 4
14. Sp. 6
15. Sp. 9
16. Sp. 10
17. Ht. 7
18. S.I. 3
19. S.I. 4
20. S.I. 19
21. U.B. 2
22. U.B. 40
23. U.B. 58
24. U.B. 60
25. Ki. 1

26. Ki. 3
27. Ki. 5
28. Ki. 7
29. Ki. 8
30. Pe. 6
31. T.B. 3
32. T.B. 5
33. T.B. 17
34. G.B. 8
35. G.B. 14
36. G.B. 20
37. G.B. 21
38. G.B. 34
39. G.B. 39
40. G.B. 40
41. Li. 3
42. Li. 8
43. G.V. 14
44. G.V. 20
45. G.V. 26
46. C.V. 4
47. C.V. 12
48. C.V. 17
49. E.P. Yin Tang
50. E.P. Tai Yang

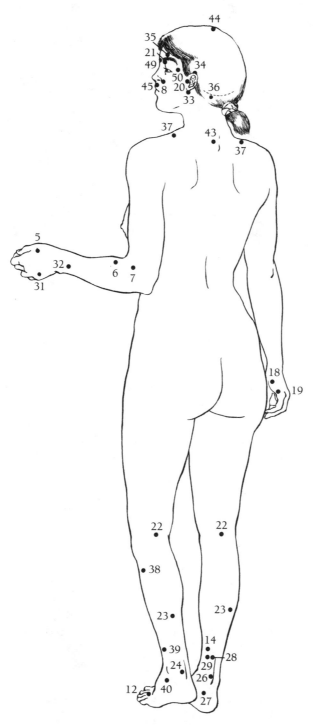

Fifty First Aid Acupressure Points

proximately three to five body units away from *Lu. 5*, or slightly less than halfway between the elbow and wrist crease.

3. *Lu. 7*—on the inner aspect of the forearm, on the thumb side, adjacent to the upper edge of the wrist bone, about two body units from the wrist crease, between the artery and the bone of the forearm.
4. *Lu. 9*—on the inner aspect of the forearm, on the thumb side, in the hollow between the wrist bone and the crease of the wrist.

Large Intestine Channel (L.I.):

5. *L.I. 4*—on the top of the hand, in the hollow of the muscle between the thumb and the index finger.
6. *L.I. 10*—on the top of the forearm, on the thumb side, in the hollow formed between two muscles when the arm is bent at a right angle and the hand is made into a fist, about two body units from the crease of the elbow.
7. *L.I. 11*—on the outside of the arm, in a hollow formed between the end of the elbow crease and the elbow when the arm is bent at a right angle.
8. *L.I. 20*—beside the nose, in the nasal groove, one-half body unit away from the nostril.

Stomach Channel (St.):

9. *St. 25*—on the abdomen, about two body units from the edge of the navel, at the level of the navel.
10. *St. 36*—on the outside of the leg, with the leg slightly bent, three body units below the lower edge of the kneecap (patella) and one body unit from the edge of the shinbone (tibia).
11. *St. 43*—on the foot, in the hollow formed between and behind the knuckles of the second and third toes.
12. *St. 44*—on the foot, in the hollow of the web between and in front of the knuckles of the second and third toes.

Spleen Channel (Sp.):

13. *Sp. 4*—on the inner aspect of the arch of the foot, in a hollow one and one-half body units behind the knuckle of the big toe.
14. *Sp. 6*—on the inner aspect of the lower leg, three body units (four fingerbreadths) from the upper edge of the inner ankle bone, in the muscle just behind the edge of the tibia (shinbone). (Directly opposite *G.B. 39.*)
15. *Sp. 9*—on the inner aspect of the leg, below the knee, in a hollow behind the tibia (shinbone) and one body unit below the crease of the knee. (Directly opposite *G.B. 34.*)
16. *Sp. 10*—in the hollow of the muscle, on the inner aspect of the thigh,

with the leg slightly bent, three body units above the upper edge of the kneecap (patella) just under the thigh bone (femur).

Heart Channel (Ht.):

17. *Ht. 7*—on the distal crease of the wrist (closest to the base of the palm), on the side of the little finger, in the hollow next to the bone.

Small Intestine Channel (S.I.):

18. *S.I. 3*—on the outer edge of the hand, in a hollow behind the knuckle of the little finger and just below the bone when making a loose fist.
19. *S.I. 4*—approximately two body units behind *S.I. 3*, in a hollow in front of the bone at the base of the hand.
20. *S.I. 19*—in front of the tragus of the ear, in a hollow formed when the mouth is open.

Urinary Bladder Channel (U.B.):

21. *U.B. 2*—in the notch at the inner end of the eyebrow, directly above the inner corner of the eye.
22. *U.B. 40*—with the knee slightly bent, in a hollow in the middle of the crease between two muscles at the back of the knee.
23. *U.B. 58*—on the outside of the leg, seven body units above the upper edge of the external ankle bone, just behind the edge of the fibula.
24. *U.B. 60*—on the outer aspect of the ankle, in the hollow between external ankle bone and the Achilles tendon.

Kidney Channel (Ki.):

25. *Ki. 1*—on the bottom of the foot, one-third of the distance from the base of the second toe to the back of the heel, on the midline of the sole, in a hollow when the toes are flexed.
26. *Ki. 3*—on the inner aspect of the ankle, in the hollow between the inner ankle bone and the Achilles tendon.
27. *Ki. 5*—on the inner aspect of the foot, two body units below *Ki. 3* in a hollow in the center of the heel.
28. *Ki. 7*—on the inner aspect of the leg, two body units above *Ki. 3*, in a hollow between the muscle and the Achilles tendon.
29. *Ki. 8*—on the inner aspect of the leg, one body unit above the upper edge of the inner ankle bone, just behind the edge of the tibia, directly in front of *Ki. 7*.

Pericardium Channel (Pe.):

30. *Pe. 6*—on the midline of the inner aspect of the arm, two body units from the crease of the wrist, between two tendons.

261

Triple-Burner Channel (T.B.):

31. *T.B. 3*—in a hollow just behind and between the knuckles of the fourth (ring) and fifth (little) fingers, with the fingers slightly bent.
32. *T.B. 5*—in a hollow on the outer aspect of the forearm, between the two bones (radius and ulna), about two body units from the bend of the wrist, with the arm and hand lying across the abdomen.
33. *T.B. 17*—in the hollow beneath the earlobe, formed when the mouth is open, between the mandible and the mastoid bone.

Gallbladder Channel (G.B.):

34. *G.B. 8*—on the side of the head, just above the tip of the ear when the ear is folded over.
35. *G.B. 14*—in a small hollow directly above the pupil of the eye when looking forward, about one-half body unit above the eyebrow.
36. *G.B. 20*—in a hollow at the lower edge of the base of the skull on the border of the large muscle that attaches to the base of the skull about two body units from midline of the spine.
37. *G.B. 21*—in the center of the muscle (trapezius) midway between the base of the neck and the tip of the shoulder.
38. *G.B. 34*—on the outer aspect of the leg just below the head of the fibula in a hollow between the muscle and the tendon. (Directly opposite *Sp. 9*.)
39. *G.B. 39*—on the outer aspect of the leg, between the muscle and the edge of the fibula, three body units above the outer ankle bone. (Directly opposite *Sp. 6*.)
40. *G.B. 40*—on the outer aspect of the ankle in a hollow in front of the external ankle bone, between the ankle bone and the top of the foot.

Liver Channel (Li.):

41. *Li. 3*—in a hollow behind and between the knuckles of the big toe and the second toe.
42. *Li. 8*—in a hollow on the inner aspect of the knee between the end of the crease of the knee and the head of the tibia when the knee is bent at a forty-five-degree angle.

Governing Vessel (G.V.):

43. *G.V. 14*—at the base of the neck on the midline of the spine in the space between the seventh cervical and the first thoracic vertebrae.
44. *G.V. 20*—in a small hollow on the top of the head, on the midline of the skull halfway between the tips of both ears.
45. *G.V. 26*—in the groove at the juncture of the nose and the upper lip.

Conception Vessel (C.V.):

46. *C.V. 4*—on the midline of the abdomen, two body units above the pubic bone and three body units below the navel.
47. *C.V. 12*—on the midline of the abdomen halfway between the navel and the lower edge of the sternum (chest bone).
48. *C.V. 17*—on the midline of the abdomen, on the sternum approximately at the level of the nipples or one and one-half body units above the lower edge of the sternum.

Extra Points (E.P.):

49. *E.P. Yin Tang*—on the front of the head, just above the root of the nose, exactly between the eyebrows.
50. *E.P. Tai Yang*—in the hollow of the temple, about one body unit behind the external end of the eyebrow.

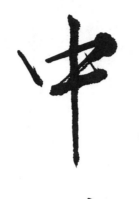

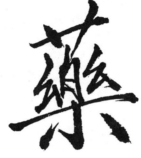

Chinese Herbs

CHAPTER FOURTEEN

THE CAULDRON
OF CHINESE HERBS:
WISDOM YOU CAN SWALLOW

Gingerly the acrid brew enters my lips.
Gnarled tenacious tendrils
Nourished in deep musty earth
Strengthen my root.
Ingesting stalks, flowers, and
Skins of caterpillars
I become the butterfly.

THE HISTORICAL ROOTS OF MODERN PHARMACOLOGY WERE EMBEDDED in herbal medicine. Aspirin was originally derived from the bark of willow trees, morphine from the seeds of poppy flowers, penicillin from fungus, quinine from the bark of the cinchona tree, and digitalis from the leaves of foxglove. Pharmaceutical laboratories continue to extract active ingredients from plant materials (a quarter of modern prescription drugs include plant extracts) as well as prepare wholly synthetic compounds. Yet by the time we see the white aspirin tablet imprinted with a brand name, or a vial of morphine, the willow tree and poppy field have slipped from view and been forgotten. About three-quarters of the world's people still rely on traditional medicine.

On the shelves of Chinese herbal pharmacies jars of barks, roots, flowers, and seeds are visible, sitting alongside rows of glass bottles filled with herbal formulas compressed into pills. Most Westerners feel like strangers to the apothecary herbs of China, yet some of these herbs, like chrysanthemum, magnolia, forsythia, honeysuckle, gardenia, hawthorn, quince, and mint, inhabit our own gardens. Others are known to us by their common name (like licorice), but not by their Mandarin equivalent (*gan cao*) or the Latin botanical name (*Glycyrrhiza uralensis*). Even when the name and reputation of an herb are familiar, like ginseng, its use within the framework of Chinese medicine remains puzzling to many. This chapter offers some essential keys for decoding the enigma, a passing curiosity for some and the initiation of a lifelong quest for others.

IN SICKNESS AND IN HEALTH

Western pharmaceutical drugs capitalize on a single biologically active ingredient to produce a specific physiological effect. This accounts for their potency and also for their secondary or side effects. Although drugs may control symptoms, they often do not treat the pathological process (for example, antibiotics may eliminate bacteria but do not improve a person's resistance to being infected; diuretics rid the body of excess fluid yet do not improve kidney function; aspirin controls arthritic pain without altering the degenerative course of the disease). Sometimes further aggravations or adverse side effects result (for instance, yeast infections may follow a course of antibiotics; kidney damage may result from long-term use of diuretics; lengthy use of aspirin may cause the lining of the stomach to erode, triggering internal bleeding).

With herbs, active ingredients are enfolded within the whole plant; this tends to buffer their side effects. Also, herbs are often blended together to counteract undesired effects and enhance intended results. Chinese herbs address the underlying condition as defined by traditional diagnosis and, when used properly, rarely cause disagreeable consequences.

Here are some examples in which Chinese herbs either complement or provide an effective alternative to Western drugs. For years Gus had been on Tagamet and antacids for a chronic gastric ulcer. His Western physician could not explain the source of the ulcer but could help him control his pain. Medication often allayed his acute discomfort but failed to improve his condition, provoking unwanted side effects like headaches, aching joints, and tiredness. Weary of medicine-induced problems and in search of a more lasting remedy, he came to us. Gus needed herbs that would clear the *Heat* and *Dampness* from his *Stomach*, relax his *Liver*, decongest stagnant *Qi*, and increase the circulation of *Blood* and regeneration of tissue. After using Chinese herbs, his pain dissipated and his ulcer healed.

Zoe had lifelong asthma, and since her theophylline and bronchodilator weren't always sufficient, she needed to rely on steroids, which caused her to retain pounds of excess fluid. She longed for an alternative. Chinese herbs helped her eliminate phlegm by strengthening the *Qi* of her *Spleen* and *Lung* and dispel fluid and build up her resistance by supporting her *Kidney*. She was able to manage her asthma with lower doses of medication and without further need for steroids.

Carlos had allergies. He constantly took antihistamines, which left him too sleepy to perform optimally at work and caused episodes of dizziness and high blood pressure. With herbs that cleared *Wind*, *Heat*, and *Dampness* from the head and sinuses while moisturizing and decongesting the *Qi* of the *Lung*, *Stomach*, and *Intestines*, he was able to control his symptoms.

Liz had insomnia, sometimes for weeks at a time, and was on the edge of becoming addicted to Valium. Herbs that harmonized the *Kidney* and *Heart* and nourished the *Blood* enabled her to regain a natural sleep cycle and reduce her level of anxiety.

Many herbs are nutritive and cannot be distinguished from food. Like food, they can be eaten because they are good for you, rather than because there is something wrong and you feel ill. Other herbs do not taste particularly pleasant and function in ways we do not associate with food, such as ridding the body of something unwanted, like *Heat* (antiinflammatory) or *Dampness* (diuretic). Herbs tend to have greater concentrations of nonnutritive compounds (glycosides, resins, alkaloids, polysaccharides, and terpenes), which contribute to their effectiveness as medicine—that is, a substance capable of promoting a desirable biological process or altering a pathological one.

Within our own household, Chinese herbs have become as fundamental as the potatoes and rice in our pantry. Spreading across our kitchen counter, small dark bottles and neatly wrapped packages bearing Chinese characters multiply as prolifically as the shrubs in our garden.

We use herbs for both prevention and cure—like vitamins or food supplements, they maintain our health, and used medicinally they redress acute and chronic ailments. Our day begins with a blender brew of juice and nutritive herbs that awaken and supplement *Qi*. In addition, we choose from many formulas according to our daily needs—our son relies on a *Qi* tonic, I on a formula that harmonizes *Spleen* and *Liver*, and Efrem uses a formula that harmonizes the *Kidney* and *Heart*. Remedies from Chinatown herb shops travel with me in my purse as instant health insurance: *Yin Chiao* ("yin chow") tablets to halt a sore throat and sniffle before they become a full-fledged cold and Curing Pills to check indigestion, nausea, and headaches related to an upset stomach. Oblivious of boundaries, our herbs nestle comfortably in our kitchen, medicine cabinet, and clinic pharmacy.

THE CHINESE STORE OF HERBAL KNOWLEDGE

Twenty-three hundred years ago, the mythic sage Shen Nung harvested, tasted, and codified wild-growing medicinal herbs. Since then Chinese herbal medicine has mushroomed from a rudimentary empirical practice to a sophisticated, systematic method of classification and prescription including more than six thousand substances, about three hundred of which are in everyday use.

The store of herbal knowledge in China today is stocked from many sources. One is the unschooled know-how of common people whose cultural

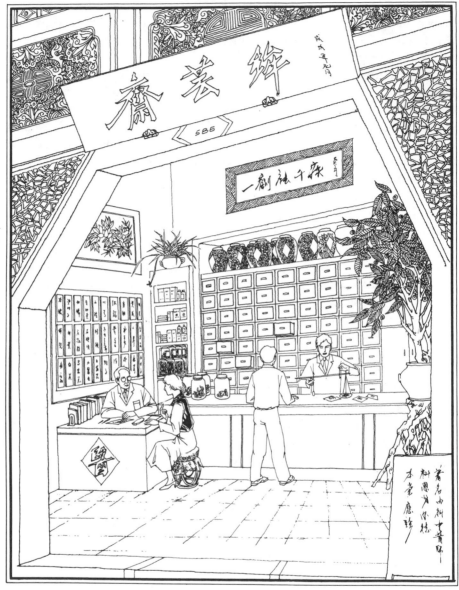

A Chinese Herbal Pharmacy

inheritance includes an herbal lore derived from personal experience with local resources. Folk healing is passed on through generations by stories about roots and seeds that grow on nearby mountainsides or sit in neighborhood shops. Another is a vast body of written commentary scrutinized by erudite scholars who possess an encyclopedic command of hundreds of herbs and a familiarity with the intellectual history of their use. Yet another is modern pharmacology and clinical research that focuses on the biological mechanisms by which herbs mediate stress, enhance immunity, and treat myriad degenerative diseases.

Branching as it does into diverse streams of thought, this herbal tradition has resisted becoming homogeneous or fixed and continues to evolve in many directions as it adapts to changing health care practices on its native soil and in the West. Out of the dense thicket of information and theory, almost as many paths through Chinese herbalism exist as there are herbalists. To clear a trail for the American reader we have selected a conceptual language that clarifies, simplifies, and demystifies how herbs are defined, combined, and prescribed. Our purpose here, as with a short course in music appreciation, is to confer understanding, to tune the ear to a new scale, not to teach composition or technique.

Mastery of herbal medicine is incredibly intricate. Yet its everyday use can be stunningly simple, something some Chinese children are practically born knowing. Without an education in horticulture, anyone with a plot of earth can dig it up, plant it, and watch carrot stalks sprout and daisies flower. Just as we can roam barefoot in our gardens, so we can all be "barefoot doctors" when it comes to cultivating Qi. More and more, people are pursuing benign alternatives to steroids, antacids, inhalers, diuretics, and painkillers. We can just as readily acquire an appetite for the exotic substances dispensed from the wooden drawers of Chinese apothecary shops as we have for soy sauce and chow mein.

HOW CHINESE HERBS ARE CLASSIFIED: QUALITIES AND PROPERTIES

Herbs are plant, mineral, and animal substances that the body assimilates through its digestive, respiratory, and cutaneous tissues. They reorganize the body constituents (Qi, Moisture, and Blood) within Organ Networks and oust the Adverse Climates (Wind, Heat, Cold, Dryness, Dampness).

The qualities most pertinent in categorizing herbs include their

- nature: warm, cool, or neutral
- taste: sour, bitter, sweet or bland, spicy, salty
- configuration: shape, texture, moisture

- color
- properties: tonifying, consolidating, dispersing, and purging (properties represent the potential of an herb to produce particular results within the body)

QUALITIES

The *nature* of an herb refers to its warming or cooling character, how it acts upon contact with the mouth, skin, or stomach. Warm, cool, or neutral herbs are matched with the warm or cool nature of individuals and their conditions. Cooling herbs treat conditions of *Heat*, warming herbs treat *Cold* conditions, and neutral herbs can be used in either case. Hot (cinnamon bark) or cold (isatis leaf) herbs have stronger effects than those that are only slightly warm (magnolia bark) or cool (chrysanthemum flower).

Configuration refers to the shape, moisture, and texture of an herb. What is known as the "doctrine of signatures"—similarities of pattern between plants and the human body—is one of the oldest principles of herbal healing and an early example of correspondence thinking. The shape, color, or texture of an herb may mimic certain parts of the body or attributes of certain diseases. Deer antler, which contains the richest marrow of the deer, is correspondingly used to nourish our own *Essence*, muscle, and bone. Steamed rehmannia—dark, sticky, sweet, and gelatinous like congealed blood—nourishes *Blood* and supplements *Moisture*, relieving anemia and *Dryness*. Walnuts, because they look like the cortex of the brain and kidney, are considered an excellent tonic for the reproductive and central nervous systems. Ginseng root, shaped like a human body with head, arms, and legs (named *ren shen* or "man root"), strengthens the *Qi* of the whole body and extends life.

Color as well as configuration suggests therapeutic correspondence. Yellow herbs tend to affect the *Organs* of *Earth* (*Stomach* and *Spleen*) and the *Adverse Climate* of *Dampness*. Bitter yellow roots like coptis and *Scutellaria* clear *Damp Heat* through their eliminative action, resolving yellowish conditions like jaundice and purulent infections. Sweet yellow herbs like licorice and polygonatum generate *Moisture* and invigorate *Qi* through their nutritive action.

Taste corresponds with each of the *Five Phases* and implies certain actions. Sourness (*Wood*) has an astringent action that concentrates *Qi*, bitterness (*Fire*) has an eliminative action that discharges *Qi* downward, sweetness or blandness (*Earth*) has a nourishing and harmonizing effect that slows *Qi* down, spiciness (*Metal*) has a stimulating action that accelerates and raises *Qi*, and saltiness (*Water*) has a softening action that dissolves congealed *Qi*. Strongly aromatic herbs such as musk and camphor dispel *Wind* and phlegm, clearing the senses and reviving consciousness. The odor and flavor of herbs in a formula direct or "lead" its action to particular parts of the body. Pungent and spicy herbs go to the *Lung*, musty and salty to the *Kidney*, fermented and sour to the *Liver*, acrid and bitter to the *Heart*, and fragrant and sweet to the *Spleen*.

Ginger, familiar to us all, illustrates how configuration, color, taste, odor, and nature correlate with use. Ginger is yellow, fragrant, and sweet, which corresponds to *Earth* (*Stomach* and *Spleen*), and pungent and spicy, which corresponds to *Metal* (*Lung* and *Large Intestine*). It has a warm nature and juicy texture, so it warms and moisturizes, making it suitable for *Cold* and *Dryness*-based digestive and respiratory conditions (such as a flu with thirst, dry cough, chills, and diarrhea). The spiciness of raw ginger decongests *Qi* (relieving symptoms such as cramps, nausea, and indigestion, including motion and morning sickness) and dispels *Wind* and phlegm (relieving symptoms such as fever, cough, and dizziness). When roasted, it has a greater warming and drying action, eliminating *Cold* and *Dampness* from the body's core (relieving symptoms like chilliness, water retention, and poor circulation).

PROPERTIES

Four basic properties—dispersing, consolidating, purging, and tonifying—represent an herb's potential for achieving a particular outcome. Properties are deduced from observing the effects herbs evoke. Dispersing circulates, consolidating condenses, purging eliminates, and tonifying strengthens. Whereas dispersing and consolidating alter the distribution and density of *Qi*, *Moisture*, and *Blood*, purging and tonifying alter the amount.

To *disperse* means to move. Dispersing redistributes *Qi*, *Moisture*, and *Blood* throughout the body, disseminating them from one part to another, relieving patterns of stagnation and overconcentration. Herbs in this category assist internal circulation (carthamus) and peripheral circulation (cinnamon), promote fluid metabolism (poria) and peristalsis (saussurea), eliminate muscle spasm (gastrodia), and remove air trapped in the chest and abdomen (aurantium). They also help dispel noxious accumulations or intrusions of *Heat* (honeysuckle), *Cold* (ginger), *Dampness* (coix), and *Wind* (sileris). Without significantly increasing or reducing body constituents, these herbs relax, invigorate, and loosen what feels otherwise tense, sluggish, and tight.

To *consolidate* means to gather together. Consolidating concentrates *Qi*, *Moisture*, and *Blood*, relieving patterns of slackness and leakage. This is done to prevent the loss of normal substances by inhibiting excess sweating (wheatberry), mucus discharge (ginkgo), hemmorrhage (sepia), urination (raspberry), or diarrhea (nutmeg). The goal is to astringe by restraining and tightening without drying or hardening, giving tissue more tone. Like isometric excercise that does not necessarily increase the size of muscle while enhancing its efficiency, these herbs do not alter quantity, but rather enhance quality—they help the body "keep it together."

To *purge* means to expel. Purging vigorously rids the body of accumulations that have become obstructive, evicting noxious substances, and counters severe or chronic patterns of stagnation. Herbs in this category work primarily through the lungs, nose, skin, bowels, stomach, uterus, and bladder. These include detoxifying, antiinflammatory, antiphlogistic herbs (scrophularia, scutellaria, forsythia) and those that stimulate discharge of menstrual blood (motherwort), urine (grifola), sweat (ephedra), phlegm (pinellia), undigested food (radish), and feces (senna). Such herbs are employed in situations where chronic accretions persist (such as cysts, boils, tumors, or other hardening of tissue) or when the gentler method of dispersing has been ineffective. Purging is used cautiously in frail, *deficient* individuals and is often combined with tonifying or consolidating herbs that ameliorate its potentially weakening effects.

To *tonify* means to augment, support, replenish, and strengthen. Tonifying nourishes the body, relieving patterns of emptiness and insufficiency. The herbs in this category have a potent effect on absorption and metabolism, increasing the total competence, adaptability, and resistance of the organism. They generate *Blood* (rehmannia), *Moisture* (*Dendrobium*) and *Qi* (codonopsis), overcoming conditions like anemia and malnutrition, dehydration, and fatigue. In a sense, all other therapies are preliminary to this since these herbs increase what benefits and constitutes the organism (*Qi*, *Moisture*, and *Blood*), sustaining health and preserving life. Tonifying herbs are often added to dispersing and purging prescriptions to protect the *Righteous Qi* of the body.

Herbal Correspondences

Tonify (to augment, nourish, build)

Qi:	Moisture:	Blood:
astragalus rt. (w), ginseng rt. (w), atractylodes rhz. (w), black dates (n) dioscorea rhz. (n), eleutherococcus hb. (n), codonopsis rt. (n), licorice rt. (n), polygonatum rhz. (n), pseudostellaria rt. (n)	polygonatum rhz. (n), dendrobium hb. (c), raw rehmannia rt. (c), ligustrum fr. (c), glehnia rt. (n), American ginseng rt. (c), pseudostellaria rt. (c), ophiopogonis rt. (c), lily bulb (c), anemarrhena rhz. (c)	cooked rehmannia rt. (w), angelica rt. (w), milettia stem (w), cooked pseudoginseng rt. (w), longan fr. (w), lycii fr. (n), donkey gelatin (n), red dates (n), white peony rt. (c), morus fr. (c)

Consolidate (to gather, astringe, condense)

Qi:
nutmeg sd. (w), astragalus rt. (w), atractylodes rhz. (w), cuscuta sd. (w), aquilaria wood (w), lotus sd. (n), euryales sd. (n), dioscorea rhz. (n), rose hips (n)

Moisture:
schizandra fr. (w), cornus fr. (w), rubus fr. (w), astragalus rt. (w), rice rhz. (n), ephedra rt. (n), dioscorea rhz. (n), euryales sd. (n), triticum fr. (c)

Blood:
pseudoginseng rt. (w), artemisia leaf (w), dipsacus rt. (w), agrimony hb. (w), lotus stamen (n), donkey gelatin (n), calamus gum (n), rubia rt. (c), eclipta hb. (c), white peony rt. (c)

Disperse (to circulate, distribute, move)

Qi:
tangerine or orange pl. (w), saussurea rt. (w), ginger rt. (w), perilla fr. (w), magnolia bk. (w), litchi sd. (w), platycodon rt. (n), hawthorn fr. (n), aurantium fr. (n), cyperus rt. (n)

Moisture:
raw ginger skin (w), atractylodes rhz. (w), cinnamon twig (w), corn silk (n), poria fungus (n), eupatorium hb. (n), coix sd. (n), agastache hb. (n), benineasa peel (n), alisma rhz. (c)

Blood:
carthamus fl. (w), ligusticum rhz. (w), turmeric rhz. (w), millettia stem (w), pseudoginseng rt. (w), myrrh resin (n), achyranthes rt. (n), bugleweed hb. (n), moutan peony bk. (c), motherwort hb. (c)

Purge (to rid, eliminate, evict)

Qi:
magnolia bk. (w), lindera rt. (w), apricot sd. (n), areca peel (n), radish sd. (n), unripe aurantium fr. (n), peach sd. (n), rhubarb rhz. (c), melia fr. (c), glauber's salt (c)

Moisture:
knotgrass hb. (n), lobelia hb. (n), mung bean (n), areca peel (n), polyporus fungus (n), akebia stem (c), dianthus hb. (c), plantain sd. (c), stephania rt. (c), lygodium spores (c)

Blood:
carthamus fl. (w), corydalis rt. (w), pseudoginseng rt. (w), peach sd. (n), sparganium rt. (n), bugleweed hb. (n), red peony rt. (c), curcuma rt. (c), salvia rt. (c), motherwort hb. (c)

Purge Adverse Climates

Phlegm:	*Wind*:	*Cold*:	*Heat*:	*Dampness*:
pinellia rhz. (w), magnolia bk. (w), mustard seed (w), citrus pl. (w), platycodon rt. (n), trichosanthes fr. (c), sargassum hb. (c), laminaria hb. (c), fritillary bulb (c), loquat leaf (c)	sileris rt. (w), gastrodia rhz. (n), unicaria stem (n), tribulus fr. (n), pueraria rt. (n), mulberry lf. (c), chrysan-themum fl. (c), peppermint leaf (c), *Haliotidis* shell (c), magnetite ore (c)	cinnamon bk. (h), evodia fr. (h), red pepper (h), dry ginger rhz. (h), long pepper fr. (h), curculigo rhz. (w), clove bud (w), trigonella sd. (w), fennel sd. (w), cardamom sd. (w)	honeysuckle fl. (c), forsythia fr. (c), gardenia fr. (c), prunella spike (c), dandelion rt. (c), scutellaria rt. (c), bupleurum rt. (c), isatis rt. (vc), coptis rt. (vc), gypsum mineral (vc)	(See disperse and purge *Moisture*) Key: rhz. = rhizome (tuber) rt. = root bk. = bark pl. = peel fl. = flower fr. = fruit sd. = seed (h) = hot (w) = warm (n) = neutral (c) = cool (vc) = very cold

HERBAL PROPERTIES AND THEIR EFFECTS: FOUR EXAMPLES

Herbal properties are identified according to the theory of correspondence. If a lack of *Qi* manifests as inertia, fatigue, and shallow breathing, then an herb that improves these symptoms is one that tonifies *Qi*. If, furthermore, this *deficiency* of *Qi* accompanies a pattern of *Spleen* weakness, manifesting as indigestion, bloating, and flabbiness, and this same herb also benefits these complaints, it is recognized as one that tonifies *Qi* and strengthens the *Spleen*. All herbs affect *Qi*, *Moisture*, and *Blood*, but not all herbs have specific influences on particular *Organ Networks*. Ginseng globally tonifies the *Qi*, whereas codonopsis particularly tonifies *Qi* of the *Spleen* and *Lung*. Coptis is an herb that purges *Heat* from all parts of the body, whereas *Scutellaria* especially clears *Heat* from the *Liver* and *Lung*. An herb is known by its effects, that is, what it can do—its presumed power to influence unseen events in the living organism. A few examples illustrate how an herb estab-lishes properties and claims its place in this system of correspondence.*

*For further information on individual herbs, the reader is referred to the *Materia Medica* prepared by Bensky and Gamble called *Chinese Herbal Medicine*. This text details the traditional properties and functions of more than four hundred herbs, summarizing abstracts regarding modern phar-macological and clinical research.

ASTRAGALUS MEMBRANACEUS (HUANG QI)

Astragalus tonifies *Qi*. When *Qi* is depleted, a person feels weak, tired, apathetic, breathless, and clammy and is vulnerable to infection. Grown in the wilds of Outer Mongolia, this fibrous yellow root strengthens metabolism, respiration, and immunity. It warms the limbs and muscles, dispels *Cold* and *Dampness* from the internal organs, and fortifies the *Spleen, Lung,* and *Kidney*. Modern research studies speak about astragalus as a "biological response modifier" that increases the adaptive function of the adrenal cortex and the production of white blood cells (particularly macrophages and T-cells), red blood cells, hormones such as interferon, and protective proteins called immunoglobulins. Because it inhibits the depression of bone marrow and extends the reproductive life of healthy cells by 50 percent, astragalus is used to support immune-compromised patients such as those undergoing radiation and chemotherapy and those with ARC or AIDS. It protects the liver from fatty degeneration caused by poisons like carbon tetrachloride, promotes diuresis, lowers blood pressure, and increases overall stamina and endurance.

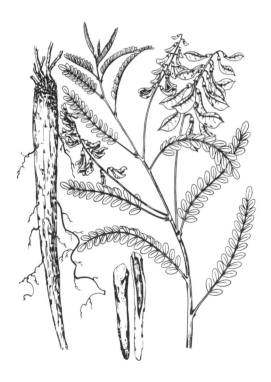

Astragalus: Root, Herb, and Plant

ANGELICA SINENSIS (DANG GUI)

Angelica root tonifies *Blood*. When *Blood* is *deficient*, a person feels limp, restless, irritable, dry, weak-hearted, cold, and fragile. Known as *dang gui* ("dong gway"), angelica root is regarded as the sovereign herb for women because of its power to restore the *Blood*, regulate menstrual rhythm, and strengthen the womb. It builds *Blood* the way astragalus builds *Qi*, bringing warmth and nourishment to the viscera as well as the skin, muscles, and flesh. By quickening and enriching *Blood*, it banishes *Cold*, *Wind*, and *Dampness*. It benefits the *Liver*, *Heart*, and *Spleen* and drives away the pain of obstructive stagnation. Pharmacological research documents that angelica stimulates and regulates uterine contractions, increases utilization of oxygen by the liver, calms the central nervous system, and relieves pain associated with neuralgia, ischemia (for example, angina), and rheumatic or osteoarthritis. Because angelica nourishes *Blood*, mobilizes circulation, generates tissue, dispels *Wind*, and alleviates pain, it is used to treat anemia, abdominal pain, menstrual cramps, and heart disease and to promote the healing of wounds, ulcers, and inflammations.

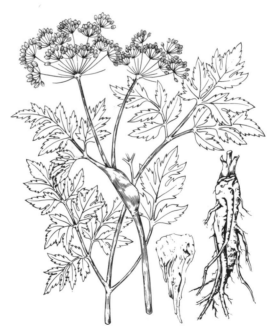

Angelica: Plant, Herb, and Root

SCHIZANDRA CHINENSIS (WU WEI ZI)

Schizandra consolidates *Moisture*. When the capacity to retain or generate *Moisture* is lost, a person feels parched, flushed, withered, ravenous, without reserves, as if her life force is tenuous and fickle. Schizandra fruit, "the seed of five flavors," fosters the generation and storage of *Essence*, awakening sexual potency and sensitivity. It calms the *Spirit*, strengthens the area called the *Sea of Qi* that lies two fingerbreadths below the navel, and supports the *Lung*, *Kidney*, and *Liver*. Contemporary research demonstrates that schizandra is an adaptogenic substance, like ginseng and astragalus, conferring nonspecific resistance, enhancing the total physiological competence of the organism. It both stimulates and relaxes the central nervous system, activates respiration, counteracts the effects of CNS-depressant drugs (like opiates), and promotes recovery from nonicteric hepatitis (without jaundice). It also eases childbirth by strengthening uterine contractions, promoting dilation of the cervix, and allaying fatigue. Schizandra alleviates chronic cough and asthma, insomnia, diarrhea, thirst, fatigue, sexual debility, and memory loss; it regulates blood sugar and assists recovery following prolonged fever or illness.

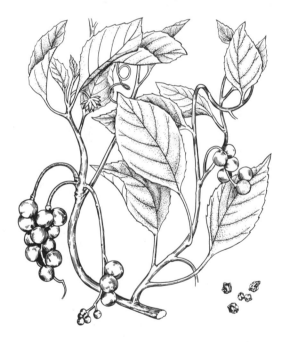

Schizandra: Plant and Berry

PORIA COCOS (FU LING)

Poria disperses *Moisture*. When *Moisture* accumulates and stagnates, a person feels heavy, puffy, lethargic, sore, tender, and vexingly soggy, sticky, and dry. Poria, a fungus that grows on the moist underground roots of pine trees, restores the proper distribution of body fluids, assisting the *Heart* and *Lung*, balancing the *Spleen* and *Kidney*. The outer skin, central pulp, and base of this bulbous fungus correspond respectively to its three powers: discharging surplus fluids via the *Kidney* and *Bladder*; aiding the transforming work of the *Spleen* and *Stomach*; and soothing the *Lung* and *Heart*. Pharmacological investigation of poria reveals that it is diuretic, reduces blood sugar, relaxes the intestines, has a mild sedative effect, and contains polysaccharides that inhibit cancer. Poria is used to treat abdominal distension, dyspepsia, edema, difficult urination, diabetes, and diarrhea. Brewed by itself or cooked with food, poria is a nutritive tonic for the young, weak, or elderly.

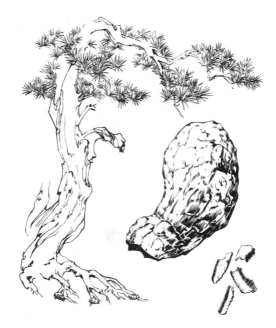

Poria: Fungus and Herb

FORMULATING HERBAL PRESCRIPTIONS

FOR PARTICULAR PEOPLE

A formula fits a patient the way a key opens a lock, mirroring and correcting patterns of disorganized *Qi*, *Moisture*, and *Blood*. A locksmith impressions a key from a blank, and the herbalist forms an impression of the patient, a diagnosis, from which he crafts the prescription. He translates symptoms and signs into patterns of disharmony, which are then matched with the therapeutic properties of herbs. Ideally the formula is a perfect reflection of the condition and needs of the patient.

Caroline, a thirty-eight-year-old patient, complains of chronic weariness, puffy eyes, a distended belly, poor concentration, hands that swell, and feet that feel cold at night. The herbalist interprets this configuration of tiredness, swelling, chilly feet, distension, and muddleheadedness as signs of depleted *Qi*, excess *Moisture*, insufficient warmth at the core, and *Spleen deficiency*. Caroline requires herbs that supplement and move her *Qi* while evicting *Dampness* and *Cold*.

The formula for Caroline matches her needs: astragalus, atractylodes, and poria tonify *Qi*, disperse *Moisture*, consolidate surface (defense) *Qi*, and strengthen the *Spleen*. Polyporus and stephania purge *Dampness*. Fresh ginger and red date invigorate *Qi* and warm her insides. By improving digestion and regulating fluids, these herbs promote the function of her *Spleen* and *Kidney*. After using this formula for two weeks, Caroline has more energy, reduced fluid retention in her face and hands, warmer feet, and a more comfortable belly.

> astragalus rt.
> white atractylodes rhz.
> poria fn.
> polyporus fn.
> stephania rt.
> ginger rhz.
> red dates

Jack, a forty-nine-year-old patient, seeks help for his stiff and weak lower back, dry eyes, thinning hair, diminished sexual enthusiasm, and inability to sleep restfully. A famous recipe from the Sung dynasty, *Liu Wei Di Huang Wan* ("loo way dee hwong wan") corresponds to Jack's pattern. Declining libido, lumbar distress, and hair loss signal diminished *Kidney Essence*. *Kidney Essence* maintains tissue and blood, elasticity of skin and muscle, agility of mind, and clarity of the senses. Dry eyes plus unsatisfying sleep suggest that depleted *Kidney* reserves have precipitated a *deficiency* of the *Blood* of the *Liver* and *Heart*.

This *Liu Wei* formula tonifies the *Kidney*, improving its capacity to supply and store *Essence*. The herbs rehmannia, dioscorea, and cornus replenish *Blood*, *Qi*, and *Essence*. Poria nurtures *Qi* and distributes *Moisture* while moutan peony and alisma eliminate *Heat*, *Dampness*, and stagnation. While rehmannia, cornus, moutan peony, and alisma benefit the *Kidney* and *Liver*, dioscorea and poria strengthen the *Spleen*. Because of this, the symptoms of anemia, dryness, irritability, a stiff and sore back, restless sleep, and impotence or infertility are relieved. This formula is often used to reinforce immunity, retard aging, and increase stamina.

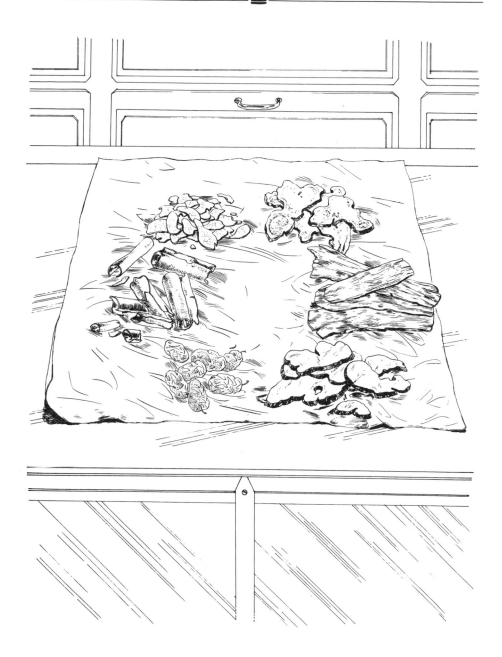

Herbal Formula to Be Prepared As Tea

cooked rehmannia rt.
dioscorea rt.
cornus rt.
poria fn.
moutan peony rt.
alisma rhz.

For Caroline the herbalist formulates a prescription unique to her pattern; for Jack, the herbalist relies on a classic formula that seems to meet his needs.

FOR SPECIFIC PROBLEMS

To formulate a prescription for a specific syndrome or complaint, an herbalist must differentiate between ingredients that have similar effects. To illustrate the selection process, we will construct several formulas for treating angina—chest pain that results from diminished cardiac blood flow. Since there are many herbs to choose from in the treatment of a symptom such as chest pain, picking the most appropriate ones depends on matching herbal properties with the underlying pattern of disharmony, so sometimes the same symptom may be diagnosed and treated differently, depending upon the person within whom it occurs.

It is axiomatic in Chinese medicine that pain arises from stagnation of *Qi*, *Moisture*, and *Blood*. In the case of angina, blood circulation is impeded, leading to a pattern of *Blood* stagnation, so herbs that disperse or purge *Blood* are considered. Next it is important to determine whether the *Blood* stagnation coexists with *Heat*, *Cold*, *Qi* stagnation, *Qi deficiency*, Blood *deficiency*, or *Moisture* stagnation (*Dampness* or phlegm). Choosing the best herbs depends on evaluating these coincident factors.

Ilex, a cold *Blood*-moving herb, also eliminates the phlegm congestion associated with high cholesterol and obesity. Angelica (*dang gui*), a warm herb that both circulates and nourishes *Blood*, is also good for strengthening someone who is underweight, frail, anemic, and chilly. Pseudoginseng promotes coronary circulation, arrests bleeding, counteracts coagulation, and reduces inflammation and cholesterol, so it is often used to treat pain associated with coronary thrombosis, myocarditis, or pericarditis.

All three herbs can be used to alleviate pain of the *Heart* due to *Blood* stasis: ilex treats *Blood* stasis with phlegm, angelica treats *Blood* stasis with *deficiency*, and pseudoginseng treats *Blood* stasis with coagulation or inflammation.

If signs of all these conditions coexist, then all three herbs to move *Blood* may be combined with others that disperse *Moisture* and *Qi* and tonify *Blood* and *Qi*. Supplementary herbs are again selected on the basis of differentiating symptoms and signs—the context in which the problem occurs.

281

Since *excesses* and *deficiencies* arise together and coexist, one transforming into the other, *Heat* can lead to *deficiency* of *Moisture*, *Dampness* can obstruct the circulation of *Qi* and *Blood*, lack of *Blood* can generate *Wind*, stagnated phlegm and *Blood* can produce *Heat*, and lack of *Qi* can create *Cold* and *Dampness*. By anticipating the ways in which disease progesses, the herbalist countervails against the tendency of one pathogenic process to convert to another.

Angina often exists within the context of an overall condition of *Damp Heat* in which the accumulation of phlegm eventually interferes with the movement of *Blood* and *Qi*. A person with this condition might be middle-aged, overweight, short of breath, and have high cholesterol, high blood pressure, a productive cough, a puffy face, a red tongue with thick sticky yellow fur, and a full, uneven soft pulse. The urgent, primary complaint of chest pain must be treated simultaneously with the underlying condition of phlegm accumulation due to *Damp Heat*. In addition to using ilex and salvia, two of the often used herbs to treat angina, we would add ligusticum to circulate *Blood* and *Qi* plus aurantium, trichosanthes, and pinellia to disperse *Qi* and purge phlegm and *Heat*. This way the herbs address not only the angina arising from stagnation of *Blood*, but also the associated conditions of *Heat*, phlegm, and *Qi* stagnation.

> ilex rt.
> salvia rt.
> ligusticum rhz.
> trichosantes fr.
> pinellia rhz.
> unripe aurantium fr.

For another person with angina there might be an altogether different pattern of *Blood* stagnation associated with *Coldness* and a *deficiency* of *Qi* and *Blood*. This is a common syndrome for weak elderly people with chronic coronary heart disease who are subject to chilly and numb arms and legs and shortness of breath or perspiration upon slight exertion and who have a pale, swollen face and tongue, and a weak, thready, uneven pulse. In this instance pseudoginseng and angelica (*dang gui*) could be selected to treat the stagnation of *Blood* because they are warm herbs that tonify as well as move *Blood*; and ligusticum, ginseng, dried ginger, atractylodes, and honey-baked licorice would circulate *Qi* and *Blood*, consolidate and tonify *Qi*, warm the body, and eliminate *Dampness*.

> pseudoginseng rt.
> angelica rt.
> ligusticum rhz.

ginseng rt.
white atractylodes rhz.
dried ginger rhz.
baked licorice rt.

Although the symptom of angina is the same, the person or context in which it occurs can account for altogether different formulas.

TRANSLATING SYMPTOMS INTO PATTERNS

Anyone who can reach for an aspirin for a headache can reach for an herbal headache remedy. But depending on the complexity or severity of a particular complaint, more knowledge may be necessary to pursue an effective herbal solution than simply identifying a symptom—it may be necessary to understand its source.

The same problem can be analyzed in a variety of ways: a headache can be thought of as congested *Qi* or *Blood*, as a symptom of a *Liver* weakness, or as a consequence of a disharmony of the *Liver-Spleen* relationship. We hope to engage you here in the actual process of diagnostic and therapeutic thinking. There is not necessarily one right description of a problem, one right answer, one right remedy, one right approach. There are patterns that are themselves dynamic, organic phenomena that can be viewed from multiple angles. The thinking of Chinese medicine gives you another point of view about what your dynamic is and how to adjust it, if need be. We provide a lot of information in the coming pages about herbs and differential diagnosis, some of which may go beyond your stage of interest or understanding. Look at the material and play with it at the level of your curiosity. Some readers will be content with learning how to think about themselves the way an herbalist does; others will want to discover how Chinese herbs make them feel.

Chinese medicine views illness as an imbalance of body constituents (in that ailments arise when there is insufficient *Qi*, *Moisture*, or *Blood* or when these constituents are too dense, too sluggish, or too unruly) and an ensuing dysfunction of *Organ Networks*. The logic of patterned thinking means correlating symptoms (patterns of distress) with categories of interpretation (patterns of disharmony). For example, in Chinese medicine if . . .

- Deborah is tense, tired, irritable and has dry skin and brittle hair symptoms—this is because she is *deficient* in *Blood*, which undermines the function of the *Liver* and *Heart* and disturbs the *Spleen*.
- Peter is restless, anxious, and prone to sharp pains in his upper abdomen and chest—this is understood as stagnant *Blood*, which interferes with the function of the *Heart* and *Liver*.

- Vinny is lethargic and worried, his face is puffy, his abdomen bloated, and he has chronic herpes—these symptoms arise from *Qi* stagnation, *Dampness*, and *Heat* affecting the *Liver*, *Spleen*, and *Kidney*.
- Marsha is timid, chilly, weak, and lacks libido; her hips frequently ache, and she often sleeps late without feeling refreshed—this translates as a lack of *Qi*, warmth, and *Essence*, which has weakened her *Kidney* and *Liver* function.
- Michael is erratic, moody and suffers bouts of dizziness, wheezing, and overheating alternating with episodes of headache, nasal congestion, and cold extremities—*internal Heat* and *Wind* combined with stasis of *Qi* and *Blood* are disturbing the harmony of his *Liver* and *Lung*.

At the very least, we hope to give you a more complete sense of how Chinese herbs are used and what benefits they hold—you will be a better-informed consumer who can more readily comprehend the prescriptions and advice given by a doctor of Chinese medicine. At the very most, we hope this chapter and the following one on herbal cuisine will encourage you to take the initiative to seek Chinese herbs to address some of your own health problems.

TRANSLATING PATTERNS INTO MODULAR FORMULAS

To simplify how to educate people about herbal medicine and encourage its greater use, we devised an alternative system for prescribing. Our goal was to preserve the most important aspects of traditional herbal medicine yet streamline its use. To do this meant conceiving of a method in which formulas could be made to conform to individual patterns while bypassing the years of study necessary to acquire detailed knowledge of hundreds of herbs and traditional formulas. This would make it feasible for people without extensive prior training to employ Chinese herbs, so long as they understand the principles of Chinese medicine.

The American penchant for innovation fused with the specificity and complexity of age-old Chinese practice spurred the design of a Chinese modular pharmacy—formulas composed of simple herbal combinations that can be mixed and matched to correspond to symptom patterns. These modules act upon

1. the body constituents (*Qi*, *Moisture*, and *Blood*) and *Adverse Climates* (*Cold, Heat, Wind, Dampness* [phlegm]).
2. the *Organ Networks* (*Liver, Heart, Spleen, Lung, Kidney*).

3. the relationships between *Organ Networks* (*Liver-Lung, Lung-Heart, Heart-Kidney, Kidney-Spleen, Spleen-Liver*).

A particular module can be used by itself or as a building block in formulating a more complex prescription. What is required is an identification of symptom configurations within the vocabulary of Chinese medicine. What is the state of your *Qi, Moisture,* and *Blood?* Is it depleted or congested? Are you burdened by the penetration or accumulation of *Wind, Cold, Heat, Wind,* or *Dampness?* On the basis of that assessment, the therapeutic strategy is to match such patterns with the actions of the formulas (to tonify, consolidate, disperse, purge, warm, cool). How well do your *Organ Networks* function? Are there patterns of *deficiency?* How harmonious is the interaction among your *Organ Networks?* On the basis of that evaluation, individual *Organ Networks* are supplemented and protected, and *Organ Network* relationships are harmonized.

MODULES FOR QI, MOISTURE, AND BLOOD

If someone is tired, irritable, dizzy, pale, and sleeping poorly, these symptoms correspond to the pattern of depleted *Blood.* The module to tonify *Blood* is appropriate. It is composed of a combination of herbs that act upon *Blood*: angelica generates and moves *Blood,* rehmannia assists angelica by nourishing *Blood* and *Moisture,* astragalus provides the transforming *Qi* necessary to generate *Blood,* peony relaxes nerves and blood vessels and dispels *Heat,* and zizyphus is nutritive for both *Qi* and *Blood.*

> cooked rehmannia rt.
> astragalus rt.
> white peony rt.
> angelica rt.
> red zizyphus fr.

If someone is weak, listless, chilly, pale, wants to sleep all the time, and gets frequent colds, this person has a lack of *Qi.* The module that tonifies *Qi* matches these symptoms. It is concocted from herbs that affect *Qi*: astragalus strengthens the surface *Qi,* codonopsis fortifies the interior *Qi,* dioscorea and atractylodes build the *Nutritive Qi,* and licorice harmonizes and nourishes *Qi.*

> astragalus rt.
> codonopsis rt.
> dioscorea rt.
> white atractylodes rhz.
> licorice rt.

Building Multipurpose Formulas

Each module is an herbal blend that addresses conditions of depleted or congested *Qi*, *Moisture*, or *Blood*. With the modules as foundation blocks, it is possible to build multipurpose formulas that conform to more complex individual patterns. For instance, the module to disperse *Moisture* is suitable for relieving the water retention that sometimes precedes a woman's men-

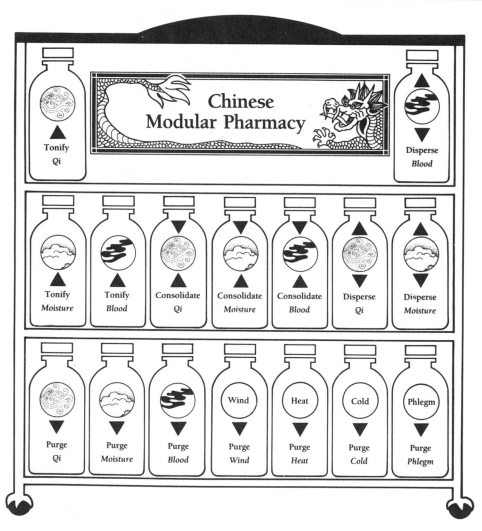

Chinese Modular Pharmacy

We have given the name *Chinese Modular Pharmacy* to our system. It constitutes a complete herbal dispensary organized around the combination of formulas rather than the blending of individual bulk herbs. The modular

strual period. However, in more severe conditions, such as chronic edema, there can be dehydration accompanying the water retention because so much fluid is suspended in the tissue that it is unavailable for cellular metabolism. In this instance, to avoid becoming too dry while eliminating excess fluid, the module to consolidate *Moisture* would be combined with the one that purges *Moisture*. That way *Dampness* is cleared while preserving essential body fluids.

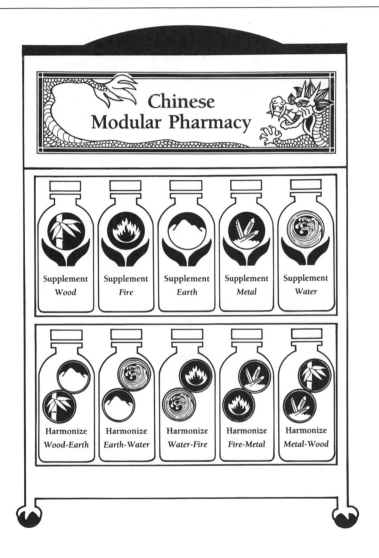

formulas have been manufactured and made available in both the United States and Europe. Further information about these products is available in the Resource Guide at the back of this book.

module to purge *Moisture*
module to consolidate *Moisture*

In general, herbs with complementary properties are combined to create balanced, effective formulas. Herbs that tonify are usually complemented by those that disperse—absorption of rich, nutritive, tonic herbs is enhanced by dispersing herbs that mobilize circulation. Congestion tends to occur with *deficiency*, so the same people who need strengthening often need better circulation of *Qi*, *Moisture*, and *Blood*. Herbs that purge are joined with herbs that consolidate or tonify to avoid weakening people whose excess is accompanied by depletion. Herbs that disperse are supplemented by those that consolidate to prevent overstimulation; conversely, herbs that consolidate are moderated by those that disperse to prevent overconcentration.

Since tonifying and dispersing herbs are combined to deal with the diminished circulation that occurs when people are weak, enriching herbs like codonopsis, polygonatum, and rehmannia are combined with dispersing herbs like tangerine peel, poria, and ligusticum, which move *Qi*, *Moisture*, and *Blood*, to avoid symptoms of congestion such as indigestion, stuffiness, and headache. Otherwise, when someone is weak, tonification without proper circulation could contribute to rather than relieve stagnation. To tonify *Blood* without aggravating congestion, the module to tonify *Blood* would be joined by the module to disperse either *Blood* or *Qi*. To tonify *Moisture* without generating *Dampness*, the module to tonify *Moisture* would be combined with either the module to disperse *Qi* or the module to disperse *Moisture*.

Many people experience conditions of depleted *Qi* and *Blood*. This may come as a result of overwork or simply of getting older. Common complaints that people bring to us are feeling tired, lacking the energy they used to have, and a litany of minor problems like indigestion, aches and pains, puffiness around the eyes and ankles, and declining sexual vigor. For this syndrome of middle age, a combination of modules would replenish *Qi* and *Blood*, enhance circulation, and eliminate *Dampness*. Such a formula would include equal parts of the modules to tonify *Qi* and *Blood* and half a part each of the modules to disperse *Qi* and *Moisture*. If a tendency to chill easily were a part of the picture, then a half part of the module to dispel *Cold* would be added.

module to tonify *Qi*
module to tonify *Blood*
module to disperse *Qi*
module to disperse *Moisture*
(option: module to dispel *Cold*)

Depleted or Congested *Qi, Moisture, Blood*: Signs and Symptoms

	Depleted Qi	Congested Qi
signs:	lethargy, low resistance and spirit, pale, dull, flaccid muscles	tension, uneasiness
symptoms:	weakness, poor appetite, lack of endurance, chilly	fullness in head, chest, abdomen belching, flatulence, distension diffuse, intermittent, migratory pain

	Depleted Moisture	Congested Moisture
signs:	flushing, sweating (especially at night)	puffy face, sticky perspiration, tender flesh
symptoms:	dry parched mouth, skin, and throat thirst, dry stool, scant urine unstable blood sugar	heavy and/or full feeling in head and limbs, pain and/or swelling of abdomen, joints, muscles

	Depleted Blood	Congested Blood
signs:	restless, irritable, pale, anemic, withered dry skin, hair, nails, eyes	nervousness
symptoms:	weak, pale, poor sleep, fatigue, heals poorly, bruises easily, cold hands and feet	headache, cramps, stabbing pain, numbness, paralysis, lumps, swollen breasts

FORMULAS FOR ORGAN NETWORKS

An herbalist also chooses herbs based on their affinity with *Organ Networks*—the capacity of an herb to promote the specific functions of an *Organ Network*. For example, the function of the *Heart* is to house the *Spirit* and propel the *Blood*: zizyphus calms the mind by nurturing the *Blood* of the *Heart*, while salvia cools the *Heart* and disperses the *Blood*. The *Spleen* transforms food and distributes *Nutritive Qi*: dry ginger warms the *Spleen* and activates digestion, and poria helps the *Spleen* by disseminating *Moisture* and *Nutritive Qi*. The *Lung* mobilizes *Qi* and *Moisture*: platycodon disperses *Lung Qi*, removes phlegm, and opens the chest; fritillary nurtures and moistens the *Lung* and dissolves phlegm. The *Kidney* stores *Essence* and adjusts fluid balance: cornus generates and consolidates *Kidney Essence*, and alisma regulates the *Kidney* by dispersing accumulated fluid. The *Liver* stores *Blood* and regulates *Qi*: white peony helps the *Liver* to store by consolidating *Blood* and counteracting spasm, while bupleurum cools the *Liver* and decongests its *Qi*.

An herb with a strong affinity for an *Organ Network* will shift the influence of other herbs to that *Network*. Ginseng, astragalus, and licorice all tonify *Qi*. When combined with cornus and alisma they will benefit the *Kidney*; with platycodon and fritillary they aid the *Lung*; with zizyphus and salvia they strengthen the *Heart*; and so on. It is on this basis that herbal formulas particularly benefit each *Organ Network*. Their composition takes into consideration the healthy dynamic of the *Organ Network* as well as the typical ways in which that dynamic becomes distorted.

Herb Affinities With *Organ Networks*

Liver	Heart	Spleen
carthamus fl. (w)	longan fr. (w)	pinellia rhz. (w)
ligusticum rhz. (w)	polygala rt. (w)	sausseurea rt. (w)
lycii fr. (n)	pseudoginseng rt. (w)	ripe citrus pl. (w)
cyperus rt. (n)	zizyphus sd. (n)	atractylodes rhz. (w)
gastrodia rhz. (n)	biota sd. (n)	poria fn. (n)
prunella spike (c)	ganoderma fn. (n)	licorice rt. (n)
chrysanthemum fl. (c)	ilex rt. (c)	codonopsis rt. (n)
unripe citrus pl. (c)	ophiopogon rt. (c)	dioscorea rhz. (n)
peony rt. (c)	coptis rhz. (c)	red and black dates
bupleurum rt. (c)	salvia rt. (c)	(n)
		polygonatum rhz. (n)

Lung	*Kidney*	key:
coltsfoot fl. (w)	psoralea sd. (w)	rt.=root
asaram hb. (w)	eucommia bk. (w)	hb.=herb
ephedra hb. (w)	trigonella sd. (w)	fl.=flower
astragalus rt. (w)	schizandra fr. (w)	rhz.=rhizome
fritillary blb. (n)	cornus fr. (w)	fn.=fungus
platycodon rt. (n)	cuscuta sd. (w)	fr.=fruit
coix sd. (n)	cooked rehmannia rt.	sd.=seed
American ginseng rt.	(w)	bk.=bark
(n)	lotus sd. (n)	pl.=peel
scutellaria rt. (c)	alisma hb. (c)	(w)=warm
bamboo shavings (c)	ligustrum fr. (c)	(c)=cool
		(n)=neutral

Herbal Support for Organ Networks

The following combinations illustrate how a few herbs can be used to maintain the integrity of the *Organ Networks* by supporting their proper function and protecting them against adverse processes that lead to dysfunction.

Liver Network

Therapeutic goal:	tonify *Blood* disperse *Blood* and *Qi* relax nerves and muscles dispel *Wind* and *Heat*

Herbs:	white peony rt.	tonify *Blood*, relax nerves and muscles, clear *Heat*
	lycii fr.	tonify *Blood*
	bupleurum rt.	disperse *Qi*, clear *Heat*
	ligusticum rhz.	disperse *Blood* and *Qi*, dispel *Wind*
	unripe aurantium fr.	disperse *Qi*, counteract spasm

Heart Network

Therapeutic goal:	tonify and disperse *Blood* dispel *Heat* tonify *Qi*, *Moisture*, and *Essence* calm *Spirit*

Herbs:	zizyphus sd.	tonify *Blood*, calm mind
	salvia rt.	disperse *Blood*, clear *Heat*, calm mind
	schizandra fr.	tonify *Essence*, calm mind
	ginseng rt.	tonify *Qi* and *Essence*, calm mind
	poria fn.	tonify *Qi*
	lopatherum hb.	purge *Heat*

Spleen Network

Therapeutic goal:	warm and tonify *Qi* disperse *Qi* and *Moisture* counter prolapse

Herbs:	poria fn.	tonify *Qi*, disperse *Moisture*
	astragalus rt.	tonify *Qi*, lift viscera
	white atractylodes rhz.	tonify *Qi*
	red dates	tonify *Qi*, nurture *Blood*
	dried ginger rhz.	warm, disperse *Qi*
	ripe aurantium fr.	disperse *Qi*, lift viscera

Lung Network

Therapeutic goal:	tonify *Qi* and *Moisture* disperse *Qi* and open the chest dispel *Wind* and phlegm

Herbs:	fritillary blb.	tonify *Moisture*, loosen phlegm
	astragalus rt.	tonify and consolidate *Qi*, disperse *Moisture*
	platycodon rt.	disperse *Qi*, dispel phlegm, open chest
	licorice rt.	tonify *Qi*, soothe tissue
	fresh ginger rhz.	disperse *Qi*, dispel *Wind* and phlegm

Kidney Network

Therapeutic
goal:

> tonify *Qi*
> disperse *Moisture*
> tonify and consolidate *Essence*

Herbs:

dioscorea rhz.	tonify *Qi*, consolidate *Essence*
cooked rehmannia rt.	tonify *Yin Essence*
poria fn.	tonify *Qi*, disperse *Moisture*
cornus fr.	tonify, consolidate *Essence*
eucommia bk.	tonify *Yang Essence*
alisma rhz.	disperse *Moisture*

Organ Network Distress: Signs and Symptoms

Organ	Signs	Symptoms
Liver:	tense, irritable, impulsive, indecisive lusterless, soft, weak, or brittle nails tenderness beneath ribs	uneven sensations of heat, cold, or pressure, fullness beneath ribs, photophobia or blurred vision, cramps, and/or spasms of muscles or viscera
Heart:	anxiety, restlessness, sensitivity, uneven heart rhythm, easy flushing, pallor of face, palms, soles	insomnia, palpitations, easy perspiration, sensitive to heat and cold
Spleen:	worried, obsessive, insecure, lethargic, prolapse of veins and organs	poor digestion with gas, bloating, or loose stool, muscle weakness, water retention, a feeling of heaviness, easy bruising or swelling
Lung:	melancholic, sentimental, self-pitying, dryness or coarseness of skin, lack of perspiration	emotionally numb, coughing, sneezing, wheezing, breathlessness, excessive mucus in sinuses, nose, throat, or bronchi, vulnerable, sensitive skin and mucous membranes

293

| *Kidney:* | suspicious, cynical, despairing, inert, early aging or diminution of mental and sensory acuity, swelling or edema of face, hands, ankles, or feet | stiffness or soreness of low back, hips, knees, infertility, impotence, diminished libido, weak bladder |

CONSTITUTIONAL FORMULAS

People are not simple, nor are their diseases. Formulas are often complex, combining many ingredients to address a multiplicity of contending needs. To be truly comprehensive, prescriptions address not only the complaints people have, but also their constitutional dynamics. Sometimes it is not possible to solve all problems simultaneously, so the herbalist sets priorities and chooses a path of action. In the example that follows, one formula deals directly with a patient's urgent condition (disease specific) and a second one with the fundamental, underlying conflicts (constitutional pattern) out of which his health difficulties arise.

Michael, a ruddy-faced forty-seven-year-old engineer, sought herbal medicine after a routine medical exam alerted him to high blood pressure (150/95). Before prescribing antihypertensive medication, his physician allowed him a few months to reduce his blood pressure, suggesting exercise, dietary changes, and stress reduction. He had sore, red-rimmed eyes, occasional but severe sinus headaches, bouts of dizziness, a red tongue, a taut, rapid pulse, and tender, tight neck and shoulder muscles.

His condition suggested a pattern of pressure and congestion in the *Liver Network*. It is not unusual for excess *Liver Qi* to rise swiftly, changing into *Heat* and *Wind* as it reaches the face and head. In this case *Heat* manifested as sinusitis, sore eyes, and a red tongue, and *Wind* became dizziness and pain. If Michael's jammed-up *Liver Qi* could dissipate and cool, his blood pressure would normalize. The herbal strategy was to purge the excess *Heat* and *Wind* (*Yang*) while tonifying *Moisture* and *Blood* (*Yin*).

Some of the herbs that treat Michael's condition are contained in the module for purging *Heat*, which includes bupleurum and scutellaria, which eliminate *Heat* from the *Liver* and *Lung*. Another module—for dispersing *Blood*—contains motherwort and ligusticum, which improve coronary and cerebral circulation by decongesting *Blood* and *Qi*. These two modules are combined with the one to supplement the *Kidney*, which contains eucommia, rehmannia, and alisma to nurture *Yin* (*Essence* and *Blood*) and disperse *Moisture*. Strengthening *Yin*, clearing *Heat*, and dispersing *Blood* help control the *excess* of *Yang* that is manifesting as high blood pressure, muscle tension, dizziness, sinusitis, and sore eyes. After taking this formula for three weeks, Michael was relieved of dizziness and sore eyes, his blood pressure decreased to a safe level, and he felt more relaxed.

The underlying constitutional dynamic for Michael is a pattern of conflict between the *Liver* and *Lung*. Disharmony develops between these *Networks* when *Liver Qi* becomes congested and rises too vigorously, blocking the descent of *Lung Qi* and increasing tension in the neck and head. Michael had been under pressure at work to complete a difficult project on a tight deadline, consumed a few more drinks than usual to relax at night, and had been eating foods that were probably too rich for him. Mental aggravation or overconsumption of alcohol and fatty foods exaggerated his predisposition to this disharmony. This disharmony produced feelings of discontent, pressure in the chest or abdomen, or cramps in the arms and legs due to a restricted blood flow. After Michael's blood pressure normalized, he was given a constitutional formula to reconcile the *Liver-Lung* relationship.

HARMONIZING ORGAN NETWORK RELATIONSHIPS

Different people have different patterns of conflict that reflect their constitutional dynamics. Key problems often arise between the *Five Phases* along the *ke* sequence—this refers to distorted interactions occurring between the *Lung-Liver*, *Liver-Spleen*, *Spleen-Kidney*, *Kidney-Heart*, and *Heart-Lung*. Since we define problems within the context of these relationships, we designed constitutional remedies called "harmonizing formulas" to reconcile these primary conflicts.

In the healthy individual, the role and function of the *Organ Networks* are complementary—that is, they balance each other and maintain the necessary tension that keeps us active and alive. However, if tension develops into friction, what was complementary becomes antagonistic. *Heart (Fire)* and *Kidney (Water)* should complement each other so that warmth *(Yang)* and moisture *(Yin)* are evenly distributed throughout the body. If friction or conflict ensues, warmth will turn to *Heat* in the upper regions, leading to *Dryness* and thirst, and *Moisture* will accumulate below, leading to *Dampness* or *Cold* in the lower regions. Reorganizing these patterns of conflict is the purpose of the harmonizing formulas, the usefulness of which is clearer after having read the typology section of this book, which elaborates upon the psychological and physiological manifestations of *Organ Network* disharmonies.

METAL-WOOD: LUNG-LIVER

To harmonize *Lung-Liver* is to reconcile *Metal* and *Wood*. This is accomplished by tonifying *Blood* and *Moisture*, dispersing *Blood* and *Qi*, and purging *Heat* and *Wind*. This formula contains bupleurum, white peony, and cyperus, which keep the *Liver* cool, relaxed, and decongested. These same herbs relieve spasm of blood vessels, nerves, and muscles, especially in the diaphragm, and fullness or pain of the liver and gallbladder. Chrysanthemum and *Morus* resolve inflammation and congestion of the upper-respiratory tract and eyes; and platycodon, fritillary, and licorice soothe and moisturize the *Lungs* and eliminate phlegm.

Therapeutic goal:

> tonify *Blood* and *Moisture*
> disperse *Blood* and *Qi*
> purge *Heat*, *Wind*, and phlegm

WOOD-EARTH: LIVER-SPLEEN

This formula harmonizes *Liver-Spleen* and makes peace between *Wood* and *Earth*. The herbs used here regulate digestion, blood circulation, and the distribution of *Nutritive Essence*, the source of *Qi* and *Blood*. The herbs bupleurum, peony, and angelica relax *Liver Qi* and nurture and distribute *Blood*. Ripe citrus and saussurea warm and activate the *Spleen* and *Stomach*, promote digestion, and relieve accumulated *Moisture*. Peppermint and licorice dispel *Wind* and *Heat* and counteract spasm and tension. This formula adjusts and subdues the appetite and corrects indigestion associated with gas, acidity, and queasiness. It also relieves constipation due to tension in the abdomen and allays the irritability, bloating, and lethargy of premenstrual distress.

Therapeutic goal:

> tonify *Blood*
> disperse *Qi*, *Blood*, *Moisture*
> disperse food accumulation
> purge *Wind* and *Heat*

EARTH-WATER: SPLEEN-KIDNEY

The formula to harmonize *Spleen-Kidney* stabilizes *Earth* and *Water*. By redistributing *Moisture* and promoting circulation of *Qi* and *Blood*, the herbs in this formula help to overcome stiffness, swelling, and inertia. Poria, atractylodes, and ripe citrus rid the *Spleen* of *Dampness* and circulate *Qi*, while alisma and cinnamon remove surplus fluids (*Moisture* and *Blood*) from cavities, joints, and tissue. Astragalus and euryales support the *Qi* of both *Spleen* and *Kidney* and protect them from being overly drained. This formula relieves dryness of skin and mouth, soreness of the joints, puffiness of the face, hands, and feet, the feeling of heaviness in the head and limbs, diarrhea, and difficult urination.

Therapeutic goal: consolidate *Moisture (Essence)* and *Qi*
                   disperse *Qi*, *Moisture*, and *Blood*
                   purge *Moisture (Dampness)*

WATER-FIRE: KIDNEY-HEART

To harmonize *Kidney-Heart* a formula must reunite *Essence (Jing)* and *Spirit (Shen)*, *Water* and *Fire*. Cooked rehmannia and schizandra nurture and consolidate *Essence*, *Blood*, and *Moisture*, while salvia and polygala soothe the *Spirit* and vitalize the *Blood*. As assisting herbs anemarrhena protects *Yin* by supplementing *Moisture* and clearing *Heat*, while motherwort and cardamom respectively encourage the downward flow of *Blood* and stabilize and warm the *Qi*. This rectifies the lack of concordance between *Heart* and *Kidney* that results in problems like insomnia, sexual and emotional anxiety, excessive perspiration and nervousness, lumbar weakness, fatigue, and intense mood swings.

Therapeutic goal: tonify *Blood* and *Moisture*
                   consolidate *Moisture (Essence)*
                   disperse *Blood*
                   purge upper *Heat*, lower *Cold*
                   calm *Spirit*

FIRE-METAL: HEART-LUNG

The *Heart-Lung* harmonizing formula soothes and cools the friction that antagonizes *Fire* and *Metal*, calming the mind and freeing the breath. Lily bulb, trichosanthes fruit, and licorice lubricate and moisturize the *Lungs*, skin, eyes, nose, throat, and intestines. Ganoderma, polygala, and schizandra quiet the psyche, settle the nerves, nurture the *Blood*, stabilize the *Qi*, and regulate perspiration. To give support, ripe citrus, platycodon, and pinellia mobilize and disperse *Qi* and phlegm from the chest and throat, reducing congestion, constriction, and pain. This formula eases mental stress, adjusts body temperature by adjusting perspiration and respiration, stops coughing, aids expectoration, and quenches thirst. It also relieves dryness and inflammation of the skin, throat, bronchi, and intestines.

Therapeutic goal: tonify *Blood* and *Moisture*
                   consolidate *Qi* and *Moisture*
                   disperse *Qi* and *Blood*
                   purge *Heat* and phlegm

297

Organ Network Disharmonies: Key Patterns

Organ Disharmony	Psychic Patterns	Somatic Patterns
Liver-Spleen	emotionally overreactive and ambivalent, impulsive and vacillating, irritable and yielding, unpredictable periods of intense activity or sudden lethargy	variable appetite, indigestion, irregular elimination, uncontrollable or vague cravings, distension and cramping of stomach or intestines, body or headache with feeling of pressure, swelling, and heaviness
Spleen-Kidney	competing desires for closeness and isolation, sharing and acquisitiveness, involvement and escape, activity and passivity	flabby muscles, weakness of spine, low back, ankles, or feet, swollen or enlarged ovaries or prostate, edema around abdomen, hips, legs, or ankles and difficulty losing weight, sensitive to dryness, humidity, and cold
Kidney-Heart	the desire for affection, intimacy, and excitement contends with the need for solitude, detachment, and quietude, unpredictable periods of heightened and diminished libido	occasionally excessive or scanty urination, variable requirements for a lot or very little sleep, hands and feet swell in hot weather and ache in cold weather
Heart-Lung	sometimes spontaneous, excitable, and anxious, sometimes melancholic, subdued, and inhibited	frequent bowel movements or constipation, frequent or scanty urination, dry cough or irritation of nose, sinuses, or pharynx without mucus or phlegm, dry skin yet perspires easily or frequently, sometimes extremely hungry or thirsty, especially for cold foods and liquids, difficulty gaining weight

| Lung-Liver | alternately spontaneous, impulsive, volatile or inhibited, prudent, and diffident; shifting moods: grouchy, sensitive, reactive, morose, defensive, unresponsive | wheezing or constriction of chest, tightness and pain of diaphragm and ribs, irritable colon or irregular bowel movements, lack of peristalsis: difficulty swallowing, distension of stomach, or constipation, allergic inflammation of sinuses, throat, ears, bronchi |

SELF-ASSESSMENT PROFILE

Some of you may find this chapter most useful after you have begun working with a practitioner—you will then be motivated to understand the thinking behind the choices that have been made in your treatment. Others of you may choose to educate yourselves in advance of working with a professional and will appreciate being able to increase your self-understanding with the aid of the charts that follow.

SYMPTOM PATTERNS OF DEPLETION AND CONGESTION

Patterns of Depletion: Deficiency and Slackness

Symptoms of Deficiency
General: weakness, fatigue, malaise, sensitivity, poor resistance

Deficient Qi:
____ weakness, lethargy, or weariness
____ lowered libido
____ decreased motivation
____ dull thinking, sensing, or feeling (lack of affect)
____ poor appetite
____ weak digestion
____ susceptible to colds or flus
____ prolonged recovery following illness
____ pasty, pale complexion
____ limp hair
____ shortness of breath
____ averse to talking

_____ perspires easily with exertion
_____ weak muscles
_____ chills easily
_____ frequent, profuse urination
_____ infertility
_____ miscarriage
_____ dull, soft nails
_____ pale, enlarged tongue with thin fur
_____ weak, soft, slow pulse

Therapy: herbs to tonify *Qi*

Deficient Moisture:
_____ dry and thirsty
_____ dryness of mucous membranes
_____ scant secretions and urination
_____ constipation
_____ uncomfortable feeling of heat in the body
_____ restlessness and insomnia
_____ low fever in the afternoon or evening
_____ parched and cracked skin
_____ emotional lability
_____ hot flashes
_____ night sweats
_____ constant hunger, sometimes with loss of weight
_____ unstable blood sugar
_____ persistent dry cough
_____ dry or sore throat
_____ dry, brittle nails
_____ flushed face with dry skin and lips
_____ dry, reddened tongue without fur
_____ rapid, thin, or weak pulse

Therapy: herbs to tonify *Moisture*

Deficient Blood:
_____ restless fatigue
_____ irritability
_____ poor sleep
_____ itching, prickling skin or scalp
_____ dryness without thirst
_____ blurred or weak vision
_____ loss or thinning of hair
_____ dizziness

_____ dry or hard stool
_____ premature aging of skin
_____ dry skin, eyes, hair
_____ anemia
_____ numbness of hands and feet
_____ muscle cramps
_____ lack of semen
_____ scanty or irregular menstruation
_____ pale, waxy, sallow complexion
_____ easy bruising
_____ poor skin healing
_____ palpitations
_____ postpartum weakness or anemia
_____ pale, opaque, thin, weak nails
_____ pale pink or orange tongue and lips
_____ weak, thin, or irregular pulse

Therapy: herbs to tonify *Blood*

Symptoms of Slackness

General: lack of tone (prolapse, flaccidity), lack of focus, dissipation (wasting or ebbing of strength), loss of tissue integrity, vulnerability, instability

Slack Qi:

_____ atony or prolapse of stomach, intestines, anus
_____ fecal incontinence or constant diarrhea
_____ hemorrhoids
_____ dizzy or weak after meal or bowel movement
_____ loose or flaccid muscles
_____ flabby tongue
_____ very weak or disappearing pulse

Therapy: herbs to consolidate *Qi*

Slack Moisture:

_____ excess secretion from eyes, nose, mouth, skin, vagina
_____ seminal incontinence or premature ejaculation
_____ frequent urination, enuresis, or incontinence
_____ dizzy or weak following sex
_____ very buoyant but thin pulse

Therapy: herbs to consolidate *Moisture*

Slack Blood:

_____ excessive or prolonged bleeding from skin, nose, lungs, stomach, intestines, bladder

_____ ulcers of skin, mucous membrane, stomach, intestines

_____ excessive bleeding during menses, pregnancy, or postpartum

_____ bleeding hemorrhoids

_____ anemia associated with inflammation of stomach, small intestine, or large intestine

_____ very thin and irregular pulse

Therapy: herbs to consolidate *Blood*

Patterns of Congestion: Stagnation and Obstruction

Symptoms of Stagnation

General: soreness, tenderness, spasms, retention, irregularity

Stagnant Qi:

_____ head feels stuffy

_____ distension or fullness in chest or abdomen

_____ mild nausea

_____ gas pains, cramps, tension in stomach or intestines

_____ hiccups, belching, or flatulence

_____ constipation with gas

_____ vague or migratory pains

_____ taut pulse

Therapy: herbs to disperse *Qi*

Stagnant Moisture:

_____ soft or loose stool

_____ bloating with water retention

_____ puffy eyes, face, hands, or ankles

_____ frequent but scanty urination

_____ feels swollen, tender, lethargic in humid weather

_____ soft swellings or enlarged lymph nodes

_____ premenstrual soreness and swelling of breasts

_____ soft pulse

Therapy: herbs to disperse *Moisture*

Stagnant Blood:

      _____ mottling or chilliness of limbs from poor circulation

      _____ sharp pains in head, eyes, joints, internal organs

      _____ irregular or painful menses

      _____ premenstrual pain and hardness of breasts

      _____ painful hemorrhoids or cysts

      _____ elevated cholesterol

      _____ uneven pulse

Therapy: herbs to disperse *Blood*

Symptoms of Obstruction

    General: severe pain and discomfort, emotionally distraught

Obstructed Qi:

      _____ generalized discomfort, fullness, pressure in the head, chest, limbs, or abdomen

      _____ belching and flatulence

      _____ wheezing

      _____ difficulty swallowing

      _____ stitch or acute pain in abdomen

      _____ thickened tongue fur

      _____ fullness under ribs

      _____ tense, full pulse

Therapy: herbs to purge *Qi*

Obstructed Moisture:

      _____ swollen or heavy head, limbs, or abdomen

      _____ tender muscles and joints

      _____ thick or sticky saliva or phlegm

      _____ sticky perspiration

      _____ lumps, nodules, and cysts

      _____ sticky or slimy stool

      _____ scanty urine

      _____ generalized water retention

      _____ edema of hands and feet

      _____ thick nauseated feeling in mouth and stomach

      _____ congestion in the eyes and sinuses

      _____ enlarged or swollen tongue with thick, cheesy fur

      _____ slippery or soft, large pulse

Therapy: herbs to purge *Moisture*

Obstructed Blood:

_____ traumatic bruises, swellings, and sprains

_____ persistent localized, stabbing, or throbbing pains (especially in joints or viscera)

_____ pain aggravated at night or from inactivity

_____ severe cramping, numbness, or paralysis

_____ severe headache

_____ dark red complexion

_____ red or purple lesions on skin and mucous membrane

_____ angina

_____ severe menstrual cramps with dark blood or clots

_____ pain worse from pressure or massage

_____ hard, fixed lumps

_____ purplish or dark red tongue or spots on tongue

_____ strong or tense, intermittent pulse

Therapy: herbs to purge *Blood*

Patterns of Penetration or Accumulation of Adverse Climates

Heat:

_____ fever, associated with infection or inflammation

_____ pain, soreness, swelling, or dryness accompanied by a sensation of heat or burning

_____ sores or infections with green or yellow pus

_____ yellow or green mucous discharges from ears, nose, throat, anus, vagina, or urethra

_____ extreme thirst with a craving for cold foods and liquids

_____ reddening of eyes, ears, nose, lips, face, skin, mucous membrane, or tongue

_____ yellow tongue fur

_____ worse from exposure to heat or dryness

_____ red tongue and/or yellow fur

Therapy: herbs to purge *Heat*

Cold:

_____ cold feeling in the limbs, head, chest, or abdomen

_____ inertia or weakness with pallor, cold or clammy face, hands, or feet

____ loose stool after eating raw or cold foods

____ profuse urination or swelling of face or limbs upon exposure to cold climate or after drinking cold liquids

____ craving for warm, cooked foods and hot drinks

____ pain in head, chest, limbs, or joints when exposed to cold air

____ pale skin, nail beds, lips, mucous membrane, or tongue

____ thickened, white tongue fur

____ soft or tense, slow, and deep pulse

____ purplish tongue and/or thick white fur

____ very slow and/or tense pulse

Therapy: herbs to purge *Cold*

Wind:

____ erratic spasms, cramps, or contractures of skin, nerves, vessels, muscles, and viscera

____ itching, prickling, twitching, and other discomfiting sensations in the skin and muscles

____ migrating pains appear or retreat suddenly and unpredictably

____ dizziness, uncoordinated movement, and disequilibrium

____ itchy, painful ears, eyes, nose, sneezing, headache, muscle soreness, or shivering when exposed to wind or drafts

____ trembling or shaking of the hands, feet, head

____ spasm or quivering of tongue

____ taut or wiry pulse

Therapy: herbs to purge *Wind*

Phlegm (congealed Dampness):

____ dizziness or fullness in head with mucus congestion or nausea

____ nausea or difficult breathing with fullness in upper abdomen or chest

____ thick, sticky secretions or discharges from the skin, mucous membrane, ears, eyes, nose, throat, mouth, anus, vagina, or urethra

____ soft, mobile lumps or enlarged lymph nodes

____ worse in humid environment or from eating sticky, greasy, fatty foods, milk products, eggs, or sugar

____ sticky or oily tongue fur

____ full, sliding pulse

Therapy: herbs to purge phlegm

Symptom Patterns of *Organ Network Deficiency* or Disturbance

Liver Network:

—— easily irritated*

—— sensitive to wind, noise, strong odors, and tastes

—— muscle tension or cramps, especially in neck, shoulders, lower abdomen, hips, calves*

—— weak or blurry vision

—— dry eyes

—— coarse brittle nails or hair

—— numbness or tingling in limbs when asleep or inactive

—— easy chilling of arms, hands, legs, feet*

—— difficult elimination, dry stool, tense colon*

—— weak, dizzy, flushed from hunger, tension, or anger*

—— irregular and/or scanty menstruation

—— nausea or queasiness from hunger or fatigue*

—— genital organ hypersensitivity

—— stitching pains in ribs, beneath diaphragm, groin, and pelvic region*

—— cravings for sour, spicy, fatty foods

—— tinnitus characterized by whistling or ringing

—— PMS characterized by symptoms marked above with asterisk*

—— aggravations from heat, wind, and drafts

—— very tense or wiry pulse

Therapy: herbs to supplement and protect the *Liver*

Heart Network:

—— easily confused

—— fatigue with anxiety and restlessness*

—— slight exertion or excitement causes heat, perspiration*

—— insomnia or palpitations when nervous, worried, or overtired*

—— frequent urination and bowel movements from nervousness

—— burning, sensitivity, or irritation of mouth, tongue, urethra, vagina, or anus*

—— dry mouth or throat with craving for cool drinks and juicy foods

—— easy blushing of face and ears

—— easily hot, easily cold*

—— anxiety and fatigue cause light, restless sleep and vivid dreams or nightmares*

—— cravings for spicy, hot, and sweet foods

—— PMS characterized by symptoms marked above with asterisk*

____ aggravations from heat and dryness

____ large or bounding pulse

Therapy: herbs to supplement and protect the *Heart*

Spleen Network:

____ easily worried

____ upset by changes*

____ overwhelmed by details*

____ lethargy and inertia*

____ slow digestion of food

____ frequent abdominal gas and bloating*

____ lingering hunger after meals

____ cravings for sweets and starchy foods*

____ heaviness of head and limbs*

____ water retention and puffiness*

____ loose stool from eating raw or cold foods and liquids

____ tender muscles*

____ easy or frequent bruising

____ lack of muscle tone or strength, especially of abdomen, back, or neck

____ prolapse of stomach, intestines, uterus, vagina, bladder

____ hemorrhoids

____ frequent but scanty urination

____ PMS characterized by symptoms marked above with asterisk*

____ aggravations from cold and dampness

____ full and soft or sliding pulse

Therapy: herbs to supplement and protect the *Spleen*

Lung Network:

____ frequent colds

____ frequent rhinitis or sinusitis*

____ cough with or without phlegm

____ frequent throat clearing or laryngitis*

____ morning attacks of coughing or sneezing with clear phlegm or mucus discharge*

____ sensitive to wind, cold, and dryness*

____ dry skin and mucous membrane, especially of face, nose, and mouth*

____ shortness of breath, chest pain, or wheezing in chest from fatigue or exertion

____ easily disappointed or offended*

____ craves spicy, juicy, sweet foods and stimulants

_____ PMS characterized by symptoms marked above with asterisk*

_____ aggravations from heat, cold, and dryness

_____ tense and buoyant pulse

Therapy: herbs that supplement and protect the *Lung*

Kidney Network:

_____ sore throats from fatigue*

_____ frequent or difficult urination*

_____ puffiness or swelling of feet and ankles*

_____ puffiness around eyes*

_____ dull hearing

_____ tinnitus characterized by low humming

_____ low back pain or soreness*

_____ weakness or soreness of hips, knees, ankles, or feet*

_____ diminished libido*

_____ diminished motivation*

_____ lack of sexual secretions

_____ infertility or difficulty conceiving and/or going to term

_____ loss or thinning of pubic hair

_____ loss of stamina

_____ needs to sleep a lot*

_____ easily depressed and disgruntled*

_____ anemia

_____ amenorrhea

_____ menopause or PMS characterized by symptoms marked above with asterisk*

_____ forgetful and dull-minded

_____ aggravations from cold, sex, and lack of rest

_____ deep and small or firm pulse

Therapy: herbs that supplement and protect the *Kidney*

Symptom Patterns of *Organ Network* Relationships

Liver-Spleen Disharmony:

_____ cold hands and feet

_____ hot flashes

_____ indigestion with nausea, bloating, flatulence, belching

_____ erratic elimination with constipation or diarrhea

____ spasm of esophagus

____ dryness and water retention

____ thirst for alternately cold and hot liquids

____ sensitivity and/or aversion to strong flavors

____ cravings for fatty, sour, sweet, or sticky foods

____ erratic appetite with difficulty knowing what to eat or feeling dissatisfied with food

____ tenderness, tension, or heaviness in muscles, especially head, neck, shoulders, jaw, arms, and legs

____ fullness or pressure in head or behind eyes

____ headaches with nausea, visual disturbances, or dizziness

____ sensitivity or aversion to light, noise, heat, and humidity

____ abdominal tension or distension with belching or flatulence

____ vascillates between assertiveness and ambivalence

____ alternates between nervous tension and languid lethargy

____ sometimes irritable and hostile, sometimes tolerant and sympathetic

Characteristic health problems:
   hypoglycemia
   diabetes
   cirrhosis
   jaundice/hepatitis
   eating disorders
   food allergies
   hives
   colitis
   migraine

Therapy: herbs that harmonize *Liver* and *Spleen*

Spleen-Kidney:

____ slow digestion and sluggish intestines

____ weak gums and loose teeth

____ dryness of skin and mouth

____ sore or swollen joints or muscles, especially of face, hands, or feet

____ heaviness of head or limbs

____ weakness or soreness of low back and sacrum

____ feet, legs, and back tire easily

____ diarrhea or dry, small stools with bloating

____ frequent, scanty, or difficult urination

____ alternately strong and diminished libido

____ easy chill of back, legs, and arms

____ constipation and water retention follow overeating

309

_____ craves salty or sweet foods

_____ nervous and distractible

_____ apathetic and insecure

Characteristic health problems:
    edema
    rheumatism
    adrenal insufficiency (Addison's disease)
    leucorrhea
    chronic gingivitis
    chronic cystitis or urethritis
    prostatic hypertrophy or prostatitis

Therapy: herbs that harmonize *Spleen* and *Kidney*

Kidney-Heart:

_____ insomnia or restless sleep alternating with heavy slumber followed by difficulty awakening and arising from bed

_____ nervousness and mood swings along with fatigue and lumbar weakness

_____ easily overheated or chilled

_____ hot chest, head, and hands with cold buttocks and feet

_____ easily excited but difficult to sustain effort and enthusiasm

_____ strength easily dissipated by hyperactivity

_____ depressed or melancholy after sustained mental or physical activity

_____ sexually excitable but unable to sustain desire or achieve satisfactory release

_____ lack of muscle tone and joint mobility

_____ anxiety and apathy

_____ tension and weakness of muscles along the spine

_____ nausea, diarrhea, urinary frequency associated with anxiety

_____ craves salty, spicy food and stimulants (nicotine, caffeine)

Characteristic health problems:
    manic-depressive syndrome
    ileitis (Crohn's disease)
    bulimia
    phobias
    chronic endometritis/cervicitis/urethritis
    chronic sleep disturbances
    hyper-/hypothyroid syndrome

Therapy: herbs that harmonize *Kidney* and *Heart*

Heart-Lung:

- ____ sensitive to changes in temperature and humidity
- ____ easily overheated but can't sweat
- ____ dry cough
- ____ flushes when coughing
- ____ coughing when nervous or embarrassed
- ____ anxiety with laryngitis, chest pain, or wheezing
- ____ heat triggers sneezing, itchy throat, or rashes
- ____ dry skin with cracking, redness, and itching, especially upper back, elbows, knees, and hands
- ____ light sleeper and wakes easily
- ____ itching and inflammation of vagina or urethra without discharge
- ____ alternately euphoric and melancholic
- ____ emotionally hypersensitive yet reserved
- ____ craves spicy, hot foods and stimulants

Characteristic health problems:

acne or dry eczema
sun allergy
psoriasis
asthma
hyperthyroidism
hysteria
chronic pharyngitis/rhinitis
chronic vaginitis

Therapy: herbs that harmonize *Heart* and *Lung*

Lung-Liver Disharmony:

- ____ tension and stiffness of muscles of neck, shoulders, chest, abdomen, and hips
- ____ irregular bowel movements
- ____ irregular, heavy, or shallow breathing
- ____ wheezing or sighing
- ____ sensitive, easily inflamed skin or mucous membranes of upper respiratory or genitourinary tissues
- ____ sensitivity and/or aversion to heat, dryness, wind, and droughts or sudden changes in weather
- ____ awkward and stiff expression of personal feelings
- ____ unpredictably reactive or indifferent, angry or sad, friendly or distant
- ____ craving for fatty and spicy foods

Characteristic health problems:
acne
asthma
irritable bowel syndrome
generalized pruritus
allergic sinusitis or rhinitis
seasonal hay fever
bursitis
headaches involving eyes and sinuses
severe or chronic torticollis (neck spasm)
depression characterized by quiet melancholy or
passive rage

Therapy: herbs that harmonize *Lung* and *Liver*

PREPARING HERBAL TEA

Herbal formulas may be taken as tea, concentrated fluid extracts, syrup, tablets, powder, or in combination with food. Although freshly brewed medicinal herbs are gradually giving way to industrial methods of extraction and tableting, drinking a decoction or infusion is still an effective way to derive the benefit of herbs. The ritual of personally cooking the herbs may be laborious, but it can be worth the investment of time and energy—herbs are easily assimilated in this form, producing rapid results. Some formulas are bitter, so Americans unaccustomed to drinking beverages that do not taste pleasant have the option of ingesting these same formulas as powders or pills.

To make an herbal tea (a water extract or decoction), the herbs are boiled in a glass, ceramic, or stainless-steel container so that the metal or plastic in iron, aluminum, or nonstick cookware does not spoil the tea. A formula usually consists of $1/2$ to 2 ounces of herbal material.

To cook the herbs, simmer them in 4–6 cups of water (depending on the quantity of ingredients) for 30–60 minutes in a covered vessel until 1 cup of liquid remains after straining. Repeat the cooking process using the same herbs with 1 cup less water. Combine the 2 cups from both boilings and drink the liquid while warm in four equal doses over the course of two to four days. The tea can be refrigerated for up to four days and reheated as needed. It is best to drink herbs in the morning and evening $1/2$ hour before or $1\frac{1}{2}$ hours after a meal.

Varying the quantity and frequency of an herbal tea determines the force of its effects. This controls the rate and intensity of the healing process according to individual needs and tolerances. People who are generally healthy and robust can tolerate stronger tea more often than those who are chronically ill or debilitated. Young and middle-aged adults can handle a higher dosage and greater frequency of herbal medicine than infants, children, or the elderly; and those with serious complaints may require more aggressive treatment than those who have mild or transient disturbances. Children under age four have ¹/₄ the standard dose; those from age five to twelve have ¹/₂ the standard dose. Dose (concentration) can be altered either by giving a smaller amount or by diluting with water and giving the same amount: adding an equal quantity of water reduces the concentration by half, adding twice as much diminishes it by three-fourths, and so on. Dilution may also improve the palatability of the tea.

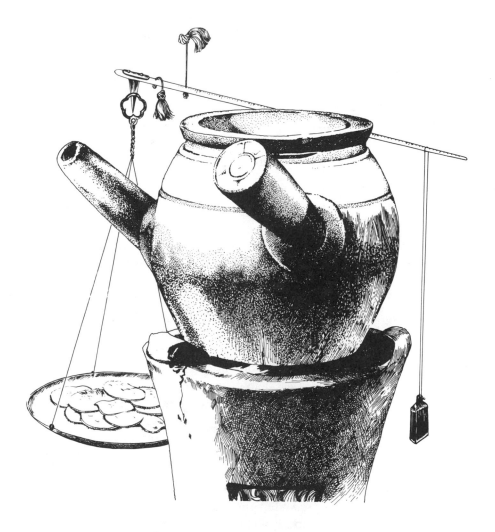

Chinese Herbal Teapot and Scale   313

Cold (refrigerated), greasy, spicy, and sour foods should generally be avoided during the process of taking medicinal herbs, especially in acute or debilitating illnesses, since they may undermine or neutralize the effects of the herbs. The simpler and more moderate the diet during the treatment process, the greater the benefit of the herbs.

USING CHINESE PATENT MEDICINES

Herbal prescriptions are either tailored to fit the individual patient or designed to fit general conditions. Ready-made formulas for general conditions are called patent medicines. As with footwear or clothes before the advent of factories, a shoemaker or dressmaker drew a pattern from the individual and cut the leather and cloth to match that shape, customizing each shirt, skirt, trouser, and boot. Then mass production developed, and as general sizes and shapes became available to the public, people chose what best fit them.

Chinese pharmacists still measure single ingredients on hand-held scales, mixing formulas for individual patients to take home and brew into tea. But herbal pharmaceutical factories also compress raw ingredients or extracts into pills, which are then bottled and sold in apothecary shops, side by side with individual herbs. Because they are ready to use without brewing, patent medicines are convenient. Because individualized prescriptions conform exactly to the problem and person being treated, they are sometimes indispensable. The use of patent medicines demands some familiarity with their indications, while formulating a prescription from scratch usually requires knowledge of the properties and qualities of many individual herbs.

When I traveled to the Chinese city of Guangzhou in 1985, a Chinese friend who had owned his own herbal factories in 1946 (which were nationalized following the revolution in 1949) invited me to observe the processing, extraction, and manufacture of herbal patent medicines at three factories that his nephew now managed.

In the factory, chemists and workers dressed in snowy white aprons, hats, masks, and slippers worked below towering stainless-steel vats in which extracts were made from cooking herbal decoctions. In another area, tumblers resembling Laundromat dryers mixed powdered raw herbs with honey into a thick paste to be shaped into pellets. The factory managers were very proud of the sophisticated packaging equipment that stamped out the finished product. I was as impressed by how tasty some of these medicines were—like a sort of licorice-molasses candy. At lunch, some of the same herbs in the pellets were served at the restaurant. The taste of some herbs allow their inclusion in soups, whereas others demanded ingestion as pills.

Patent medicines are marketed worldwide from factories in Hong Kong,

Japan, Taiwan, and the People's Republic of China. Hundreds of remedies are available in Chinatown herb shops, the vast majority of which are based on traditional formulas. Gradually, however, industrious American herbalists and entrepreneurs are developing and manufacturing their own products. Remedies exist for a vast array of disorders ranging from high cholesterol to arthritis, PMS, migraine, infertility, and the common cold. A number of the most useful and available Asian and American products, their recommended uses and sources, are listed at the end of this chapter.

Since some products from Asia are made from extracts and others from raw herbs, the dosage varies from as few as 3–5 pills for extracts to 10–20 pills at a time for formulas using raw materials. The American tablets tend to be somewhat larger (500–750 grams) than their Asian counterparts in order to decrease the number of tablets for each dose: generally 2–4 tablets at a time, 1–3 times per day. Dosages for fluid extracts are about 1–4 milliliters (¼–1 teaspoon), depending on the concentration, 2–3 times per day.

As with herbal teas, pills or fluid extracts are usually taken on an empty stomach ½ hour before or 1 to 2 hours after eating. They are most effective swallowed with warm water since cold drinks inhibit the digestive function of the stomach. Dosages for children are proportionately less than for adults.

Intelligence, effort, and history permeate these piquant mixtures, and it is part of the alchemy of herbs that the body assimilates their value through sight, skin, and smell as well. In any form, Chinese herbal medicine provides wisdom you can swallow.

NO HOME SHOULD BE WITHOUT HERBAL FIRST AID

No home should be without certain formulas that help people overcome common problems like coughs, sore throats, stomachaches, bruises, fever, insomnia, and headaches. Chinese first aid can replace the need for many Western over-the-counter pharmaceuticals and remove the worry of their unpredictable adverse effects. Chinese herbs can be considered differently: they can do us good, along with getting rid of what bothers us. Using herbs is a positive gesture toward health as well as a means to soothe discomfort. For this reason some formulas can be used generously, like nutritional supplements, whereas Western pharmaceuticals are to be used sparingly and with caution.

For example, *Yin Chiao Chieh Tu Pien* ("yin chow chee dew peein"), a formula developed during the Ching dynasty and still popular today, is appropriate for symptoms such as sneezing, sniffles, and a sore, swollen throat associated with the common cold. Generally, symptoms of a cold or flu are regarded as an invasion of *Wind* and *Heat* attacking the surface, and *Yin Chiao* is a purging formula that expels *Heat* and *Wind* from the skin, muscles, upper-respiratory tract, and head.

Honeysuckle and forsythia are the primary herbs in *Yin Chiao*, used   315 together for their powerful antitoxic and antiinflammatory effect. They are assisted by arctium, lophatherum, and soja (fermented black soybeans), which also clear *Heat* and relieve thirst, muscle ache, sore throat, and swollen glands. Peppermint and schizonepeta clear *Wind* and promote perspiration, allaying headache and dizziness. Platycodon relieves cough and dispels phlegm. Licorice harmonizes these herbs, soothes the throat, and counteracts toxins. Since the *Lung* governs the skin, respiration, and perspiration, these herbs assist it in warding off noxious external influences like *Wind* and *Heat*.

This formula is used during the first stages of acute illnesses like colds and allergies, which are characterized by fever, headache, nasal congestion, thirst, cough, chills, sore throat, itching, and rashes. Many patients have been impressed by the quick demise of a cold after taking this remedy. They are pleased not to experience any of the unpleasant effects of pharmaceutical antihistamines or decongestants, like drowsiness or drying of the mucous membranes.

COMMON COLD

Taken at the very first signs of a runny nose or scratchy throat, six tablets of *Yin Chiao* or *Gan Mao Ling* ("gon mow ling"), repeated every three hours, can avert a cold before it has taken root. These remedies can really impress the novice who has not yet tried Chinese herbs. Once a cold or flu is in progress, if symptoms are primarily chills, body soreness, and headache, then the same dosage of *Zhong Gan Ling* ("jong gan ling") is appropriate. With nausea and diarrhea, Lopanthus Anti-Febrile pills (also known as *Huo Hsiang Cheng Chi Pien* ["hwa shang chung chee pien"]) are used. For a dry cough, or thirst with the cold or flu, a delicious instant beverage tea called *Lo Han Kuo* ("low han gwo") will soothe the throat, relieve the dryness, and assist expectoration. For coughs with sticky or yellow phlegm, Pinellia Expectorant (also known as *Qing Qi Hua Tan Wan* ["ching chee hwa tahn wahn"]) plus Fritillary-Loquat cough syrup are appropriate.

TRAUMA: INJURY OR SURGICAL

The Chinese province of Yunnan produces a secret "herbal treasure" of international fame called *Yunnan Pai Yao* ("you nahn bye yow"), known to be a lifesaving remedy for wounds, hemorrhages, shock, and infections. On many occasions we have given two capsules, three times a day, to our patients who undergo surgery or suffer traumatic injury. Several women took *Yunnan Pai Yao* following extensive cosmetic surgery, and the surgeon remarked on the low incidence of bruising and swelling and the rapidity of their recovery. This was also true for patients who had prostate, abdominal, foot, and dental surgery. In each case the attending Western physician was impressed by speedy recuperation and diminished loss of blood during the operation. This remedy is also useful for gum infections, menstrual cramps, hemorrhoids, ulcers, sprains, and other sorts of pain or inflammation. It can be taken two days before surgery to prevent postoperative swelling and infection; for seven to ten days after trauma or surgery; and during the period for menstrual cramping or excess bleeding. *Yunnan Pai Yao* should be used short-term for acute problems; it is not suitable during pregnancy or as a long-term tonic.

INDIGESTION

Curing Pills, both benign and versatile, are suitable for indigestion, diarrhea, hangovers, motion sickness, nausea, headache, reactions to MSG contaminated food, or overeating, and are indispensable for the traveler as a buffer against dysentery, jet lag, and the consequences of irregular sleeping and eating. For travelers in places where the water is of questionable quality, a vial with each meal can be taken prophylactically, along with the ordinary precautions. We have given this remedy to patients coming down with symptoms of stomach flu, and in many cases their nausea and headache have cleared within ten minutes. The appropriate dosage, one to three vials (as needed), strengthens digestion, clears congestion, detoxifies, and facilitates elimination. Each vial costs about fifteen cents. Curing Pills are a sort of digestive cure-all—a simple wonder in terms of versatility, low cost, and effectiveness.

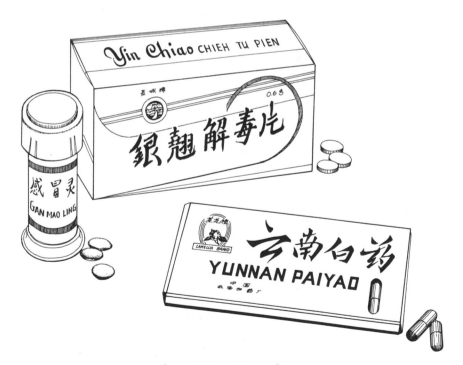

Some Patent Remedies

WOMEN'S PROBLEMS

To ameliorate menstrual and other reproductive problems, *Wu Chi Pai Feng Wan* pills ("woo chee bye fung wan") address many common complaints, including fatigue, water retention, moodiness, cramps, irregular cycle, and anemia. This formula can be used as a tonic before ovulation to replenish *Blood* and *Qi*, after ovulation to disperse premenstrual buildup of fluid and tension, and during the menstrual flow to relieve cramps and distension. For acute symptoms, ten pills four times a day is appropriate, whereas ten pills two times a day is adequate for long-term tonification.

ALLERGIES

For respiratory allergies with sneezing, itchy eyes and nose, cough, wheezing, postnasal drip, sore throat, and headache, *Bi Yan Pian* ("bee yan pien") is invaluable. In acute crisis, use six tablets four times a day until symptoms are relieved. To prevent attacks, use six tablets twice a day. This has helped countless people when pollen and grasses abound, in some cases, reducing or eliminating sensitivity to environmental irritants.

Fifty Common Patent Herbal Remedies and Their Uses

Colds

Two of the best cold remedies, especially good for head colds and sore throats	*Yin Chiao Chieh Tu Pien* *Gan Mao Ling*
Flu with headache, body ache, fever, chill	*Zhong Gan Ling*
Flu or cold with nausea, diarrhea, or digestive upset	Curing Pills
Upper-respiratory symptoms and gastrointestinal symptoms combined	Lopanthus Anti-Febrile *Huo Hsiang Cheng Chi Pien*
Thirst and dehydration	*Lo Han Kuo* tea

Coughs

Dry cough	*Lo Han Kuo* tea or *Lo Han Kuo* Cough Juice
Cough with profuse phlegm	Pinellia Expectorant Pills and Fritillary-Loquat syrup

Headaches

With colds or chills	*Chuan Xiong Chao Tiao Wan*
With hay fever-sinusitis	*Bi Yan Pian*
With indigestion	Curing Pills
With fever	*Yin Chiao Chieh Tu Pien* or *Zhong Gan Ling*
Migraine	Corydalis *Yan Hu Suo* Analgesic *Head-Q (HC)
Muscle tension-spasm	*Hsiao Yao Wan*
Mental tension or cerebral allergy syndrome	*Cyperus 18 (SF)

Digestive

Overeating, nausea, stomach upset, gas, dysentery, acute diarrhea or mild constipation, motion sickness	Curing Pills
Constipation (habitual)	Fructus Persica
Constipation with cramps, gas, or bloating	*Mu Xiang Shen Qi Wan*
Chronic diarrhea	*Liu Jun Zi Wan* and *Wu Ling San*
Dysentery or food poisoning	Curing and *Huang Lian Su*
Ulcers	*Bao He Wan*
Ulcers with pain	Add *Wei Te Ling*
Ulcers with bleeding	Add *Yunnan Bai Yao*

Insomnia

With anxiety and fatigue	Healthy Brain Pills
With tension-stress	*Schizandra Dreams (HC)

Genitourinary

Acute cystitis, prostatitis, urethritis	*Lung Tan Xie Gan Wan*
Chronic-recurring prostatitis	*Kai Kit Wan*
Chronic-recurring urethritis	*Passwan*
Acute vaginitis	*Yu Dai Wan*
Chronic-recurring vaginitis	*Chien Chin Chih Tai Wan*

*American-manufactured products:
HC = Health Concerns; SF = Seven Forests

Rheumatic Pain

With muscle or joint pain   *Qi Ye Lien* Analgesic
With numbness or nerve pain   *AC-Q(HC)

Pain

Of internal organs   Corydalis *Yan Hu Suo* Analgesic
Due to trauma or infection-   *Yunnan Pai Yao*
  inflammation

Hemorrhoids

Painful   Fargelin High Strength
Bleeding   *Yunnan Pai Yao*

Trauma

Postsurgical recovery, injury,   *Yunnan Pai Yao*
  sprain, fracture, inflammation,
  infection, menstrual pain with
  excessive bleeding, hemorrhage,
  shock, pain

Allergies

Generalized   *Cyperus 18 (SF)
  hay fever, sinusitis   *Bi Yan Pian*
Food sensitivities   Lopanthus Anti-Febrile pills (*Hou Hsiang Cheng Chi Pien*)

Menstrual Problems

Irregularity, scanty or excessive   *Wu Chi Pai Feng Wan* (condensed)
  flow and weakness
PMS   *Hsiao Yao Wan*
Generalized abdominal-pelvic-   *Qi Ye Lian*
  lumbosacral pain   Corydalis *Yan Hu Suo* Analgesic
Acute uterine cramps

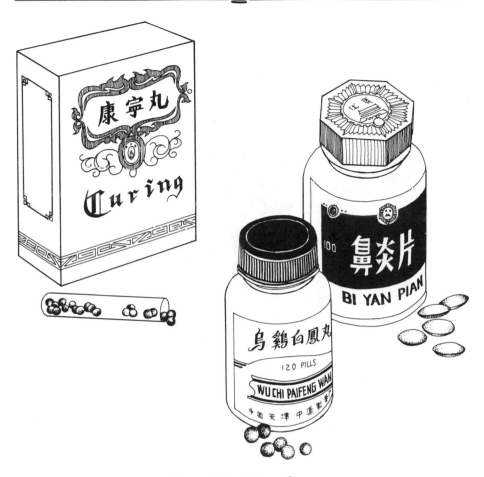

Some Patent Remedies

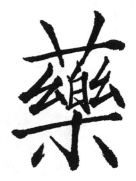

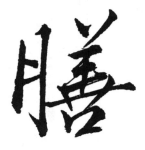

Culinary Alchemy:
Herbal Food, Kitchen Medicine

CHAPTER FIFTEEN

CULINARY ALCHEMY: HERBAL FOOD, KITCHEN MEDICINE

In the misty era before the Han tribes coalesced into the beginnings of the Chinese race, the first mythical hero to emerge was Fu Hsi. The main activities of this god-like fabled figure were hunting and fishing, and to him is attributed the invention of the kitchen and cooking. The next legendary figure in early Chinese mythology was Shen Nung, the Divine Husbandman. To him goes credit for the plow, the hoe and the care of farm animals. Huang Ti, the Yellow Emperor and the patron saint of Taoism, is worshipped still for the conception of planting grain and the invention of the pestle and mortar to crush it to make flour. The hunter, the husbandman and the farmer—it is no accident that the first three objects of worship of the ancient Chinese should all have to do with food.

China: The Beautiful Cookbook

REGARDLESS OF WHAT ELSE WE MAY OR MAY NOT DO TO MAINTAIN OUR health, we all need to eat, regularly. Like amoebas, we human animals are digesting tubes. We move through the world by eating it. We swallow it, taking bits and pieces for ourselves, and push the rest out. One of the principal organizing processes of a living organism is its eating behavior. Food is the means by which we re-create the world as ourselves. Through eating we embody sun and rain, heat and cold, dryness and wetness, we feed the cosmic interaction of *Yin* and *Yang* that we are regenerating our *Essence* and *Spirit*. Our own nature interacts with the properties of the foods we eat. This relationship is the subject of this chapter.

FOOD IDEOLOGY WEST AND EAST

In the West the value of food is determined by the presence of proteins, carbohydrates, fats, vitamins, and minerals. Foods that contain similar quantities and proportions of these nutrients are considered equivalent in bio-

323

logical value. According to this principle, a bowl of spaghetti with tomato sauce is equivalent in protein and calories to a two-egg omelet, and a peanut-butter-and-jelly sandwich is equivalent to a chocolate éclair with a glass of milk. In addition, people are assumed to be the same physiologically, so the choice of diet is simply a matter of preference within these quantitative guidelines. Health-conscious Americans also evaluate their diet on the basis of whether foods are fresh, unrefined, without artificial ingredients, or too high in cholesterol, calories, sugar, and salt.

In Chinese medicine, who we are determines what is most beneficial for us to eat. And what we eat is considered to affect the expression of who we are. Both food and people are understood within the language of *Yin-Yang* and *Five Phases*. Foods are selected on the basis of their correspondence with individual patterns, modified by the climate, the season, and acute illness. People who are cold and dry need warm, moisturizing food; people who are hot and damp need cool, drying food; people with congestion need decong-esting food; and people who are depleted need replenishing food. The appropriateness of a food cannot be established without knowledge of the context—not everyone will benefit equally from foods that contain the same measure of nutrients. In other words, "one man's meat is another man's poison" means there is not a universal standard of what constitutes "good food."

A diet consisting mainly of raw fruits and vegetables cools *(Yin)*, not because these foods have been refrigerated, but because they promote the loss of body heat and the secretion of fluid. For a person who is *Cold, Damp*, and depleted, this diet exaggerates *internal* climate, aggravating symptoms of chilliness, puffiness, phlegm, fullness, and fatigue. Similarly, a diet consisting of fried, broiled, fat-rich, and spicy foods warms *(Yang)*, since these foods have absorbed the heat of cooking and because they generate body heat and stimulate circulation. For a person who is *Hot, Dry*, and congested, these foods exacerbate existing problems such as nervousness, sweating, tension, pain, constipation, and thirst. The same salads and juicy fruits that undermine an already cool, moist person are therapeutic for someone who is hot and dry; and the warm stimulation of spicy, broiled, and enriching foods that congest one person strengthen another.

Another factor that guides food selection is a person's particular condition at a given time. When someone is recovering from a flu, diet should counterbalance the sickness: for a high fever with parched mouth and throat, moisturizing, cooling foods are appropriate, whereas for a fever with aches and chills, foods that are warming and stimulating are helpful. Climate may also play a role: a cooling diet of raw, juicy foods is more appropriate in the summer when it is hot and dry, whereas in the winter, when it is damp, windy, and cold, a warming, enriching diet stokes our internal fire and protects us.

To the majority of Americans these considerations are alien. Our diet conforms more to the dictates and demands of the marketplace—we eat quick, easy, tasty meals and buy what advertising sells us. We've lost touch with what feels good or is good for us. We have a distorted relationship to food: starving ourselves to cast off unwanted weight and overeating as a substitute for real pleasure and satisfaction. To meet our demand for intense, constant productivity, we relentlessly overstimulate our bodies with high-protein, high-fat, high-sugar foods that have become associated with affluence and the good life.

In reaction to this, within the holistic health movement, there's been an overemphasis on purification and elimination through fasting, juice diets, and raw foods. Here, too, we've disconnected from how this makes us feel long term, relying more on our belief that this is good for us. These cleansing regimens often promote prolonged or intense discharge through sweating, purging the bowels, and increasing urination. This program is based on the premise that a "clean machine" is a well-running machine, that "cleanliness is next to godliness," and that "toxicity" is the primary culprit in poor health.

In the Chinese view what is considered "toxicity" in the popular holistic vocabulary (mucus, cholesterol, yeast, infection, or chemical pollution) is defined as *excesses* of undesirable influences such as phlegm, *Heat*, and *Wind*. Chinese food therapy emphasizes restoring wholesome digestion, increasing *Qi*, *Moisture*, and *Blood*, and reinvigorating *Organ* function. Especially where weakness exists, the priority is to use supplementing herbs and foods to restore and strengthen *Qi* and only later to use eliminative therapy if our organism hasn't already detoxified itself.

In the alternative health movement and in mainstream Western medicine, dietary recommendations are applied in a standardized, uniform way without particular regard for individual differences. A variety of systems offer the "perfect diet" for everyone, regardless of one's condition. Pritikin protects you from heart disease, cancer, and aging; raw food advocates rescue you from a life that is "dead," "toxic," and unnatural; and macrobiotics aspires to transform you from an aggressive, overexcited, greedy person into a peaceful, altruistic, righteous one. Each disagrees with the other about how to go about this: Pritikin recommends pure and fresh foods high in fiber and low in fat, salt, and sugar; hygienic raw-fooders insist on only uncooked organic fruits and vegetables; and macrobiotic followers eat primarily cooked grains and vegetables flavored with salty or pickled condiments and eschew many fruits and all concentrated sweets. There is substantial merit in each of these diets; each has helped some people some of the time. But each program is limited by a narrow and fixed way of thinking. Although ideology and method differ, the principle is the same: Feed everyone according to the same rules.

When modern medicine considers diet in the case of special diseases   325 like diabetes and hypertension, sugar or salt are excluded, but aside from that food is not regarded to contribute therapeutically. In Chinese medicine, in keeping with *Yin-Yang* thinking, it's crucial to discern whether a person with diabetes is weak or strong, heavy or thin, *Hot* or *Cold*, *Damp* or *Dry*. A diet high in complex carbohydrates, excluding simple sugars, and low in protein and fat decongests an overweight diabetic with excess *Heat* and *Dampness*, whereas a diet rich in protein and high-quality fats may be necessary for a weak, emaciated, *Dry* diabetic. Diabetes is understood to arise from *deficiency* of *Moisture* and *Essence (Yin)* of either the *Lung*, *Spleen*, or *Kidney* or all three. Herbs and foods that nourish *Yin* as well as clear *Heat*, dispel *Dampness*, and replenish *Qi* are an integral part of the treatment for a diabetic.

People with hypertension are advised to eliminate salt and saturated fats to reduce water retention and prevent arteriosclerosis. But again a person with high blood pressure can be strong or weak, congested or depleted, *Hot* or *Cold*, with disturbances of the *Heart*, *Spleen*, *Liver*, or *Kidney Network*. The proper diet for these individuals must incorporate all of these considerations to be truly effective as a therapeutic aid. The general strategy is to decongest *Blood*, strengthen the *Kidney*, and eliminate *Wind*, *Heat*, and *Dampness* from the *Liver*, *Heart*, and *Spleen*.

Because macrobiotics uses *Yin-Yang* terminology to classify foods and people, it appears to be similar to Chinese medicine. It shares the words but not the thinking, neglecting the relational, interactive paradigm. In Chinese medicine foods cannot be classified as being *Yin or Yang* except in relation to the person and circumstance. Just like people, foods have a character and a set of tendencies depending on the context.

A raw carrot tends to be a little sour, moisturizing, cooling, and dispersing and because of this is good for decongesting *Qi* and *Heat* in the *Liver* and *Stomach*. A cooked carrot becomes relatively sweet, warming, and consolidating and is good for replenishing *Qi* of the *Spleen*, *Lung*, and *Kidney*. A

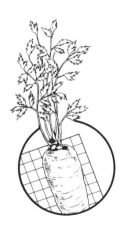

raw or cooked carrot is *Yang* compared with a watermelon and *Yin* compared with an egg. Cooked carrots are included in supplementing food recipes that are either warming or cooling because they are neutral in this context. For someone who is very *Cold* and depleted, even a cooked carrot may need to be combined with cardamom or dried ginger, stir-fried or broiled to make it more warming. Foods are adaptable, depending on how they are combined and prepared. Ordinary foods familiar to your kitchen can serve therapeutic ends, especially by including edible herbs that enhance potency and specificity.

HOW IS YOUR DIGESTION?

Evident from a hungry infant's shrill cry and the contented calm that follows after suckling, there is a primal sense of satisfaction and security that comes from adequate nourishment. Throughout our lives, food is basic to our comfort as well as our survival. Yet in our culture we are educated to ignore messages from our body, to be indifferent to the sensations of our internal organs unless they give us pain. We mask signs of poor digestion rather than seeking their cause. If our breath smells, we chew mints. If gas erupts from our stomach or bowels, we swallow antacids. We either endure constipation or resort to a laxative; and for loose bowels we gulp milk of magnesia between meals. We'd rather take medications than change our diet. However, by examing the situation more carefully, we can determine the signs of digestive comfort and discomfort and take appropriate action to sustain our health.

EATING: DIGESTION OR CONGESTION

In Chinese medicine, healthy digestion is synonomous with a happy *Spleen*. A good diet supports the work of the *Spleen* and counters idiosyncratic patterns of disharmony. An unsuitable diet will give rise to or aggravate the effects we saw above for poor digestive function. What is the role of the *Spleen Network*? How can particular foods restore our equanimity?

DIGESTION

The role of the *Spleen* is to transform and absorb food in order to generate and distribute *Qi*, *Moisture*, and *Blood*. The *Spleen* governs all activities along the digestive tube from the mouth to the large intestine, including those functions of the liver, gallbladder, and pancreas that enter into the process of digestion and assimilation. This *Organ Network* is differentiated into a *Yang* aspect, the *Stomach*, which tends to be warm, dry, and moves *Qi* downward, and a *Yin* aspect, the *Spleen*, which tends to be cool, wet, and send *Qi* upward. Food enters into this dynamic balance and either supports or sabotages its harmony.

The *Spleen* is like a crucible, a cooking pot, warmed by the living fire from the body's core, the *Kidney*. The *Spleen* depends on the ascension of heat from below to convert food to *Qi* and *Blood*. The refined *Qi* from food rises from the *Spleen* to the *Lung*, where it joins with the *Qi* from air. This pure essence of food and air then begins its journey through the channels and viscera. Denser, unrefined *Qi* descends from the *Stomach* by way of the *Small Intestine* to the *Kidney* and *Large Intestine*. The *Kidney* further purifies the liquid portion, storing some and eliminating the rest by way of the

---

Here are some signs of good digestion:

- No discomfort in your stomach or intestines.
- Regular, easy elimination, feeling better after than before.
- Satisfaction after meals, without lingering hunger or craving.
- Feeling alert and clear-headed after eating rather than lethargic or spaced out.
- A pleasant taste in your mouth and fragrant breath.

Here are some signs of indigestion:

- Discomfort in stomach and intestines.
- Belching and flatulence.
- Foul taste in mouth and offensive breath.
- Unpleasant odor of urine and feces.
- Difficult bowel movements and urination.
- Fatigue, depression, irritability, and fuzzy-headedness after meals.
- Lack of satisfaction with what you eat or not knowing what to eat to gain satisfaction.
- Uncontrollable cravings or lingering hunger for stimulants and fats or cold, spicy, salty, sweet, or sour foods.
- Headaches, nausea, nasal and sinus congestion, sudden perspiration, sores in the mouth, skin eruptions, unpleasant hot or cold sensations.

Of all these factors, the most important dietary rule to keep in mind is to eat only what you can digest effectively. This means you feel better after eating than before.

Bladder, while the *Large Intestine* receives the coarse, solid, unusable products of digestion and discharges them.

The function of the *Spleen Network* can be impeded by incompatible food, overeating, emotional turmoil, stress, or extreme hunger. This interrupts the rhythmic movement along the digestive tube, which is the same as saying that the *Qi* of the *Spleen* and *Stomach* is obstructed. Obstructed *Qi* leads to congested foods and fluids, which in turn can generate conditions of *deficiency* and *excess.* Congestion prevents the *Spleen* from doing its job well: when the *Spleen* cannot generate *Qi* and *Blood,* this results in weakness; when it cannot distribute *Qi* and *Blood,* stagnation occurs, which creates *excesses* such as *Heat, Cold, Dampness,* and *Wind.* Either of these outcomes will aggravate the other *Organ Networks.* For example, stagnant *Qi* in the *Spleen* agitates the *Liver;* an accumulation of *Heat* overstimulates the *Heart;* congestion of fluids produces phlegm in the *Lung;* and *excess Cold* depresses the fire of the *Kidney.*

CONGESTION

Congestion and disharmony of the *Spleen-Stomach Network* may give rise to a variety of physical complaints. This can be viewed in relation to the flow of *Qi* and *Blood,* which must move upward and downward through the center of the body, the province of the *Spleen* and *Stomach.* The *Spleen* helps raise *Qi,* and the *Stomach* helps bring it down. With congestion, *Qi* cannot move up and down properly. The warm dry *Qi* of the *Lung* and *Heart* cannot descend, and the cool moist *Qi* of the *Kidney* cannot rise. Sometimes this accounts for the fact that the upper body becomes overheated and dehydrated while the lower body becomes cold and waterlogged. This may make a person crave cool, moistening foods to counteract the upper body's discomfort, and warm, drying foods to remedy discomfort in the lower body. When *Qi* is blocked, it follows the path of least resistance, sometimes reversing patterns of proper movement. When the *Stomach* is overly hot, dry, or congested with food, *Qi* rises instead of descending, and belching, hiccups, difficult swallowing, or heartburn occur. When the *Spleen* is too *Cold* and *Damp, Qi collapses* downward instead of ascending, and distension, prolapse, flatulence, and diarrhea occur. The solution is to avoid congestion so that the *Qi* can travel freely. For this reason, the Chinese suggest that a person never eat until they are full but instead always leave some space in the *Stomach* for the movement of *Qi.*

Foods that move *Qi,* remove *Heat* from the *Stomach* and *Cold* from the *Spleen,* and tonify *Qi* and *Moisture* are good for the *Spleen Network.* Vegetables and fruits with abundant roughage such as cabbage, beets, radishes, apples, pears, mushrooms, and whole or sprouted grains move *Qi* and ease the passage of food. Sweet, starchy vegetables and grains like yams, barley, and rice, and fruits like dates, figs, papaya, and coconut increase *Qi* and *Moisture.*

The *Stomach* tends to become *Hot* and *Dry*, whereas the *Spleen* tends to become *Cold* and *Damp*. So the *Stomach* likes cooling foods that dispel *Heat* and replenish *Moisture*, and the *Spleen* likes warm foods that dry *Dampness* and generate *Qi*. Generally, eating a variety of foods—cool and warm, moist and dry, nourishing and decongesting—is what pleases the body.

Often food cravings are the result of *Spleen-Stomach* disharmonies. If the *Spleen* is undermined by *Cold* and *deficiency*, cravings for foods like coffee, chocolate, and alcohol are likely to occur. These are warming, bitter foods that stimulate the *Liver* and *Heart*, producing a temporary feeling of increased energy and circulation. If the *Stomach* is overheated and congested, cravings for iced drinks and ice cream are likely. Ice cream and frozen yogurt are cold, sweet foods that relax and expand the *Stomach*, relieving feelings of tension and agitation. It is common for people to have both *deficiency* of the *Spleen* and *excess* of the *Stomach*, so depending on which condition is most prevalent, these cravings alternately demand satisfaction. Fulfilling these desires may do more harm than good. If the *Spleen* is already weak and *Cold*, ice cream will steal its warmth and squelch the fire of the *Kidney*, exacerbating symptoms like poor circulation and water retention in the legs and feet. Because the *Kidney*'s moisture becomes confined to the lower body, the inner membranes of the chest, neck, and head become dry and sticky, manifesting as irritation and mucus congestion of the nose, throat, and bronchi. If the *Stomach* is already overheated and congested, roasted cocoa or coffee bean will create more heat or, if mixed with sugar and milk, more phlegm. This increased heat dries up the body's moisture, which weakens the *Kidney*, *Liver*, *Heart*, and *Lung*. Alcohol's extreme heat especially overexcites the *Liver* and *Heart*, which generates *Wind*, exhausts the *Blood*, and undermines the *Spirit*. This is why alcohol can cause high blood pressure, stroke, impotence, and dementia.

ESTABLISHING THE CONDITION OF EARTH: STOMACH AND SPLEEN

The overall body picture does not always reflect the status of the *Stomach* or *Spleen*. Someone might be depleted and have a congested *Stomach* or *Spleen*, overheated in general, but have a *Cold Spleen*, and retain excess fluids yet have a *Dry Stomach*. Restoring the warmth (*Yang*) of the *Spleen* or the moisture (*Yin*) of the *Stomach* harmonizes the center. This has a ripple effect throughout the organism as a whole.

If there is a conflict between the *Organs* of *Earth* in which the *Stomach* is *Hot* and the *Spleen Cold*, the *Stomach Dry* and the *Spleen Damp*, then each needs remedying without exacerbating the other. Faced with this dilemma, identifying which pattern is more chronic or severe, and which most fits the overall state, helps someone decide what to eat: otherwise, foods with a neutral nature (not too cooling warming, juicy, or dry) are used.

Changes in weather and season can mask the prevailing *internal* climate. Even though a person with *Cold-Damp Earth* may feel less chilly and lethargic as the sun beats down in the heat of summer, and even though there is a strong urge then to eat raw, juicy, cooling foods, a predominantly warming, drying diet is best. Similarly, someone with *Hot-Dry Earth* should resist the temptation to consume hot, spicy, rich foods, even during a wet, snowy winter. Eating in accord with the climate and season is appropriate when compatible with the existing *Stomach-Spleen* pattern.

Combinations of patterns such as *Hot-Damp* and *Cold-Damp* can occur within the same person, as can depletion and congestion. Someone who is weak and depleted needs thicker, more enriching food (avoid thin soups), whereas someone who is congested and agitated needs to avoid sticky and rich foods (dairy products, fats, casseroles). Reflect on how different foods (or the same foods prepared differently) make you feel. This will train your instincts and help you to follow them.

DEFINING THE RELATIONSHIP BETWEEN FOOD AND FUNCTION

Plump apple, smooth banana, melon, peach
gooseberry . . . How all this affluence
speaks death and life into the mouth . . . I sense . . .
Observe it from a child's transparent features

while he tastes. This comes from far away.
What miracle is happening in your mouth?
Instead of words, discoveries flow out
from the ripe flesh, astonished to be free.

Dare to say what "apple" truly is.
This sweetness that feels thick, dark, dense at first;
then, exquisitely lifted in your taste,

grows clarified, awake and luminous,
double-meaninged, sunny, earthy, real—.
O knowledge, pleasure—inexhaustible.

Rainer Maria Rilke
(Stephen Mitchell, trans.)

To determine what foods best suit us, it is helpful to know how our *Qi*, *Moisture*, and *Blood* are behaving within the parameters of *Yin-Yang* and *Five-*

Phase correspondence. The basic guidelines for food therapy are generated by how the qualities and properties of foods affect the quality and quantity of *Qi*, *Moisture*, and *Blood*. Foods are classified loosely on the basis of

- texture and density: crunchy, soft, heavy, light
- flavors: sour, bitter, sweet, spicy, salty
- nature: warm, cool, dry, moist
- properties: supplementing (replenishes *Qi*, *Moisture*, and *Blood*) or decongesting (eliminates stagnation of *Qi*, *Moisture*, and *Blood* and dispels *Heat*, *Cold*, *Wind*, *Dryness*, and *Dampness*)

As with herbs, the medicinal use of a food is determined by the relationship between its observable qualities and its experienced effects.

A cooked yam is yellow, moist, soft, slightly sticky, and sweet. Yams are considered to be excellent food for supplementing *Qi* and strengthening the *Spleen* and *Stomach*. Because they are so nourishing and digestible, they are good food for relieving weakness, fatigue, and building tissue. Cooked eggplants are dark purple, rich, pungent, gelatinous, and moist. Eggplant is eaten to enrich and move the *Blood* and especially benefits the *Kidney* and *Liver*. A radish is white, crisp, juicy, and pungent and feels fresh and cooling in the mouth and stomach. Radishes disperse *Qi* and phlegm, relieving congestion in the throat, chest, and digestive tract. Radishes promote the function of the *Lung* and *Large Intestine* by precipitating *Moisture* and *Qi* downward. Because raw celery and green pepper are green, crunchy, juicy, and sour, they moisturize, consolidate, cool, and relax the *Qi*, which benefits the *Liver*, *Stomach*, and *Gallbladder*. Cooked asparagus is pulpy, slightly salty, and sweet and has a strong diuretic effect, which makes it good for eliminating *Heat* and *Dampness*, benefiting the *Heart* and *Kidney*.

Characteristics and effects do not always fit neatly together to designate the property of a food. It is difficult to definitively pin down specific properties for most foods, but some do cross over the line between food and herb because of specificity and potency: lycii berries nurture *Blood* and *Essence*, red dates build *Qi* and *Moisture*, pearl barley (similar to the herb coix seed) builds *Qi* and eliminates *Dampness*, seaweed clears phlegm, and black fungus disperses *Blood* and lubricates the intestines.

It is possible to generalize and say that one person will benefit from a supplementing diet, another a decongesting one, that warm foods are better for one person, moist and cool ones for another, but it is more likely that combinations of food will be appropriate for each of these people, and that what is right at one time may not be so on a permanent basis. Variety accommodates changing needs. The same flavor or food that feels good in moderation may be damaging in excess.

Sweet foods generally supplement *Qi* and *Moisture* but in excess produce

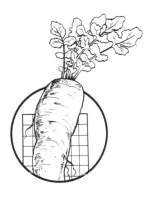

phlegm and *Heat*. Bitter foods clean and empty but in excess dissipate *Qi* and *Moisture*. Spicy foods activate and decongest *Qi* and *Blood* but in excess exhaust them. Salty foods supplement *Blood* and *Essence* but in excess congeal them. Sour foods tone the viscera and nerves but in excess cause cramping and pain. A sweet, nourishing food like milk "does a body good" if the body is *Dry* and weak but can do another body harm if it is *Hot* and *Damp*, producing mucus congestion and inflammation. Yams or rice are sweet and nourishing, yet rich cake is so sweet that it tends to create more *Dampness* and *Heat* than *Qi* and *Blood*. Our interaction with food is affected by the flavor and nature of what we eat, its concentration and quantity, as well as by our preexisting internal environment.

Flavors

Understanding the effects of various flavors is one guide in choosing appropriate foods.

> salty—densifying, concentrating
> sour—astringent, contracting
> bitter—eliminating, descending
> sweet—expanding, relaxing
> spicy—accelerating, dispersing

WHAT SHOULD I EAT?

The answer to the question, "What should I eat?" is based on an evaluation of your current status. It is programmatic rather than dogmatic. The first step is to determine if you are *Cold*, *Wet*, *Hot*, or *Dry*. Do you show signs of congestion or depletion or both? What combination of traits and signs characterize you? The following chart is designed to aid you in making these determinations.

Patterns of Dysfunction

Yin

Cool	Damp	Depleted
little thirst; uncomfortable in cool environment; slow, passive, yielding; craves spicy and hot food and liquids, sometimes in large quantities	lack of thirst; copious saliva or mucus in mouth, throat; oily skin and hair; clammy, sticky perspiration; uncomfortable in humid environment; frequent, scanty urine; lethargic, heavy, slack; craves dry, stimulating foods	sensitive, weak, tires easily; lacks motivation and perseverance; frequent, abundant urine; diarrhea; aversion to prolonged, intense activity; requires rest and quiet; craves stimulating, astringent (tart or binding), rich foods and beverages; prefers small, frequent meals

Yang

Warm	Dry	Congested
thirst; uncomfortable in warm environment; impulsive, reactive, provocative; likes to be active and stimulated; craves cold foods and liquids	thirst; dry mouth, skin, and hair; uncomfortable in arid or windy environment; infrequent, concentrated, scanty urine; easily irritated and difficult to soothe; craves tart, juicy, mucilaginous, and oily foods	uneasy fullness or pressure in head, chest, or abdomen; constipation and gas; difficult urination; restless, difficult finding comfort or satisfaction; worse after eating or drinking, better after fasting or skipping a meal; craves stimulants and simple foods and beverages; seeks carminatives (gas expelling) or laxatives

(For further self-assessment, refer back to self-evaluation charts on depleted or congested *Qi*, *Moisture*, and *Blood* in chapter 14, on page 299.)

Basic Strategies

Once you have determined your condition, you can work out a strategy and means of implementation. The basic strategies are

for *Heat*, cool
for *Dampness*, dry
for *deficiency*, fill
for congestion, empty
for tension, relax
for slackness, tighten

Food Nature and Food Preparation Spectrum

You will also need to consider which foods are generally cooling or warming. For example, if your condition is more *Yin* according to the "Patterns of Dysfunction" chart, you will want to emphasize the more *Yang* (or warming) foods listed in "Properties of Food" on the pages that follow. The method of preparation also affects the warming and cooling effects of foods in the body.

Most Cool   Most Warm

soft,		vege-		grains		nuts		milk
juicy		tables						cheese
fruits								eggs
	drier		roots		seeds		legumes	seafood
	harder		tubers					poultry
	fruits							meat

Most Cool   Most Warm

raw	raw	steamed	sautéed	baked	fried	dry-	broiled
fresh	dried					roasted	

Properties of Food

Yin: cooling; moisturizing; decongesting; relaxing
Yang: warming; drying; supplementing; stimulating

Supplementing Qi: bland, sweet, starchy foods

	Vegetables	Fruits	Legumes-grains	Dairy-meats	Nuts-seeds-oils-sugars
Warm	sweet potato, artichoke, mustard greens	dates, coconut milk	sweet rice	butter, eel, fresh ham, lamb	sorghum, chestnuts, brown sugar, malt syrup
Neutral	yam, potato, celery, carrots, string beans, beets, winter squash, turnip, okra, shiitake mushrooms, Jerusalem artichoke	papaya, apricots, figs, grapes, raisins, currants, coconut	rice, pearl barley, black beans, kidney beans, bean curd skin, tapioca, carob, vanilla	milk, cheese, whitefish, mackerel, herring, goose, pork, beef	peanuts, almonds, cashews, pecans, white sugar, honey, maple syrup, nutmeg
Cool	watercress, lettuce, summer squash, tofu, lotus root	banana, apple, avocado	corn, barley, millet, buckwheat, wheat-berries, gluten	cottage cheese, yogurt	
Cooking herbs	astragalus rt. (w), codonopsis rt. (n), dioscorea rhz. (n), red and black dates (n)				

Supplementing Moisture: sweet, bland, sour, juicy foods

	Vegetables	Fruits	Legumes-grains	Dairy-meats	Nuts-seeds-oils-sugars
Warm		peaches, nectarines, coconut milk	sweet rice, rice milk		pine nuts, litchi nuts, malt syrup, soy oil
Neutral	string beans, carrots, potatoes, beets, Chinese cabbage, Jerusalem artichokes	grapes, pineapple, plums, apricot, blue-berries, huckle-berries, straw-berries, oranges, tangerines, olives	oats, pinto beans, black beans	milk, cheese, sardines, herring, oysters, duck, goose, pork	sesame seeds, peanuts, almonds, honey, white sugar, peanut oil, olive oil, coconut oil
Cool	cucumber, water chestnuts, spinach, asparagus, watercress, seaweed, radish, tomatoes, kudzu, agar	apples, pears, bananas, lemons, limes, mangos, melons	buckwheat, wheat-berries, gluten, tofu, bean sprouts	cottage cheese, yogurt, egg white, octopus, squid, clams, abalone	sugar cane, sesame oil
Cooking herbs	lily bulb (c), glehnia rt. (n), polygonatum rhz. (n.) American ginseng rt. (c)				

Supplementing Blood (Essence): sweet, sour, astringent foods

	Vegetables	Fruits	Legumes-grains	Dairy-meats	Nuts-seeds-oils-sugars
Warm	chives, leeks	black dates, currants, cherries, rasp-berries, black-berries	glutinous rice, nutritional yeast	butter, shrimp, mussels, salmon, eel, trout, anchovy, chicken, chicken liver, turkey, lamb, marrow bone	pinenuts, walnuts, chestnuts, vinegar
Neutral	shepherd's purse, carrots, beets, black fungus	red dates, raisins	black beans, kidney beans, aduki beans	milk, egg yolk, oysters, sardines, herring, beef, pork, beef liver, brain	sesame seeds, peanuts
Cool	spinach, eggplant, spirulina, chlorella		gluten	abalone, rabbit	sesame oil
Cooking herbs	white peony rt. (c), lycii fr. (n), cooked rehmannia rt. (w), cornus fr. (w)				

Decongesting Qi: spicy, bitter, salty foods

	Vegetables	Fruits	Legumes-grains	Dairy-meats	Nuts-seeds-oils-sugars
Warm	mustard greens and seeds, chives, onions, shallots, scallions, black pepper, fresh ginger, cardamom, coriander, parsley, fennel, anise, red cabbage	kumquats, oranges and orange peel, straw-berries, black-berries			soy oil, peanut oil, safflower oil
Neutral	peas, turnips, beets, cabbage, cauli-flower, black mush-rooms, carrots	plums, prunes, tangerines, pineapple, figs	brown rice, rice bran, rice and barley sprouts	shark, beef kidney	almonds, olive oil
Cool	rhubarb, radishes, white pepper, endive	bananas, apples	wheat bran, oat bran		sesame oil
Cooking Herbs	fresh ginger rhz. (w), tangerine or orange peel (w), radish sd. (n), platycodon rt. (n)				

Decongesting Moisture: bitter, bland, salty foods

	Vegetables	Fruits	Legumes-grains	Dairy-meats	Nuts-seeds-oils-sugars
Warm	artichoke, kohlrabi, parsley, coriander, cinnamon	grapefruit peel		butterfish, mussels, eel, shrimp, turkey	sunflower seeds
Neutral	pumpkin, celery, cabbage, corn silk	grapes, papaya, pineapple	amaranth, rice, rice bran, pearl barley, black beans, aduki beans, kidney beans, broad beans, hyacinth beans	whitefish, carp, mackerel, duck, pork and beef kidney	almonds, pumpkin seeds
Cool	asparagus, watercress, button mushrooms, seaweeds, endive, alfalfa sprouts, plantain, muskmelon	pears, watermelon and rind	barley, millet, corn, mung beans	clams, black and green tea	
Cooking herbs	skin of fresh ginger (w), corn silk (n), poria fungus (n), tangerine (peel) (n)				

Decongesting Blood: spicy, sour, and bitter foods

	Vegetables	Fruits	Legumes-grains	Dairy-meats	Nuts-seeds-oils-sugars
Warm	chives, scallions, onions, sweet basil, safflower, cayenne, turmeric	peaches, cherries			vinegar, rice wine, shrimp
Neutral	shiitake mush-rooms, saffron, black fungus, beets, eggplant, leeks	rose hips, olives	rice bran	sardines, sturgeon, shark	
Cool	swiss chard, watercress, fresh lotus root	wheat germ		crab	
Cooking herbs	carthamus fl. (w), ligusticum rhz. (w), turmeric rhz. (w), white peony rt. (c)				

Specific recipes harmonize *Qi, Moisture,* and *Blood* as well as influence each of the *Organ Networks.* The remainder of this chapter will be devoted to enumerating a selection of herbal food recipes that can be easily prepared with edible herbs and commonly available foods.

LEARNING HERBAL CUISINE

The idea of cooking with herbs is centuries old but fairly new to most Americans. Just as many people wonder how acupuncture feels, they want to know how herbal food tastes. Just as they want to know if the needles work, they want to know what eating these foods will do for them. The most accurate assessment will come from your own experience, but here are some general principles. Foods that supplement *Qi,* like yams and astragalus, have   341 a sweet, bland flavor and will energize and build resistance to colds and flus. Foods that supplement *Moisture*, like polygonatum and pears, tend to be sweet and juicy and help the body generate vital fluids and lubricate tissue. Foods that nourish the *Blood* and *Essence*, like eggplant and rehmannia, help to build and repair tissue and taste rich, sweet, bitter, or tart.

A sense of adventure and access to the ingredients are all that is needed to eat herbal cuisine. The Chinese herbs listed in this chapter can be acquired either from your local Chinatown herb shop or by mail order. Even before you use the herbs, you can begin to apply the principles of Chinese food therapy. Ask yourself what your body wants to eat, how it needs to be nourished, what foods you ought to avoid, and how your daily habits could be modified to remedy patterns of disharmony and reinforce your body's integrity. In addition to carefully noting your own physical responses to food, refer to the charts on pages 334–341 to help you identify patterns of disharmony and which foods could be beneficial. Become sensitive to your responses to a meal—both the ingredients used and the methods of preparation.

We have seen people with *Damp, Cold Spleens* miraculously improve when they stop eating raw fruits, raw vegetables, and cold, sticky dairy products and switch instead to a diet of cooked foods. People with *Hot*, congested *Spleens* feel better when they eat lots of fiber-rich vegetables and avoid fried and spicy foods. Herbal supplementation can be especially beneficial to people who have been adhering to a strict vegetarian diet or who find they have cravings for salt, fat, coffee, alcohol, or sugar. Herbal cuisine can prevent disharmonies from becoming symptoms and sicknesses—it can be healing and keep us healthy as well.

If you are unsure of your dietary needs, try a variety of these recipes. Unless a recipe makes you feel ill, you can assume that it's good for you. If you want to build your strength, rotate the supplement *Qi, Moisture,* and *Blood* recipes along with those that *harmonize* the *Five Phases*, sampling each one.

COOKING TIPS

Cooking is a matter of trusting your own sensibilities. . . . A cook's mind is supple and flexible enough to do justice to the beauty and particularity of fruits and vegetables and is always ready to warm to the task. There is a lot to think about and a lot to get done, but to be efficient does not mean to be hurried, and to be unhurried does not mean to sit in a lawn chair. Take the time to give each task its due—it comes out in the food: a generosity of spirit. Call it rejoicing, tenderness, graciousness, or simple attention to detail, the quality of caring is an ingredient everyone can taste.

> Edward Espe Brown
> *Greens Cookbook*

Preparation of Chinese Herbs

Among people concerned about healthy eating and cooking, prevailing opinion holds that foods retain more value when they are closest not only to their natural but to their raw state. Chinese herbal cuisine, however, depends on the cooking process to extract medicinal properties and make the ingredients more easily digestible, so cooking in this context enhances food value.

Ideally herbs may be soaked overnight or a few hours before cooking, but because many of us do not plan that far ahead, it is also possible to soak the herbs for a shorter period of time or not at all. If they have been soaked, save the soaking water and add this to the stock. When using dried black or shiitake mushrooms and black fungus, cover them with boiling water and soak them for ten to thirty minutes, again adding this soak water to the stock. Black fungus needs to be rinsed carefully because of occasional pebbles. Red or black dates are easier to pit if they have been soaked, although if diners are warned of the pits, they can remain unpitted. Herbs such as tangerine peel and codonopsis are also easier to cut after being soaked in boiling water, whereas dioscorea can be broken into small pieces when dry. When herbs have not been soaked, make sure they are well cooked—tender and easy to chew and swallow. This helps them to be digested easily.

Some herbs are inedible because of their fibrous or stringy texture and are therefore placed in a bag or tied with string so that they can be removed after cooking and before eating. The herb astragalus is too fibrous to be

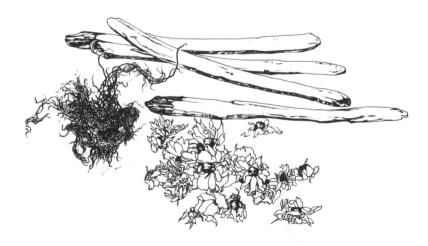

Corn Silk, Astragalus, Chrysanthemum   343

broken down by chewing—it can be identified as a slightly yellow, flat-cut root that looks a little like a tongue depressor. Another inedible herb is corn silk because it is too stringy. Chrysanthemum or honeysuckle flowers can be eaten, but we suggest that they be removed because of their texture. To make the edible herbs more appealing visually as well as easier to eat, it is best to cut them into bite-size pieces.

After adding herbs, it may take ten to twenty minutes for the stock to resume simmering—the cooking time is for simmering stock, so wait until the broth simmers again before you set the timer.

Preparing Stocks

Our recipes use either vegetable- or chicken-based stock. Although it is also possible to purchase vegetable and meat bouillon, or canned chicken stock, there are advantages to preparing your own. The more legumes and vegetables in the vegetarian stock, the richer it will be (the recipe below makes an excellent soup base). Chicken bones are inexpensive, less than fifty cents per pound, and rich in the marrow that nourishes *Blood* and *Essence*. A rich chicken stock congeals into a gel when cooled overnight; then the unwanted fat may be easily skimmed off.

Ready-made broths are usually high in salt and some include monosodium glutamate. Generally, their nutritional value is less than that of a homemade soup. It is prudent to make the stock ahead of schedule so that dinner preparation does not take an unreasonable length of time. If you plan to try many of these recipes, the stock recipe can be doubled and frozen until needed.

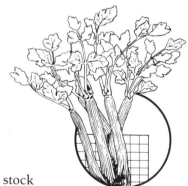

Vegetable Stock

Yield: 7–8 cups of stock

2 large carrots	1 onion	1¹/₂ inch fresh ginger
3 celery stalks	2 leeks (white part)	10 c. water
1 zucchini	2 cloves garlic	

Cube and simmer all ingredients for 1 to 2 hours over low heat, strain the broth, and discard the solid portion. Additional options: 1 tbsp. sesame oil, 1 tbsp. soy sauce, 2 beets, 1 eggplant, 1 turnip, 1 c. parsley, or ¹/₂ cabbage.

Chicken Stock

Yield: 7–8 cups stock

3½ lbs. chicken bones	2 carrots	1 inch fresh ginger
or 1 whole chicken	1 onion	12 c. water
3 celery stalks		

Cube the vegetables and simmer along with the chicken for 3–5 hours over low heat. Strain the broth, squeezing the liquid, and then discard the solid portion. Cool and remove congealed fat (this is most easily done after refrigeration). Refrigerate (up to 5 days) or freeze (up to 2 months) until ready to use. Additional options: 1 c. parsley, 1 tbsp. soy sauce.

ADAPTING RECIPES

Recipes may be varied according to taste or available foods. Feel free to experiment. When substituting ingredients, the food property lists (pages 336–341) will be helpful (for example, for a recipe to supplement *Qi*, substitute ingredients from the food category for supplementing *Qi*). Most of the

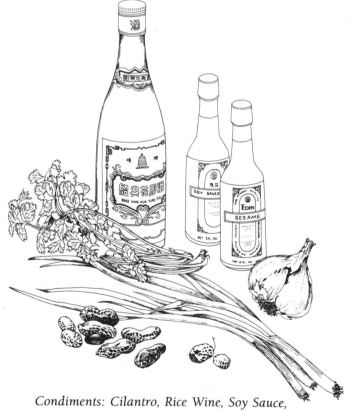

Condiments: Cilantro, Rice Wine, Soy Sauce,
Sesame Oil, Garlic, Scallions, Peanuts

following recipes are for soups that depend on the stock to extract the benefits from the herbs. But the meal can be structured in a variety of ways, depending on preference. For instance, a meal that includes lotus seeds and spinach in the listed recipe could be altered to use those items as a side dish, cooked separately: for 1 oz. of lotus seeds, use 1 cup broth, simmer for 1 hour, add spinach for 5 minutes, and season to taste. The lotus seeds and spinach can be served as a side dish, called "pearls in jade forest."

We urge you to use your imagination to devise variations that work for you and appeal to your tastes—these recipes are meant to provide an example and some direction. Fresh vegetables are available seasonally, so it may be necessary to substitute celery, mushrooms, or watercress in a recipe for decongesting *Moisture* that calls for asparagus unless you choose to use frozen asparagus spears.

For added flavor, the following condiments may be used: soy sauce, rice wine and vinegar, roasted sesame oil or seeds, ground peanuts, chopped cilantro, parsley, basil, scallions, garlic. The chopped greens are suitable for

PANTRY HERBS

	Supplementing	
Herb	*Flavor*	*Texture*
American ginseng rt. (ren shen)	mildly sweet and bitter	dense, chewy
astragalus rt. (huang qi)*	mildly sweet	hard, fibrous
black date (da zao)	sweet	soft, chewy, sticky
codonopsis rt. (dang shen)	sweet and slightly musty	chewy, starchy

color as well as flavor. The bland recipes can acquire some subtle zip from this sauce:

2 tbsp. rice wine (the Chinese product is called *Shao Xing*)
1 tbsp. soy or tamari sauce
1 tsp. roasted sesame oil

The recipes listed provide six servings. If only one person is cooking a recipe for an acute condition, then it may be wise to prepare half the recipe and eat one serving three times, twice the first day, and once the second. Or for general strengthening, prepare half the recipe and eat one serving per day over the course of three days. Adjust the amounts listed to accommodate the number of people being fed or the number of days the meal will last. Again, be guided over time by your own assessment and experience. In cases of grave weakness, appropriate recipes like an easy-to-digest congee can be eaten three times a day for as long as necessary. If these foods make you feel good, you need not worry that you are overdoing them.

	Supplementing	
Action upon Qi, Moisture, Blood, or Adverse Climates	Organ Network benefited	Effects
replenishes *Moisture* and *Qi*	Lung Kidney Heart	relieves weakness, fatigue, dryness; enhances libido, fertility, immunity
replenishes *Qi*, warms body, dispels *Dampness*	Spleen Lung Kidney	relieves weakness, fatigue, edema; enhances stamina and immunity; protects blood
replenishes *Qi*, and *Blood*	Spleen Liver	relieves fatigue, anemia; regulates appetite and promotes growth
replenishes Qi	Spleen Lung	relieves weakness, fatigue, enhances stamina and protects blood

Supplementing

Herb	Flavor	Texture
cornus fr. (shan zhu yu)	mildly sweet and tart	soft
dioscorea rt. (shan yao)	bland	soft, starchy, chewy
glehnia rt. (bei sha shen)	mildly sweet	chewy, starchy
lotus sd. (lian zi)	mildly sweet	soft, starchy
lycii fr. (gou qi zi)	sweet and slightly tart	soft
longan fr. (long yan rou)	sweet	soft, sticky
polygonatum rhz. (yu zhu)	mildly sweet	sticky, chewy, starchy
red date (hong zao)	sweet	soft
rehmannia rt. (cooked) (shu di huang)	sweet	sticky, gelatinous

Supplementing		
Action upon Qi, Moisture, Blood, or Adverse Climates	*Organ Network benefited*	*Effects*
replenishes *Blood* and *Essence*	*Kidney* *Liver*	regulates secretions and discharges; fortifies marrow and blood; strengthens bones and tendons; enhances libido and fertility
replenishes *Qi* and *Essence*	*Spleen* *Lung* *Kidney*	relieves weakness, fatigue; generates tissue; promotes growth; enhances fertility
replenishes *Moisture* and *Qi*	*Spleen* *Lung*	relieves fatigue, thirst, cough, constipation
nourishes the body, promotes growth, consolidates *Qi* and *Essence*, calms *Spirit*	*Spleen* *Kidney* *Heart*	regulates appetite, relieves weakness and slackness, stops diarrhea, relaxes mind
replenishes *Blood* and *Essence*	*Kidney* *Liver* *Heart*	relieves dryness, anemia, fatigue; softens skin; improves vision; regulates blood sugar, enhances fertility
replenishes *Blood*, calms *Spirit*	*Liver* *Heart* *Spleen*	relieves weakness, dizziness, restlessness
replenishes *Moisture* and *Qi*	*Spleen* *Lung* *Heart*	relieves weakness, thirst, cough; increases pulmonary and cardiac capacity
replenishes *Qi*, *Blood, Moisture*	*Spleen* *Liver*	relieves fatigue, dryness, anemia, nausea; regulates appetite, growth
replenishes *Blood* and *Essence*	*Kidney* *Liver* *Heart*	relieves weakness, dizziness, fatigue, anemia, dryness; strengthens tissue, marrow, and bones; enhances fertility

Supplementing and Decongesting

Herb	Flavor	Texture
black fungus (hei mu erh)	mildly sweet and salty, slightly musty	chewy, gelatinous
black mushrooms (xiang gu)	mildly sweet and salty	chewy, gelatinous
lily bulb (bai he)	mildly sweet and musty	soft, starchy
poria fn. (fu ling)	bland	soft
pueraria rt. (ge gen)	mildly sweet, a little sour	soft, starchy
white peony rt. (bai shao yao)	bland, a little sour	chewy, starchy
tangerine pl. (chen pi)	a little sweet, spicy, and bitter	soft, gelatinous

Supplementing and Decongesting

Action upon Qi, Moisture, Blood, or Adverse Climates	Organ Network benefited	Effects
replenishes *Essence*, activates *Blood*, lubricates *Intestines*	*Lung* *Kidney* *Liver*	promotes circulation; lowers cholesterol; relieves constipation; enhances immunity
replenishes *Essence* and *Blood*, activates *Blood*, lubricates *Intestines*	*Lung* *Kidney* *Liver*	similar to black fungus, but better for enhancing immunity and not as good for lowering cholesterol
replenishes *Moisture* and eliminates phlegm	*Lung* *Heart*	relieves dryness, thirst, cough, and restlessness; lowers fever
replenishes *Qi*, distributes *Moisture*, eliminates *Dampness*	*Spleen* *Lung* *Kidney* *Heart*	relieves bloating, water retention, and edema; promotes absorption and assimilation; alleviates diarrhea
dispels *Wind*, relaxes spasm, replenishes *Qi* and *Moisture*	*Spleen* *Lung* *Liver*	relieves chills, fever, muscle ache, thirst; promotes circulation, lowers blood pressure
replenishes, consolidates, and distributes *Blood*, relaxes spasm, dispels *Wind*	*Liver* *Spleen*	relieves cramps, pain, tension, dizziness, headache; lowers blood pressure; regulates menses, controls uterine bleeding
supports and activates *Qi*, dispels *Dampness* and phlegm	*Spleen* *Lung*	promotes expectoration; relieves hiccup, nausea, and gas; stimulates appetite and promotes digestion

Decongesting

Herb	Flavor	Texture
chrysanthemum fl. (ju hua)*	mildly sweet and bitter	soft, light
carthamus fl. (hong hua)*	mildly spicy and bitter	soft, light
corn silk (yu mi xu)*	bland	soft, light
corydalis rhz. (yan hu suo)	mildly spicy and bitter	soft, starchy
ginger rhz. (fresh) (sheng jiang)	spicy and mildly sweet	chewy, fibrous
honeysuckle fl. (jin yin hua)*	sweet	soft, light
ligusticum rhz. (chuan xiong)	mildly spicy and sweet, slightly bitter	soft, chewy

*These herbs are suitable for cooking but inedible because of their fibrous, stringy, or leafy texture. Place these herbs in a bag or, in the case of astragalus which is a long flat root, tie with string and remove before serving.

Decongesting		
Action upon Qi, Moisture, Blood, or Adverse Climates	Organ Network benefited	Effects
dispels *Heat* and *Wind*, counteracts toxins	*Liver* *Lung*	relieves fever, inflammation, headache; improves vision, brightens eyes; lowers blood pressure, aids in fat metabolism
activates *Blood*, eliminates *Blood* stagnation	*Liver* *Heart*	promotes circulation, relieves bruising, swelling, pain
eliminates *Dampness* and *Damp Heat*	*Kidney* *Liver* *Heart*	relieves edema, jaundice; lowers blood pressure and blood sugar
activates *Blood* and *Qi*, eliminates *Blood* stagnation	*Liver* *Heart* *Spleen*	relieves bruising, swelling, pain; promotes restful sleep; regulates menstruation
stimulates circulation of *Qi* and *Blood*, eliminates *Wind*, *Cold*, phlegm	*Spleen* *Lung*	relieves chill, cough, indigestion; counteracts nausea, dizziness, diarrhea, abdominal pain
dispels *Heat* and *Wind*, counteracts toxins	*Lung* *Heart*	relieves swelling and inflammation and dispels pus; lowers fever and relieves thirst; lowers blood pressure and cholesterol
activates *Blood*, *Qi*; dispels *Wind*	*Heart* *Liver*	promotes cerebral and coronary circulation—ameliorates angina; relieves muscle and head pain; regulates menstruation and relieves cramps and seizures

	Decongesting	
Herb	Flavor	Texture
platycodon rt. (jie geng)	sweet, slightly bitter	chewy, soft
radish sd. (lai fu zi)	spicy and a little sweet	soft, chewy
sweet almond sd. (xing ren)	sweet and a little bitter	crunchy, chewy

ITEMS FOR PREPARING RECIPES

These items would be useful in the preparation of the recipes:

- *cheesecloth or muslin bag* to place herbs that are used in the recipe but are not eaten as part of the meal
- *nonaluminum 8-quart cookware*
- *food mill, blender, or coffee grinder* to make herbal flours or powders

Fresh ginger should be available at your local supermarket. If not, see if they will order it for you. The herbs in the following recipe to supplement *Qi* (astragalus, dioscorea, lotus seeds, codonopsis, and red dates) probably win the "most often used in these herbal recipes" prize. This *Qi* recipe, along with the similar one to supplement and harmonize *Earth* later on, would be a good place to begin if you are unsure about which recipes best suit your needs.

SIMPLE RECIPES TO HARMONIZE QI, MOISTURE, AND BLOOD

Supplement Qi
    Energizes, builds vital capacity,
    and increases immunity

Decongesting		
Action upon Qi, Moisture, Blood, or Adverse Climates	*Organ Network benefited*	*Effects*
activates Qi, relaxes chest, dispels phlegm	*Lung*	relaxes bronchi, relieves cough and mucus congestion; eliminates pus and reduces inflammation
regulates and activates *Qi*, dispels *Wind* and phlegm	*Lung Spleen*	relieves indigestion, cough, gas, belching, and stomach acidity; promotes expectoration
lubricates *Intestines*, dispels phlegm	*Lung*	promotes expectoration and relaxes bronchi; relieves constipation

Invigorates *Organ Networks*, especially *Spleen, Lung,* and *Kidney*

1 oz. astragalus root
1 oz. dioscorea rhz.
1 oz. lotus seeds
1 oz. codonopsis root
12 red dates, soaked and pitted
1 inch fresh ginger root, minced

7–8 c. vegetable or chicken stock (pages 334–335)
1 turnip
2 yams
1/2 c. chopped parsley

A. To prepare as a soup or stew:

- Tie the astragalus and codonopsis in a bundle with string or place in a muslin bag.
- Simmer all the herbs in the stock for 1 hour.
- While the stock simmers, peel and cut the turnip and yams into cubes.
- After an hour, add the turnip and yams and simmer an additional 30 minutes.
- Garnish with parsley and serve.

B. To prepare as a casserole:

- Tie the astragalus and codonopsis in a bundle with string or place in a muslin bag. If the dioscorea has not been soaked, break it into ½-inch pieces.

- Peel and dice the turnip; peel and slice the yams into ⅛-inch-thick medallions.
- Add the herbs to the stock and simmer for 30 minutes. Add the red dates and continue cooking for another 30 minutes.
- Line the casserole dish with the yams and turnip.
- Preheat the oven to 350°.
- Add the herbal broth to the casserole and all the herbs except the astragalus and codonopsis.
- Cook for ½ hour in a 350° oven.
- Garnish with parsley and serve the casserole over rice with soy sauce to taste.

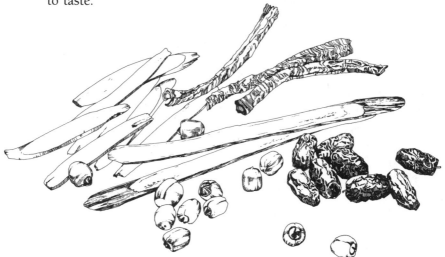

Common Cooking Herbs: *Dioscorea*, Codonopsis, Astragalus, Lotus Seeds, Dates

Supplement Moisture

Supports vital fluids, eliminates thirst, softens skin, and lubricates mucous membranes

Moisturizes *Organ Networks*,
especially the *Spleen, Lung, Kidney*, and *Heart*

1 oz. polygonatum rhz.
1 oz. American ginseng root
1 oz. lily bulbs
12 red dates, soaked and pitted

½ c. wheatberries
7–8 c. vegetable or chicken stock
(pages 344–345)
2 c. string beans

2 large thin-skinned potatoes
8 oz. tofu
4 tsp. oil

2 tbsp. soy sauce
¹/₄ c. sesame seeds

- If possible, soak the herbs and wheatberries in 1¹/₂ cups of water for at least 1 hour.
- Slice the polygonatum into ³/₄-inch lengths.
- Simmer the wheatberries and herbs in the stock for 1 hour.
- Diagonally slice the string beans in 1-inch segments, dice the potatoes into ¹/₄-inch cubes, and cut the tofu into ¹/₂-inch triangles.
- Heat 1¹/₂ tsp. oil in a wok (at high heat) or in a skillet (at medium heat), add potatoes, and sauté for 10 minutes.
- Add ¹/₃ cup of the herbal broth, cover, and cook until tender. Then remove the potatoes to a saucepan.
- Heat 1¹/₂ tsp. oil and sauté the string beans about 5 minutes. Add ¹/₃ cup of the herbal broth until it evaporates, then add the beans to the potatoes.
- Add the tofu to the beans and potatoes along with the soy sauce and 2 tbsp. of water. Cover and heat for 3–4 minutes until the tofu is warmed through.
- Serve the vegetables and herbal soup as separate dishes, and garnish both with sesame seeds as well as with seasonings (such as soy and sesame oil) to taste.

Supplement Blood

Nutrifies *Blood*, improves circulation, enhances reproductive capacity

Fortifies *Organ Networks*, especially *Kidney*, *Liver*, and *Heart*

1 oz. (cooked) rehmannia root
¹/₂ oz. ligusticum rhz.
2 oz. lycii berries
1 oz. longan fr.
12 red dates, soaked and pitted
1 in. fresh ginger sliced

¹/₂ c. black beans
7–8 c. vegetable or chicken stock (pages 344–345)
6 shiitake or black mushrooms (if dry, soaked), slivered
¹/₂ c. peanuts (with skin)
¹/₂ c. pine nuts
4 tbsp. rice vinegar

- Rinse the black beans and simmer them in 3 cups of boiling water for 1 hour.
- Combine the cooked beans and bean water with the herbs (except for the red dates) and simmer them in the stock for 1 hour.

357

- Add the dates and mushrooms to the stock and simmer for another 30 minutes.
- Roast the peanuts until golden brown in a 350° oven (about 10 minutes), and roast the pine nuts (about 5 minutes.)
- Add the peanuts, pine nuts, and vinegar to the herbal stew, and serve with white or brown rice.

Options: Spinach can be added to the above or served as a side dish with steamed carrots.

Decongest Qi

Improves digestion of protein and carbohydrates, stimulates peristalsis
Especially beneficial for *Liver, Stomach*, and *Intestines*

¹/₂ oz. radish seeds	1 c. fresh radishes
¹/₂ oz. sweet almond seeds	2 beets
2 in. fresh ginger, minced	1 c. shiitake or black mushrooms
¹/₂ oz. dried tangerine peel, soaked	(if dry, soaked), slivered
and cut in strips	4 cloves garlic, minced
3 c. vegetable stock (page 344)	3 c. chopped cabbage
3 shallots	1 tbsp. sesame oil

- Grind the radish seeds in a mortar or coffee mill.
- Simmer the radish seeds, almond pits, ginger, and tangerine peel in the stock for 1 hour.
- Dice the shallots, radishes, and beets, and sauté them with the mushrooms and garlic in sesame oil until tender, about 15 minutes.
- Add the cabbage and stock, cover, and simmer 5–10 minutes until the leaves are wilted. Serve.

Decongest Moisture

Improves circulation and discharge of fluids
Especially beneficial for *Spleen, Lung*, and *Kidney*

1 oz. corn silk	¹/₂ c. pearl barley
¹/₂ oz. tangerine peel	7–8 c. vegetable stock (page 344)
¹/₄ c. peel of fresh ginger	1¹/₂ c. asparagus
1 bunch parsley	1¹/₂ c. celery
1 oz. poria fungus	¹/₂ c. chopped parsley

- Place the corn silk, tangerine peel, ginger peel, and a bunch of parsley in a muslin bag and simmer them in the stock along with the poria and barley for 1 hour.

- Diagonally slice the asparagus and celery into bite-size pieces and add them to the herb stew, simmering this an additional 15 minutes.
- Remove the muslin bag.
- Garnish with parsley and serve.

Decongest Blood

Promotes circulation, reduces fatty accumulations, counteracts constriction

Especially beneficial for *Liver, Heart*

1 oz. white peony	2 leeks (white and pale green portions only)
1/4 oz. safflower	
1/2 oz. ligusticum rhz.	1 c. beets
3 tsp. turmeric	2 c. eggplant chunks (1 globe or 2 Japanese eggplants)
5 medallions fresh ginger	
7 c. vegetable or chicken stock (pages 344–345)	1/2 c. rice wine
	1/4 c. rice vinegar

- Place all the herbs in a muslin bag, and simmer in the stock for 30 minutes.
- Chop the leeks, peel and dice the beets, and cut the eggplant into 1-inch chunks
- Add the beets, leeks, and eggplant, and continue to simmer for 15 minutes.
- Add the rice wine and vinegar, simmer 5 more minutes, and serve.

INGREDIENTS TO ELIMINATE HEAT, COLD, WIND, AND PHLEGM

The following are some suggested groupings of ingredients to address specific conditions. You may devise your own recipes and prepare these foods in one or more different dishes.

Dispel Heat

Cools the body, reduces inflammation, neutralizes toxins

Benefits *Heart, Liver, Lung, Small Intestine, Gallbladder, Large Intestine,* and *Bladder*

2 burdock roots	1 c. mung bean sprouts
1 daikon radish	1 cucumber
1 c. tofu	

Dispel Cold

Warms the body, stimulates circulation

Benefits *Spleen, Lung, Kidney, Stomach, Large Intestine*

1 oz. fresh ginger	1 c. mustard greens
¹/₄ oz. cardamom seeds (grated)	¹/₂ c. chives
1 oz. fresh coriander	¹/₂ c. rice wine or vinegar

Dispel Wind

Soothes the nerves, relaxes the muscles, promotes perspiration

Benefits *Liver, Lung, Gallbladder*

1. oz. *Pueraria* root	2 whole scallions
¹/₂ oz. chrysanthemum flowers, steeped	1 c. celery
¹/₂ oz. peppermint or ¹/₄ oz. rosemary leaves	

Dispel Phlegm

Helps expectoration and elimination of excess mucus

Benefits *Lung, Spleen, Stomach, Large Intestine, Gallbladder*

¹/₂ oz. orange or tangerine peel (1 oz. fresh)	1 c. daikon radish
¹/₂ oz. apricot or almond seeds	2 inches fresh ginger
1 fresh pear (diced)	

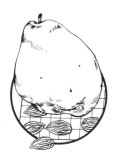

RECIPES FOR THE FIVE PHASES: SEASONS AND CLIMATES

In winter *Qi* consolidates at the core, and in summer it disperses toward the surface. In spring *Qi* mobilizes and begins to expand outward, and in fall it begins to coalesce and sink inward. Seasonal recipes promote these processes, smoothing our transition from one state to the next. Through the law of correspondence, the foods for each season benefit the *Organ Network* associated with it.

Spring recipes assist the *Liver* in moving and discharging *Qi* and *Blood*. Summer recipes help the *Heart* to circulate *Blood* and eliminate *Heat*. Fall recipes aid the *Lung* in tightening the surface (skin) and moistening the *Qi*, while winter recipes support the *Kidney* in storing, replenishing, and concentrating *Essence*. Recipes that benefit the *Spleen* are good throughout the year, since it is the job of the *Spleen* to generate *Qi* and *Blood* and harmonize the interaction of all *Organ Networks*.

Regardless of the season, foods that counteract *Wind, Heat, Dampness, Dryness,* and *Cold* protect the body from sudden changes in the weather. Spring and fall are usually associated with dramatic variations in temperature, pressure, humidity, and wind, so cooking with herbs like astragalus, white peony, dioscorea, and fresh ginger improve the body's resistance to *Wind, Dampness,* and *Cold* and defend it against the acute, infectious illness that often occur at these times. Even in the tropics, during the winter season,

Five-Phase Yin-Yang Correspondences

Phase	Wood	Fire	Earth	Metal	Water
Yin-Yang	Small Yang	Great Yang	Between Yin and Yang	Small Yin	Great Yin
Yin Viscera	Liver	Heart	Spleen	Lung	Kidney
Yang Viscera	Gall-bladder	Small Intestine	Stomach	Large Intestine	Bladder
Nature	Warm	Hot	Neutral	Cool	Cold
Adverse Conditions Most Likely	Wind Heat Dampness	Heat Dryness	Dampness Cold Heat	Dryness Heat Cold Phlegm	Cold Dampness Dryness Heat
Depleted or Congested Constituents	Qi Blood	Blood Moisture	Qi Moisture	Moisture Qi	Essence Moisture
Cooking Herbs	Carthamus Ligustium Lycii White Peony	Chinese Ginseng Lily Longan Lotus	Astragalus Condonop-sis Dioscorea Poria	Astragalus American Ginseng Glehnia Platycodon	Cornus Dioscorea Lotus Rehmannia

it is still important to eat foods like dioscorea, lotus seed, and cornus, which will help the *Kidney* to consolidate *Qi* and *Essence* but will not generate additional *Heat* and *Dampness*. The coolness of northern regions, even in the summer, may require that warming herbs and foods continue to be eaten in order to protect the body's interior from *Cold* and *Dampness* and to ensure sufficient *Qi* and *Essence* to survive an even colder winter.

The following recipes sustain the *Organ Networks* and buffer seasonal stresses. If you are unsure which one to try first, start with the recipe to supplement and harmonize *Earth*—it has a pleasant, hardy taste and is a choice general tonic.

Supplement and Harmonize Earth

Spleen congestion occurs when food and fluids accumulate, causing stagnation of *Qi* and *Moisture*. Foods that decongest *Qi*, promote peristalsis, and eliminate *Dampness* are needed.

Spleen depletion results from *deficiency* and stagnation of *Qi*, persistent *Dampness*, and accumulation of *Cold*. Foods that tonify and disperse *Qi* and eliminate *Dampness* and *Cold* are required.

Remedial principle: Tonify *Qi* and *Moisture*, disperse *Moisture*, activate digestion

1 oz. astragalus root	7–8 c. vegetable or chicken stock
1 oz. codonopsis root	(pages 344–345)
1 oz. dioscorea rhizome	1/4 c. uncooked white rice
1 oz. lotus seeds	2 carrots
1 oz. poria curls	1 yam
12 red dates, soaked and pitted	1/2 c. black or shiitake mushrooms
1 in. fresh ginger, chopped	(if dry, soaked), slivered
	1/2 c. spinach

- Place the astragalus and codonopsis in a muslin bag or tie them in a bundle with string. Break the dioscorea into half-inch pieces.
- Place the muslin bag, dioscorea, the remaining herbs, and the rice in the stock and simmer for 1 hour.
- While the stock is simmering, dice the carrots and yam and cut the spinach leaves into 1-inch sections.

- Add the carrots, yam, and mushrooms to the herbal stew, and simmer for 30 minutes.
- Remove the muslin bag. Option: After the codonopsis has cooked it can be removed from the muslin bag and cut into ¼-inch lengths and added to the stew.
- Add the spinach for 5 additional minutes, and serve.

The following variations on the basic *Earth* recipe substitutes ingredients that more particularly address specific disharmonies.

For Congested Earth

1 oz. astragalus root	7–8 c. vegetable stock
1 oz. lotus seeds	1 c. radish
1 oz. poria curls	2 beets
1 oz. white peony root	½ c. black or shiitake mushrooms
12 red dates, soaked and pitted	(if dry, soaked), slivered
½ oz. dried tangerine or orange peel, soaked and slivered	½ c. brown rice
1 in. fresh ginger	½ c. spinach

For Damp Earth

2 oz. astragalus root	7–8 c. vegetable or chicken stock
2 oz. poria curls	2 carrots
1 oz. corn silk (place in bag, along with astragalus)	½ c. turnip
1 oz. lotus seeds	½ c. black or shiitake mushrooms (if dry, soaked), slivered
12 red dates, soaked and pitted	½ c. chopped parsley or cilantro
1 in. fresh ginger	½ c. pearl barley

For Dry Earth

1 oz. polygonatum rhizome	7–8 c. vegetable stock
1 oz. lotus seeds	½ c. uncooked white rice
1 oz. poria curls	2 carrots
12 red dates, soaked and pitted	2 zucchini
1 in. fresh ginger	1 c. tofu
	½ c. fresh basil

For Cold Earth

Follow the basic recipe, but

delete mushrooms and spinach
add another inch of fresh ginger, ½ oz. cardamom, and ½ c. rice wine

Supplement and Harmonize Wood

Liver congestion occurs when *Heat* and *Wind* plus stagnation of *Qi* and *Blood* persist. Foods that clear *Heat*, moisten *Dryness*, and disperse *Qi* and *Blood* resolve this congestion.

Liver depletion occurs with *deficiency* of *Blood* and *Qi* along with stagnation of *Blood* and *Qi*, requiring foods that nourish *Qi* and *Blood* and move *Qi* and *Blood*.

Remedial principle: Tonify *Qi* and *Blood*, disperse *Blood*, dispel *Heat*.

¹/₂ oz. white peony root
1 oz. codonopsis root
¹/₄ oz. carthamus flowers
¹/₄ oz. chrysanthemum flowers
1 oz. lycii berries
12 red dates, soaked and pitted

2 bay leaves
6¹/₂ c. vegetable or chicken stock (pages 344–345)
1 leek (white and pale green portions only)
2 celery stalks
1 c. eggplant
12 black or shiitake mushrooms (if dry, soaked), slivered
4 tbsp. sesame seeds
¹/₄ c. pine nuts
1 tbsp. roasted sesame oil
¹/₄ c. rice vinegar
1 tbsp. turmeric or ¹/₈ tsp. saffron

- After soaking in boiling water to cover, chop the white peony and codonopsis in bite-size pieces. Place the carthamus and chrysanthemum flowers and bay leaves in a muslin bag and set aside.
- Simmer the white peony, codonopsis, lycii, and red dates in the stock for 1 hour.
- While that is cooking, slice the leek and celery, and cut the eggplant into cubes.
- Add the vegetables and mushrooms to the stock, and simmer an additional 30 minutes.
- Toast the sesame seeds in a 350° oven for about 8–10 minutes and the pine nuts for about 5 minutes.
- Add the herbs in the bag, sesame seeds, pine nuts, sesame oil, rice and vinegar, sesame oil, saffron or turmeric, and simmer 5 minutes. Remove the bag and serve.

For Blood *Congestion*

delete lycii berries, vinegar, pine nuts, leek
add ¼ oz. ligusticum rhizome, ½ c. rice wine, 1 c. chives

For Qi *Congestion*

delete codonopsis, eggplant, pine nuts
add ½ oz. dried tangerine peel (1 oz. fresh), 1 c. radish, ½ c. uncooked
brown rice (cook with herbs 1 hour), ½ oz. fresh ginger

For Heat

delete vinegar, saffron/turmeric, leek, eggplant, bay, pine nuts
add 2 beets, 1 c. tofu or tomato, ¼ oz. dried honeysuckle flowers, 2 tsp.
marjoram

For Wind

delete vinegar, carthamus flowers, leeks
add ¼ oz. peppermint or marjoram, 3 scallions

Supplement and Harmonize Fire

Heart congestion occurs when *Heat* and *Dryness* cause *Blood* stagnation and
agitation of the *Spirit*. Cooling, moisturizing, dispersing, and calming foods
are indicated.

Depletion of the *Heart* results from *deficiency* of Qi and *Blood* along with
stagnation of *Blood* and restlessness of *Spirit*. Foods that nourish the *Blood*
and *Qi*, activate circulation, and calm the *Spirit* are needed.

Remedial principle: Tonify Qi, *Moisture, Blood*; promote circulation of *Blood*,
clear *Heat*, soothe the *Spirit*.

1 oz. codonopsis root	6½ c. vegetable or chicken stock
½ oz. carthamus flowers	(pages 344–345)
2 oz. lotus seeds	1 c. beets
1 oz. longan fruit	1 c. carrots
1 oz. lily bulbs	1 c. corn
½ oz. lycii berries	1 tbsp. roasted sesame oil
	3 tbsp. toasted coarsely ground sesame seeds

- Tie the codonopsis with string. Place the carthamus flowers in a bag and set aside.
- Simmer all the herbs except for the carthamus in the stock for 1 hour. Remove the codonopsis, cool, cut into ³/₄-inch lengths, and return to stew.
- While the stew is simmering, cut the beets and carrots into cubes, and if the corn is fresh, remove it from the cob.
- Add the beets and carrots, and simmer for an additional 15 minutes.
- Add the carthamus, corn, and sesame oil, and simmer for 5 minutes.
- Serve, using the sesame seeds as a garnish.

For Blood *Stagnation*
delete longan, lily, beets
add 1 tbsp. turmeric, ¹/₄ oz. ligusticum rhizome, 1 c. chives, 1 eggplant

For Heat
delete longan fruit
add ¹/₂ oz. honeysuckle flowers (place in bag and simmer 5 minutes)

Supplement and Harmonize Metal

Lung congestion occurs when *Wind, Heat,* and phlegm obstruct *Qi.* Foods that clear *Wind, Heat,* and phlegm, disperse *Qi,* and replenish *Moisture* are indicated.

Depletion of the *Lung* occurs when *Qi* becomes *deficient* and *Qi* and *Moisture* become stagnant. Food that tonify *Qi* and disperse *Moisture* and *Qi* are needed.

Remedial principle: Tonify and disperse *Qi* and *Moisture*; eliminate *Heat, Wind,* and phlegm.

1 oz. astragalus	5 c. vegetable or chicken stock
¹/₄ oz. dried tangerine peel (¹/₂ oz. fresh)	(pages 344–345)
	1 turnip
1 oz. glehnia root	1 yam
¹/₂ oz. American ginseng root	1 fresh pear
¹/₂ oz. almond or apricot seeds	6 scallions
¹/₄ c. fresh ginger root, minced	¹/₂ c. uncooked white rice

- Place the astragalus and tangerine peel in a muslin bag.

- Cover the glehnia and ginseng with boiling water, soak for 20 minutes, and cut into bite-size pieces.
- Simmer the herbs in the stock for 1 hour.
- Cut the turnip, yam, and pear into ½-inch cubes, and slice the scallions.
- Add the rice to the herbal stew, and simmer another 10 minutes.
- Remove the muslin bag of astragalus and tangerine.
- Add the turnip, yam, pear, and scallions, and place in a covered casserole dish in a 400° oven for 15 minutes.
- Remove the lid and cook for an additional 15 minutes.
- Serve.

For Heat

delete ginger, scallions
add ½ oz. mint (1 oz. fresh)

For stagnation of Moisture *(Phlegm)*

delete glehnia root, yams
add 1 oz. lily bulbs, 3 carrots

Supplement and Harmonize Water

Kidney congestion occurs when *Heat* or *Cold* obstructs *Moisture*, leading to accumulation of *Dampness*. Foods that disperse *Moisture* and purge *Dampness* are used, combined with either warming or cooling ingredients.

Depletion of the *Kidney* occurs when *Essence* or vital warmth becomes *deficient*. Foods that replenish *Essence* and warm the body are needed.

Remedial principle: Tonify *Qi* and *Essence*; disperse *Moisture*; eliminate *Cold*.

½ oz. dioscorea rhizome
1 lotus seeds
1 oz. poria fungus
1 lycii berries
½ oz. rehmannia
½ oz. cornus fruit
1 inch fresh ginger, minced

1 clove garlic, minced
½ c. chopped cilantro or parsley
½ c. kidney beans
2 tbsp. ground pasilla chili (sweet)
1 tsp ground chili negro (hot)
6. c. vegetable or chicken stock or water
1 c. string beans
½ c. roasted peanuts
1 tsp. salt

- Break the dioscorea into ½-inch pieces.
- Simmer all the herbs (except the cilantro or parsley), the kidney beans, chili, and garlic in the stock or water for 1½ hour.
- While this is cooking, diagonally cut the string beans and roast the peanuts in a 350° oven for 10 minutes.
- Add the string beans and peanuts, and cook for another 15 minutes.
- Add the cilantro or parsley and salt to taste.

For congestion of Moisture

delete lotus seeds, lycii, peanuts, salt
add 1 oz. corn silk (place in muslin bag), 1 c. sliced celery

For Cold

delete ginger peel
add 1 tsp grated cardamom, 1 tsp. grated dry ginger

HERBAL BREADS AND CAKES

To demonstrate the versatility of herbal cuisine, we ground a few nourishing herbs into powder and used them like flour. These included millet, poria, dioscorea, and lotus seeds, which can be ground into flour in a food mill, if not available in powdered form. After a hardy Chinese herbal soup, wholesome baked goods are a treat. Preparing the recipes in this chapter has been a wonderful adventure: tasting them, making adjustments, and looking forward to a time when Chinese herbal cooking gains wide popularity in the West. We hope that you will be moved to re-create and embellish these recipes as well as follow them.

None of these baked desserts use wheat flour. Minimal sugar is used, lecithin is substituted for oil and gluten, and oat bran is sometimes included. Except for eggs and coconuts, these recipes are very low in saturated fats and cholesterol. And they taste delicious!

Pineapple and Coconut Lotus Cake:

Remedial principle: Supplement *Qi, Moisture,* and *Blood.*

1 c. lotus seed flour	½ c. lycii berries
1 c. corn meal flour	1 c. raisins
1 c. millet flour	½ fresh pineapple or 8 oz. canned
2 ripe bananas	1 cup shredded coconut (optional)
1½ c. coconut milk (28 oz.)	

- Combine the flours.
- Puree the banana and coconut milk in a blender, and stir this into the flour mixture.
- Add the lycii, raisins, chopped pineapple, and shredded coconut.
- Bake in two well-greased cake tins at 350° for 50–60 minutes or until done (toothpick test).

Gingerbread

Remedial principle: Warm and supplement *Qi*.

1 c. millet flour
1/2 c. dioscorea flour
1/4 c. lotus seed flour
1/4 c. poria flour
2 tsp. baking powder
2 tsp. cinnamon
1/4 tsp. cloves (powdered)

1 c. oat bran
1/4 c. lecithin (granulated)
1/2 c. orange juice
3 tbsp. fresh ginger, minced
5 eggs, separated (3 yolks, 5 whites)
1 c. molasses

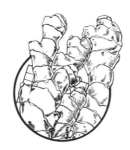

- Combine and sift the millet, dioscorea, lotus seed, and poria flours with baking powder, cinnamon, and cloves.
- Mix in the oat bran and granulated lecithin.
- Puree the orange juice and ginger in a blender.
- Separate the eggs, mixing the yolks with the molasses and the ginger-orange paste.
- Fold the dry ingredients into the wet (except the egg whites).
- Beat the egg whites until stiff but not dry, and gently fold them into the batter.
- Bake in well-greased bread tin for about 45–60 minutes in a preheated 350° oven until done.

Date-Walnut Loaf

Remedial principle: Supplement *Qi* and *Blood*.

1 c. millet flour
1/2 c. dioscorea flour
1/4 c. poria flour
1/4 c. lotus seed flour
2 tsp. baking powder
2 tsp. cinnamon
1/2 tsp. nutmeg
1/2 c. oat bran

1/4 c. granulated lecithin
1/4 c. raw sugar
3 eggs
1 c. orange juice
1 tsp vanilla
1 c. chopped dates
1/2 c. chopped walnuts

- Sift the millet, dioscorea, poria, and lotus flours with the baking powder, cinnamon, and nutmeg. Mix in the oat bran, granulated lecithin, and sugar.
- Beat the eggs and combine them with the orange juice and vanilla.
- Lightly fold the wet ingredients into the dry, and then fold in the walnuts and dates.
- Bake in a greased loaf pan in a preheated 325° oven for 45–60 minutes until done.

Lycii-Walnut Honey Spirals

Remedial principle: Supplement *Blood* and *Moisture*.

1 1/2 c. millet flour
3/4 c. dioscorea flour
1/2 c. lotus seed flour
1/2 c. poria flour
2 tsp. baking powder
2 tsp. cinnamon
1/2 tsp. nutmeg
1/4 tsp. cloves

1/2 c. oat bran
4 oz. lycii berries
1/8 c. orange juice
3/4 c. walnuts
1 c. honey
2 tbsp. liquid lecithin
1 grated orange rind

- Sift the millet, dioscorea, lotus, and poria flours with the baking powder, cinnamon, nutmeg, and cloves. Mix in the oat bran.
- Rinse the lycii berries in hot water, drain, and puree them with the orange juice.
- Chop the walnuts to a crumbly consistency in a blender.
- Warm the honey for about 4 min. over a low flame to liquefy (until it reaches a watery consistency), remove from the heat, and add the lecithin.
- Gradually add the dry ingredients to the honey mixture in parts, stirring and mixing until a soft dough is formed.
- Roll out the dough on a board sprinkled with flour into a rectangle about 1/4-inch thick.

- Spread the lycii-orange juice paste evenly on the dough, then sprinkle with crumbled walnuts and grated orange rind.
- Roll the dough into a log and carefully place on a greased cookie sheet.
- Bake in a preheated 350° oven for 20 minutes, remove from the oven, let cool for 10 minutes, and cut into serving slices.
- For crispier spirals, cut the log into 1/2-inch slices before baking and place them evenly spaced on a greased cookie sheet.

Oat Bran Lycii Muffins

Remedial principle: Supplement and circulate *Blood.*

1/2 c. millet flour	2/3 c. oat bran
1/2 c. lotus seed flour	1 egg
1/2 c. poria flour	1/4 c. liquid lecithin
1 1/4 tsp. baking powder	1/2 c. honey
3/4 tsp. baking soda	1 1/4 c. buttermilk
1/4 tsp. salt	3/4 c. lycii berries

- Sift the millet, lotus, and poria flours with the baking powder, baking soda, and salt. Mix in the oat bran.
- Beat the egg and mix it with the lecithin, honey, and buttermilk.
- Soak the lycii berries in hot water for 5 minutes and drain.
- Fold the wet and dry ingredients together along with the lycii berries until the flour is moistened.
- Bake in a greased muffin pan in a preheated 400° oven for about 20 minutes.

CONGEES AND SOUPS FOR COMMON AILMENTS

PREPARING CONGEE

Congee is a gruel or porridge made from grains. The grain is simmered one to two hours in a ratio of 1/2-cup grain to 8 cups liquid. Rice and barley are most often used, although millet or buckwheat may be substituted. In China a simple rice congee is commonly served for breakfast with slivered ginger and scallions as a garnish. Because it is easy to digest, congee is a particularly good vehicle for delivering nutrients and medicine to people who are weak or frail. Any of the herbs listed in the categories of supplementing or de-congesting *Qi, Moisture,* and *Blood* can be used, along with appropriate foods to prepare a congee targeted toward a particular therapeutic goal. Below are a few simple recipes that can serve as examples. A condiment sauce com-

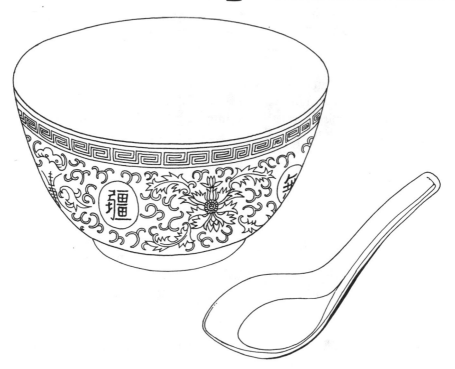

posed of 2 tbsp. rice wine, 1 tbsp. soy sauce, and 1 tsp. sesame oil is particularly tasty in some of the bland congees.

Robust Health for Babies, Kids, and Seniors

In China, dioscorea is often the first food fed to infants because it is highly
nourishing, of special benefit to the *Spleen, Stomach, Lung,* and *Kidney,* and
quite easy to digest. Dioscorea is a tuberous rhizome of a Chinese yam that
translates from Mandarin to English as "mountain medicine." This herbal
meal has a mildly sweet taste and is therefore appealing to children or adults
who have sensitive digestion or are feeling weak.

1 oz. dioscorea rhizome
1 oz. poria fungus
1 oz. lotus seeds
1 carrot or yam, peeled and cut in
cubes

$1/2$ c. white rice
8 c. vegetable or chicken stock
(pages 344–345)
1 pinch sea salt

- Break the dioscorea into small pieces.
- Simmer all the ingredients for 2–3 hours until the dioscorea and lotus
  seeds are quite soft.
- For infants, this mixture can be pureed in a blender and given 1–3
  times a day.

Warming Congee on a Cold Winter Day

1 oz. astragalus root	12 black dates, soaked and pitted
1 in. fresh ginger, minced	2 carrots, peeled and diced
1/2 tsp. powdered ginger	3/4 c. millet
2 tsp. cinnamon (powdered)	8 c. water, milk, or stock
1 tsp. cardamom seed (powdered)	

- Place the astragalus in a bag or tie with string.
- Toast the millet in the oven or in a pan until the yellow turns to light brown.
- Simmer the ingredients for 1–2 hours, until desired consistency is reached, remove astragalus, and serve with a dash of cinnamon as a garnish.

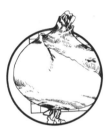

Building Stamina and Resistance

2 oz. astragalus root	3 cloves garlic, minced
1 oz. codonopsis root	1/2 c. white rice
1 oz. pueraria root	8 c. vegetable or chicken stock
1 oz. lotus seeds	(pages 344–345)
8 shiitake or black mushrooms (if dry, soaked), slivered	1 carrot, peeled and diced

- Place the astragalus in a bag or tie with string. Cover the codonopsis and pueraria with boiling water for 20 minutes and cut into 1/4-inch lengths.
- Simmer all the ingredients except the carrot for 60–90 minutes.
- Add the carrot for 12 minutes, remove the astragalus, and serve.

DEBILITY AND COMPROMISED IMMUNITY

People who feel debilitated and weary from serious illnesses (such as AIDS or chronic viral fatigue syndrome) or from chemotherapy often face compromised immune function. In Chinese medicine this reflects a profound degeneration of *Essence*, the root of *Qi* and *Blood*, stored in the *Kidney*. The wasting of the body that can characterize these illnesses is a sign of the withering of internal resources. Countering this trend depends upon strengthening the *Kidney* and *Spleen*, restoring *Essence*, and generating *Qi*. A recipe that is easy to digest, highly nourishing, and restorative is this immune-enhancing soup.

For those who want to maintain their strength, this soup is equally appropriate because it tonifies *Qi* and *Blood*, accomplishing the goal of *fu zheng* therapy, which means to fortify (*fu*) the constitution (*zheng*).

1 oz. astragalus root
1 oz. codonopsis root
1/2 oz. tangerine peel
1 oz. polygonatum rhizome
1 oz. poria fungus
1 oz. lycii berries
12 red dates, soaked and pitted

6 black or shiitake mushrooms (if dry, soaked), slivered
1/2 c. loose seaweed (nori, hijiki, kombu)
7–8 c. vegetable or chicken stock (pages 344–345)
2 yams
1 leek (white and pale green portions only)
5 scallions

- Place the astragalus, codonopsis, and orange peel in a muslin bag. Cut the polygonatum into 1-inch strips.
- Simmer all the herbs, mushrooms, and seaweed in the stock for 1 hour.
- While this cooks, cut the yams into 1-inch cubes, slice the leeks, and add them to the stock for an additional 25 minutes.
- Add slivered scallions for the last 3 minutes and serve.

Astragalus, codonopsis, poria, seaweed, and shiitake mushrooms contain immune-enhancing, adaptogenic compounds known as saponins, glycosides, and polysaccharides. Including 1/3 c. white rice in the soup thickens the broth, making it even more nutritive, or rice may be served as a side dish. Consistency of the meal depends on the preference of the diners. It is important that food be appetizing, and some people enjoy a thick porridgelike gruel, finding it easy to eat, while others prefer a clear broth with discrete, chewy vegetables. These recipes can be varied according to this sort of preference.

COMMON COLD

During the course of a cold or flu, we experience changing conditions from mild sniffles and sore throat to an entrenched, enervating cough, trailing off to a dull, lingering malaise. Appropriate medicinal foods may help to abort the sickness or hasten its demise by reinforcing our powers of recovery.

The first stage of a cold (with slight fever, chills, aching, scratchy throat, and stuffiness) is an invasion of *Wind* with either *Cold* or *Heat*, depending on whether chills or fever predominate. Herbal food should dispel *Wind*, increase surface circulation, and support *Qi*. The following broth will warm the body, promote perspiration, and supplement the defensive *Qi*.

2 oz. pueraria root
2 inches fresh ginger, minced
5 c. vegetable or chicken stock (pages 344–345)
2 celery stalks, diced

¹/₂ c. chopped parsley
5 scallions, slivered
1 c. cooked wheat or rice noodles

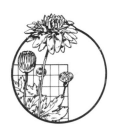

- Cut the pueraria into ¹/₂-inch lengths.
- Simmer the pueraria and ginger in the stock for 45 minutes.
- Add the celery and simmer for another 10 minutes.
- Add the parsley, scallions, and noodles for a final 3 minutes, and serve.

The following cooling broth reduces fever, promotes perspiration, soothes and moistens the throat, and supplements the defensive *Qi*.

1 oz. pueraria root
1 burdock root
5 c. vegetable or chicken stock (pages 344–345)
1 c. chard

2 tsp. miso
1 c. bean noodles or sprouts
1 oz. honeysuckle flowers
¹/₄ tsp. white pepper

- Cut the pueraria and burdock into bite-size lengths and simmer them for 45 minutes in the stock.
- Add the chard, miso, noodles, or sprouts and simmer for 5 minutes. Place the honeysuckle in a muslin bag and steep it for 5 minutes, remove the bag, add the pepper, and serve.

COUGH

If the illness progresses to a deeper stage in which cough is predominant, then food and herbs should decongest phlegm and replenish *Qi* and *Moisture*.

1 oz. glehnia root
1 oz. lily bulbs
¹/₂ orange peel

2 in. fresh ginger, minced
5 c. vegetable or chicken stock (pages 344–345)
2 pears, cut in cubes

- Cut the glehnia into ½-inch lengths. Simmer it in the stock along with the lily bulbs, orange peel, and ginger for 45 minutes.
- Add the pears and simmer for another 15 minutes, remove the orange peel, and serve.

Where there is profuse phlegm, add ½ oz. each of platycodon and apricot kernels. If the phlegm is dry or sticky, delete the orange peel.

RECOVERY

In the recovery stage people often feel weak and weary, with lingering cough or headache. This is because the body's resources of *Qi* and *Moisture* have been temporarily depleted. The following recipe replenishes *Qi* and *Moisture* while eliminating the last remnants of *Wind* and phlegm.

1 oz. pueraria root	12 red dates
1 oz. polygonatum rhizome	½ oz. orange peel
1 oz. lotus seeds	1 in. fresh ginger, minced

These herbs can be combined with:

5 scallions, sliced	⅓ c. white rice
3 carrots, cubed	8 c. vegetable or chicken stock
2 celery stalks, diced	(pages 344–345), or water
or substitute 2–3 diced pears for the vegetables	

- Slice the pueraria, polygonatum, and orange peel into small pieces.
- Simmer all the ingredients except the vegetables or pears for 2–3 hours.
- Add the vegetables or pears for the last 20 minutes and serve.

WOMAN'S CYCLE

A woman's menstrual cycle is another example of a progression of bodily events that invites particular strategies at different stages. The premenstrual phase is characterized by a buildup of *Qi* and *Blood* in preparation for conception. This temporary surplus increases susceptibility to problems of congestion such as swollen breasts, abdominal distension, increased water retention, erratic moods, and disruption of mental clarity and focus. Food becomes an ally or adversary at this time because of unusual appetites or cravings. Assuming pregnancy has not occurred, the goal is to activate *Qi* and encourage the downward flow of *Moisture* and *Blood*.

1 oz. corn silk	½ c. pearl barley
½ c. fresh ginger peel	6 c. vegetable or chicken stock
1 oz. white peony root	(pages 344–345)
½ oz. ligusticum rhizome	1 c. chopped parsley

1 c. radish, diced
1 leek (white and pale green
portions), sliced

1 carrot, sliced
1/4 c. sweet vinegar

- Place the corn silk and ginger in a muslin bag.
- Simmer all the herbs along with the pearl barley in the stock for 1 hour.
- Add the vegetables and simmer an additional 15 minutes, remove the muslin bag, add the vinegar, and serve.

During the menstrual period, the predominant activity is discharge, often accompanied by feelings of fatigue, chilliness, and vulnerability. The following recipe promotes the release of *Blood* and *Moisture* from the breasts, uterus, bowels, and bladder, while preserving the *Qi* and *Essence* of the *Kidney*, *Liver*, and *Spleen*.

1 oz. carthamus flowers
1 oz. ligusticum rhizome
1 oz. lotus seeds
1 oz. poria fungus
12 red dates, soaked and pitted
2 in. ginger, minced

7 c. vegetable or chicken stock
(pages 344–345)
1/2 c. aduki beans
8 black or shiitake mushrooms (if
dry, soaked), slivered
2 beets, cut in cubes
1 eggplant, diced

- Place the carthamus in a muslin bag and set aside. Simmer all the other herbs along with the aduki beans in the stock for 1 hour.
- Add the muslin bag of carthamus, the mushrooms, beets, and eggplant, and simmer another 20 minutes. Remove the muslin bag and serve.

With painful cramps, soreness of the back and loins, or dark clotted blood:

delete lotus seeds and beans
add 1/2 oz. corydalis, 1 tbsp. turmeric

After the flow, to restore *Blood* and *Essence* and invigorate the internal organs, use

1 oz. dioscorea rhizome
1 oz. rehmannia
2 oz. lycii berries
1 oz. lotus seeds
12 red dates, soaked and pitted

7 c. chicken or marrow bone stock
1 yam, diced
5 black or shiitake mushrooms (if
dry, soaked), slivered
1/4 c. rice wine

- Break the dioscorea into small pieces and simmer it along with the rehmannia, lycii, and lotus seeds for 1 hour.
- Add the dates, yam, and mushrooms, and simmer for another 20 minutes. Add the rice wine and serve.

The above recipe is also appropriate for a postpartum mother.

During pregnancy, this recipe nourishes the fetus, strengthens the uterus, and combats morning sickness:

1 oz. dioscorea rhizome	7 c. vegetable or chicken stock
1/4 oz. tangerine peel	(pages 344–345)
1 oz. lotus seeds	2 yams, diced
12 red dates, soaked and pitted	1 c. radish,* diced
1 1/2 in. fresh ginger, minced	1 c. spinach, chopped
	1 tsp. roasted sesame oil

- Break the dioscorea into small pieces, and slice the tangerine peel into slivers.
- Simmer the herbs for 1 hour.
- Add the yams and radish, and simmer for another 20 minutes.
- Add the spinach and sesame oil for 5 minutes, and serve.

WEIGHT AND CHOLESTEROL MANAGEMENT

To reduce weight and cholesterol levels, it is as important to avoid a diet high in fat, salt, sugar, and refined carbohydrates as it is to incorporate fresh, whole foods high in fiber, lean protein, and complex carbohydrates. This Western wisdom is a sensible beginning. Yet it is difficult for many to resist drastic measures like liquid diets and fasting in pursuit of quick, dramatic change. According to Chinese medicine, these extreme tactics can be damaging to the *Spleen*. Repeated dietary "terrorism" can make it even more difficult to regulate body weight.

Long-term strategy incorporates *Yin-Yang* thinking—matching your individual pattern with particular foods and styles of preparation. Gradual shifts in food eating patterns enable the body to integrate change and maintain stability. Determining whether you are *Cold* or *Hot*, *Wet* or *Dry*, congested or depleted, is the next step after giving up unhealthy foods and habits.

Medicinal foods tune the body, providing metabolic efficiency and power without extra mass. An herbal food solution for weight management im-

*1–2 tbsp. of the juice of fresh radish is an antidote to the nausea, acidity, and regurgitation associated with morning sickness.

proves assimilation and elimination and supplements *Qi* and *Blood*. The following are nutritive herbs that eliminate congested fluids, break down fats and proteins, and lubricate and activate the intestines. Astragalus and corn silk supplement *Qi* and eliminate fluids. All these ingredients can be brewed as a beverage or cooked in soup and combined with other foods.

2 oz. astragalus root
2 oz. poria fungus
1/2 oz. black fungus, crumbled, soaked, and drained
12 red dates, soaked and pitted
1 1/2 in. fresh ginger, minced

1/2 c. barley
7 c. vegetable or chicken stock (pages 344–345)
3 celery stalks, diced
3 beets, sliced in lengths
8 black or shiitake mushrooms (if dry, soaked), slivered
3 cloves garlic, minced
1/2 c. chopped parsley

- Place the astragalus in a muslin bag or tie it with string.
- Simmer the herbs with the barley for 1 hour in the stock.
- Add the celery, beets, mushrooms, and garlic to the stock and simmer for another 20 minutes. Remove the astragalus.
- Add the parsley, simmer for 3 minutes and serve.

Instead of fasting, eat 2–4 cups a day for several days or more. This is nutritive as well as supportive of weight loss and cholesterol reduction.

AFTERWORD

Individuality is inseparable from community . . . for in the Taoist view there really is no obdurately external world. My inside arises mutually with my outside, and though the two may differ they cannot be separated.

Alan Watts
Tao: The Watercourse Way

If I am not for myself, who will be for me? If I am for myself alone, what am I? If not now, when?

Rabbi Hillel
Ethics of the Ancestors

THE PARADIGM OF CHINESE MEDICINE ENGAGES US BECAUSE OF OUR DIS-comfort with "the way things are," socially as well as personally. We face environmental, political, economic, and health crises that are challenging our core perceptions, values, and beliefs.

We realize that cigarettes and alcohol cause major health problems, an accident in Chernobyl impacts on dairy farms in Norway, pesticides sprayed on grapes injure the children of farmworkers, military aid to El Salvador encourages the violation of human rights, eliminating steamy rain forests alters the temperature of the entire planet, and toxic chemicals dumped upstream poison the people downriver. But our ability to deal with these problems is handicapped by maintaining a worldview that ignores what we know. We name isolated problems, reducing whole puzzles to segregated pieces, ignoring the relationships between the bits. We worship nouns (things in and of themselves) and snub verbs (process).

That fifty million children are at risk of perishing in this decade from lack of food and medicine could be remedied. That one in six children live in poverty in the United States, the wealthiest country in the world, could be amended. That missiles that deliver nuclear arms are designated "peace-keepers" deserves serious questioning. Our priorities (values) and our conceptual models (paradigms) are ailing. Confronted with the dangers of war, destruction of the Earth, and inhuman practices toward each other, we have global as well as personal healing on our minds. Chinese medicine represents the remembering of a world made in a different image.

Today, as civilization escalates in complexity, our daily lives are compartmentalized. We are mandated to keep our emotions under cover at work and trained from an early age to keep our bodies hushed. Our spiritual lives are often preempted by the urgency of economic survival. Isolated from a community of support, families no longer run households or raise children collectively. Many fathers do not live in the same home as mothers, and many do not share in the life of their children. The meaning of family and community has become elusive, its integument fragile.

We are readily herded into compliance, discouraged from drawing the road maps to guide ourselves toward the cooperative pursuit of fundamental change. Education focuses upon teaching children to accept, compete, and conform rather than question, collaborate, and invent—as young people we do not receive enough practice in finding our own voice or testing the merit of what stands as given.

By choosing between mutually exclusive either-or options, we splinter our world into winners and losers, masters and slaves, superiors and inferiors, haves and have-nots. Such hierarchical divisions are reinforced by a self-serving morality. We choose between what's good for my mind *or* body, me *or* you, my business *or* the environment, my national security *or* yours, means and ends, swaggering and swearing to defend what we arbitrarily decree as the righteous side of this tissue-paper wall. Rather than honoring our gender and ethnic differences with mutual respect, we confuse equal opportunity with homogeneity, crushing our diversity and imposing upon ourselves the banality of a mass monoculture.

Instead of perceiving the world as a living organism, we see it as a machine that exists for our short-term profit and convenience. We experience ourselves as cogs in the machine rather than cells in a breathing organism. Instead of recognizing the interdependence of all living creatures and pursuing partnerships, we set up institutions whereby one species, race, or nation overcomes and dominates another.

This fragmentation in our outer world is echoed in our inner life, by how we experience ourselves. We lack interpretive systems that connect our deepest aspirations with our personalities and the shape and performance of our bodies. We lack a language for appreciating our physical, emotional, and spiritual life as one seamless, uninterrupted story. Specialists have been trained to handle our discrete parts, but no one is there to help us grapple with and grasp the relationships between them.

Feelings of being disconnected exist inside us, between us, and above us, as human beings in relation to the cosmos. Over the last centuries we have ruptured our felt connection with Nature—Heaven and Earth—depriving ourselves of the sense of belonging we once held sacred. At another time, as part of another cosmology, we knew that our personal destiny was not unrelated to the dancing of clouds, the singing of wind, the eternal tumult of ocean waves, the grandeur of chestnut boughs stretching toward the light.

Out of the absolute fissure between self and other is born the problem:

other becomes Nature; women; children; people of color. As genders, nations, and cultures we exist in dynamic tension and sensitive ecological balance. If we were to fully digest this knowledge, we would recognize that to harm another is to damage ourselves and to abuse ourselves is to injure another. Following this logic, it is no more tolerable to subjugate and exploit others than it is to hold hostage that within us that struggles for its voice. If we define freedom as integrity of relationship, then self would be understood *as* relationship, not as singular entity, and freedom would exist only for us, not merely for me.

It is becoming evident that our well-being is contingent upon healthy global conditions: we can be only partially free of disease as long as we ignore or neglect the health of our community; our freedom is incomplete as long as our privilege is dependent on the privation or domination of our neighbors; we are only partly nonviolent as long as we permit others to make war in our name; we cannot be good parents until all of our children have the family, food, and skills they need in order to thrive; and we are only semiprotectors of our environment as long as we benefit from a world economy that ravages the Earth. How can we address problems until we can name them?

Medicine not only defines health and disease, but also make implicit assumptions about what life is and what it is to be human. As such, it occupies a position of great power. In our view, Chinese medicine is not a replacement for Western medicine, but another window through which we can view ourselves, take stock of our personal and global situations, and use its insights to prompt a revolution in priorities, strategies, and choices.

Once we recognize and assume the interconnectedness of all things, how we shape our process of inquiry alters. The relevant question becomes: How is the relationship working? The lens of our intelligence, like that of the eye, is pliable: we can shift our focus from the relationship between *Spleen* and *Liver, Blood* and *Qi*, resting and doing, ingesting and eliminating, speaking and listening, citizen and government, consumer and producer, student and teacher. Cooperation and partnership are qualities of productive, healthy relationship. This means that in the body the *Liver* must be reeducated when and if it dominates the *Spleen*, the *Spleen* in turn must not tyrannize the *Kidney*, and the *Kidney* cannot bully the *Heart*. Poor relationships create patterns of disharmony. Ambition (*Wood*) cannot be permitted to overcome compassion (*Earth*), sympathy (*Earth*) must not obstruct our vision (*Water*), and the relentless pursuit of knowledge (*Water*) must not altogether exclude our innocent sense of wonder and joy (*Fire*). Dysfunctional families beget wounded children—soggy *Wood* cannot make *Fire* burn bright.

Chinese medical thinking integrates medicine, whose aim is to heal the body and mind, with philosophy, whose purpose is to guide us in living. The test of our health becomes the measure of our capacity to realize ourselves as cooperative, connected links in a fundamental chain of being who seek to serve each other and our world and not merely act as political conquerors or technological consumers of it. Health, like freedom, is not a passive commodity to be delivered or purchased, but an ongoing active process, a striving for coherence. It is about navigating our ship at sea, not about reaching port as a finite and final destination. Health is no more the mere absence of disease than freedom is the absence of interference—both involve identifying and surmounting obstacles.

The primal language of *Yin-Yang* and *Five Phases* knits together the threads of our personal, social, and transcendent experience. The momentum of transformation is inevitable and inexorable. What exists gives way to what comes after through a labor of striving and contending. Our purpose in this process is to become, to change, and to become again—to organize, disorganize, and reorganize. We cannot resist this cellular impulse, but we can participate with greater awareness, appropriately exercising our will (*Water*), determination (*Wood*), passion (*Fire*), generosity (*Earth*), and discipline (*Metal*). The mission of Chinese medicine is to evoke, provoke, and steer change.

Western either-or thinking prompts us to conceive of illness within a narrow logic that fails us by its lack of breadth. We blame the victim by asserting that people cause their own sickness; hence, with a positive attitude, they can make themselves well. So if they don't, it's their own fault. Or we assume ailments are statistical probabilities that befall people like the weather, something over which they have no control. Or patients pay doctors to tell them what's wrong and fix it; so if they're not better, it's the doctors who have failed. Illness becomes the punishment one always suspected, or an undeserved curse, or a result of professional incompetence.

Sometimes illness can be overcome, sometimes there is no way to make it vanish, and sometimes it is a tough coach and tutor, towing us along our path. We create our life and are created by it. We make our sickness and are shaped by it. We exert our intention and will to struggle against our maladies, and we are at their mercy, our final task being to capitulate gracefully to the eventual process of decay.

Our illness confronts us with an existential demand: to fight with righteous indignation against the unacceptable and to open with glad acceptance to the inevitable—only by embodying this tension can we reach the limits of what is possible. Simultaneously we must reject the complacency of the status quo and the despair that accompanies our dissatisfaction with it. We must refuse to accept what is for the sake of what could be, yet be able to embrace what exists, as it is, in order to transform and reclaim it. We are a bundle of contradictions, not governable by a simple morality or easy answers.

We hope that this book prompts the disassembling of former views,   383 frames new perspectives with which problems can be defined, and proposes some alternative strategies. Change begins with radical questioning and proceeds with unavoidable turbulence. Introducing yet another set of criteria by which to evaluate our behavior, our diet, our daily regime, is altogether unsettling. One person, after reading the chapter on food, said, "Now I don't know what to eat." Then he began experimenting with recipes, tasting how different herbs and foods made him feel. Puzzlement itself can initiate a compelling inner dialogue, an adventurous exploration, coercing us to listen to the body's expression and attend to the mind's reverberation. This is useful practice, for we probably need to question the big systems as well as the little ones. Instead of patching the world, we may need to remake it. Learning to be self-reflective, self-critical, and self-aware is just the kind of process avoided when we look entirely outside ourselves, to the "experts" to tackle our problems on our behalf yet without our participation.

To accept who we are, we need to know ourselves. Self-recognition within the language of *Five Phases* can be agonizing as well as rewarding, and there is sometimes great resistance. It remains a struggle for me to feel that embodying the qualities of *Earth* is as virtuous as if I were more like my father, a *Wood* type. Our culture extols his urgent ambition, his sense of purpose and achievement. Unlike *Earth*, he is filled with self-confidence—he knows he's right. *Earth* is self-doubting and ambivalent, seeing excellence everywhere before itself. The tiger stalks its prey without distraction, while the chameleon changes colors to melt into rock, sand, or moss. *Earth* is far from single-minded, easily diverted by contesting interests, tempted to go where need demands. *Earth* prefers to take care of people, out of the limelight, to just be there, supportive without recompense or outright recognition. Before acquiring the *Five-Phase* vocabulary, I believed that to fully evolve would mean to become more like *Wood*, fitting better within American culture: to rise heroically to challenges, be willing to compete and win a place in the sun, and single-mindedly pursue well-defined goals. It was a revelation to discover that I could aspire to become a more developed *Earth* type—I could identify my own talents rather than always come up short by measuring myself against someone else's standards.

One of my friends is a midwife. She burns with the warmth of *Fire*. She struts onto center stage like a peacock, without timidity or self-consciousness, reaching toward excitement like a moth to flame. It is precisely the intense intimacy of birth, the thrilling stimulus of it, that keeps her up night after night, year after year. She likes short, potent experience—total immersion, climax, and then, like a hummingbird, she's on to the next blossom.

Earth is less excited or exciting than *Fire*, less creative than *Water*, less logical than *Metal*, and less energetic and driven than *Wood*. Still, it was the determination of my *Wood*, the discipline of my *Metal*, the enthusiasm provided by my *Fire*, and the solitary reflectiveness of my *Water* that enabled me to produce a book. The scholarship and originality spring from my coauthor's well of *Water*; the commitment to connect with the reader comes from my *Earth*. *Earth* is a good friend, parent, and organizer—able to listen, serve, satisfy needs, and resolve problems. My friends and patients appreciate my faithful willingness to immerse myself in their affairs and lavish them with my focused attention.

I can imagine myself fitting better into a provincial village in another era when I would have worn an apron over wide hips in a household teeming with children. My home would have been located at the crossroad of this hamlet so that everyone could pass through my kitchen on their way to somewhere else. As people emptied their pockets of troubles, I would dish out generous servings of soup, administer instant counsel, offer matchmaking services, and settle disputes judiciously. Amber sunlight would splash onto my table and ripple from it into the community. And everyone who, for better or worse, was born in that valley would also die there. I would have been pleased with the security, the togetherness, even the predictable boredom. I would relish the still point while nomads would pass through and tell stories of faraway lands.

The insights of Chinese medicine can nurse our sense of ourselves, our awareness, at the same time as acupuncture and herbs can promote our direct experience of integration. Meredith asked me to make a house call—she needed help and was too weak to move. Besieged with unremitting nausea and vomiting, she was unable to hold down plain water, let alone solid food, and she wanted to avoid hospitalization and intravenous feeding. She had an inoperable tumor that had spread to her bones, and her legs and hips were in extreme pain. A combination of acupuncture treatments, an herbal fomentation on her abdomen, powdered ginger under her tongue, and rectal injections of herb broth halted the nausea and vomiting within one day and provided her with nutrition. She then progressed to eating small portions of herb broth and rice gruel. Acupuncture every six hours enabled her to discontinue the use of morphine that had been leaving her groggy and tired. She complained of feeling that her upper body felt disassociated from her lower body. Minutes after the needles were in place, she began to feel as if her abdomen and lower limbs were again joined to her upper body, returning to her the sense of connectedness that she was craving. The acupuncture not only altered her perception of pain, but seemed to soothe and lighten her consciousness. She felt more charged and a greater sense of calm.

What is it that we want? To fully experience our aliveness. To feel in our bodies a streaming, like the rush of a river over stones. To be awake, alert, and responsive in our limbs and sensitive in our fingertips to the textures we touch; to be infused with our own whispering current of wind; to feel as if our outer and inner reality is congruent and that our efforts are rewarded by a sense of satisfaction. We carve out our own identity and possess our own purpose, and yet we also yearn to shed the isolation we feel within the envelope of our skin. We desire union. We aspire to have our private lives nestle within the valley of a public world that we can affirm. We long to feel connected with each other. Like the woods that harbor wild creatures, creekbeds, and fertile pastures that rest upon a mound of earth that spreads into a vast range of mountains and plains—we want to feel a part of a community that spills into and becomes part of a larger universe. We want to be able to embrace and be embraced. We want to live the life of our bodies and want our bodies to permit us to fully live our lives.

Chinese medicine is a beginning.

ACKNOWLEDGMENTS

A book takes on a life of its own, nudged along by diverse currents and nurtured by multiple energies. This one began as a two-page brochure, which in stages grew into an eighty-page essay, and then, after realizing there was so much more to say, assumed the form of a full-fledged book.

Subhuti Dharmananda, himself author of many publications on herbal medicine, after reading our essay gave us the assignment: "Write a book." The prospect was daunting. Our friends Bernardine Dohrn, Bill Ayers, Yeshi Neumann, Evie Talmus, Linda Saraf, Mary Ashley, Michael Tierra, Trent Schroyer, Joanna Rinaldi, Kosta Bagakis, Melody James, Susan Collins, Kathy Coyne, and Susan and Malcolm Terrence assured us that we could do it and cheered us on.

We have attempted to emulate the style of provocative inquiry exemplified by Ted Kaptchuk and Michael Broffman and have been encouraged by their support. Paul Unschuld provided inspiration. His thorough, reflective examination of the history of Chinese medicine challenges the myth that it is a strictly defined orthodoxy, a fixed, unchanging entity. Instead he insists we perceive any medicine as a fluctuating mode of thinking and practice that inevitably takes on the hue and shading of its social and historical context. Indirectly he gave us permission to interpret the meaning and significance of Chinese medicine from the vantage point of our own experience and culture. We have also built upon the somatic psychology of Stanley Keleman. Our study with him helped us to develop the frame of reference from which our expression of Chinese ideas emerges.

It's one thing to write a book and another to prepare it for publication. Judy Olasov taught us that words could be processed as well as written. Throughout the writing process we relied on our free-lance editor, Deke Castleman, for his abundant good humor and camaraderie as well as his expertise. That he could consistently transform discouragement into mirth was no small feat. In reading early versions, Dan Nevel, Angus McKenzie, Ani Chamechian, Roberta Gardner, and Garry Meyers made suggestions which we valued.

Determined to bring awareness and knowledge of complementary approaches to health into greater public view, Cheryl Woodruff, our editor at Ballantine, affirmed the value of this project from the start, contributing her talent to its fruition. Our auspicious liaison with her was fostered by our agents John Brockman and Katinka Matson. We gratefully acknowledge artists Susanne Panasik, Bruce Wang, and Val Mina for creating the graphic images that accompany our text.

We owe a debt of gratitude to our family. Dr. Gayle Pierce provided lucid counsel throughout. Efrem's father, Murray Korngold, invited us to our first acupuncture seminar, engaging with us in animated dialogue about Chinese medicine ever since. The unqualified faith of Harriet's parents, Marjorie and Malcolm Beinfield, in our mission of communication buoyed our spirits and determination. Our parents may not have taught us everything we know, but from their ground our flowers bloom. Harriet's lineage of physicians— grandfathers, Harry Koster and Henry Beinfield; father, Malcolm; sister, Lynn; uncles Robert Koster and Barry Singer; cousins Harry Koster and Susie Singer; and our extended family brothers, Alan Steinbach and John Edoga—have together demonstrated several generations of devotion to the wonders and perplexities of medicine. From them we gained perspective. And our children, Natasha, Shem, and Bear Korngold, have patiently witnessed how much longer it takes to write a book than to read one. For their tolerance they deserve credit.

Countless herbal meals were shared with Nam Singh, who initiated us into the tradition of cooking Chinese medicinal food. Later, Edward Espe Brown contributed his poetic sensibility and, along with Patti Sullivan, critically tasted these creations with us.

Our teachers in Chinese medicine, Miriam Lee, Jane Tang, C. S. Cheung, Andrew Tseng, Zheng Wen Tao, Wang Weng-Jing, and Y. K. Tan, generously passed on their knowledge. No persons other than ourselves are responsible for the fallibility of our ideas or their expression.

And our patients, who, through us, have placed their trust in Chinese medicine, have guided our experience and explanation of it. Their stories about how it has altered not only their symptoms, but their deeper selves, in ways that often elude precise articulation, continue to demonstrate to us the power of Chinese medicine to shift consciousness, promote integrity of relationship, and, in that way, assist us in the perpetual remaking of our world.

ACUPUNCTURE

Aside from checking under *Acupuncture* or *Herbs* in your local phone directory, for a fee you may obtain a photocopy of the names of the registered practitioners in your area or the national list of practitioners registered with the American Association of Acupuncture and Oriental Medicine. Contact:

American Association of Acupuncture and Oriental Medicine
c/o National Acupuncture Headquarters
1424 16th Street, N.W., Suite 501
Washington, D.C. 20036

Information about professional standards and licensing requirements for acupuncturists, the addresses of the state medical boards in charge of supervising the practice of acupuncture in your state, and a list of acupuncture schools and colleges is available from another group that shares the same office:

National Commission for the Certification of Acupuncturists
c/o National Acupuncture Headquarters
1424 16th Street, N.W., Suite 501
Washington, D.C. 20036

CHINESE HERBS

For the general public:

Patent herbal formulas and individual herbs are available from Chinese herb shops located in the Chinatowns of large cities. Although they are pleased to fill orders from walk-in customers, most of these shops are unwilling to ship small quantities to retail customers.

To purchase small quantities of the herbs mentioned in this book for formulas and food recipes through the mail, contact:

Institute Herb Company
1190 N.E. 125th Street, Suite 12
North Miami, Florida 33161
(305) 899-8050

For Chinese herbal solutions, formulas for the general public developed by the authors of *Between Heaven and Earth,* contact:

Chinese Medicine Works
1201 Noe Street
San Francisco, California 94114
FAX (415) 821-7804

For health professionals:

Sizable orders of bulk herbs and prepared herbal products are available to practitioners by mail order from:

Tai Sang Trading Co.
1018 Stockton Street
San Francisco, California 94108
FAX (415) 981-2032
(415) 981-2032

Mayway Trading Co.
622 Broadway
San Francisco, California 94133
(415) 788-3646

North-South China Herbs
1556 Stockton Street
San Francisco, California 94133
(415) 421-5576

For Chinese Modular Pharmacy formulas developed for practitioners by the authors, contact:

Chinese Medicine Works
1201 Noe Street
San Francisco, California 94114
FAX (415) 821-7804

For Chinese herbal products manufactured in the United States for health practitioners, contact:

K'an Herbs
2425 Porter Street, Suite 18
Soquel, California 95073

Planetary Herbs
Box 533
Soquel, California 95073

Health Concerns
2236 Mariner Square Drive #103
Alameda, California 94501

Zand
P.O. Box 5312
Santa Monica, California 90405

Seven Forests
2017 S.E. Hawthorne
Portland, Oregon 97214

Brion
12020-B Centralia Road
Hawaiian Gardens, California
90716

Meridian
17 St. Saveur Court
Cambridge, Massachusetts 02138

Tea Garden Herb Emporium
1344 Abbot Kinney Boulevard
Venice, California 40291

East-Earth Herbs
P.O. Box 2082
Eugene, Oregon 97402

For European health practitioners, books, individual herbs, prepared herbal products, and Chinese Modular Pharmacy formulas are available from:

East-West Herbs
Langston Priory Mews
Kingham, Oxon OX7 6UP
United Kingdom
060-865-8862; FAX 060-865-8816

CHINESE MEDICINAL MUSHROOMS

Modern reasearch has shown that medicinal mushrooms which have long been a part of the Chinese pharmacopeia have potent health promoting properties including enhancement of the immune and cardiovascular systems. High quality liquid extracts of organically grown medicinal mushrooms are available from:

MycoHerb
P.O. Box 8
Graton, California 95444
(707) 829-6839 FAX (707) 823-1507

TREATMENT FOR SUBSTANCE ABUSE AND DETOXIFICATION

Clinics exist that treat the symptoms of withdrawal from substance abuse. Information about detox treatment using Chinese medicine is available through:

National Acupuncture Detoxification Association, Inc. (NADA)
3115 Broadway #51
New York, New York 10027
(212) 993-3100; (212) 579-5138

TREATMENT OF PEOPLE WITH HIV AND AIDS

A training program for health professionals in the treatment of HIV infection with Chinese medicine is available through Quan Yin Healing Arts Center in San Francisco. Affiliated treatment programs exist in New York, Boston, Santa Fe, Chicago, Austin, Miami, and many other cities. Patients interested in referrals to practitioners all over the world as well as health professionals interested in learning about treatment programs should contact:

Quan Yin Healing Arts Center
1748 Market Street
San Francisco, California 94102
(415) 861-4964; FAX (415) 861-0579

Information can also be obtained from:

National Acupuncture Detoxification Association, Inc. (NADA)
3115 Broadway #51
New York, New York 10027
(212) 993-3100; (212) 579-5138

WORKSHOPS AND LECTURES

For workshops or lectures on the material presented within *Between Heaven and Earth,* contact the authors:

Chinese Medicine Works
1201 Noe Street
San Francisco, California 94114

CHAPTER 2   PHILOSOPHY IN THE WEST: THE DOCTOR AS MECHANIC

1. The phrase *power over Nature* and the phrase *power through Nature* are used by Starhawk in *Dreaming the Dark* (see Bibliography).
2. This chapter generally draws on the story of Western thinking, science, and medicine as told by Fritjof Capra in *The Turning Point* (New York: Bantam, 1982). It also relies on the ideas of René Dubos, *Man Adapting* (New Haven: Yale University Press, 1965). Another excellent resource is Edmund Pellegrino and David Thomasma, *A Philosophical Basis of Medical Practice* (New York: Oxford University Press, 1981).
3. Daniel Garber, "Science and Certainty in Descartes," in Michael Hooker, ed., *Descartes* (Baltimore: Johns Hopkins University Press, 1978).
4. Genevieve Rodis-Lewis, "Limitations of the Mechanical Model in the Cartesian Conception of the Organism," in Michael Hooker, ed., *Descartes* (Baltimore: Johns Hopkins University Press, 1978).
5. Fred Sommers, "Dualism in Descartes: The Logical Ground," in Michael Hooker, ed., *Descartes* (Baltimore: Johns Hopkins University Press, 1976).
6. H. R. Holman, "The 'Excellence' Deception in Medicine," in *Hospital Practice* (April 1976): 11.
7. Ivan Illich, *Medical Nemesis* (New York: Bantam, 1977), 23.
8. René Dubos, *Man Adapting* (New Haven: Yale University Press, 1965), 338.
9. John Cairns, "The Treatment of Diseases and the War Against Cancer," *Scientific American* 253, no. 5 (November 1985).

CHAPTER 3   PHILOSOPHY IN THE EAST: THE DOCTOR AS GARDENER

1. Nathan Sivin, in *Traditional Medicine in Contemporary China*, comments that the eternal daily and annual rotations and revolutions of the sun, moon, and planets are resonant with cycles of human transformation. He relates that in *The Annals of Lu Pu-wei* there is discussion of the *Round Way (yuan tao),* which speaks of the cyclic processes that unite sky and earth: "Day and night make up a cycle: this is the Round Way. The threading of the moon through the twenty-eight divisions of its path, from Horn (roughly Virgo) through Axletree (roughly Corvus), belongs to the Round Way. The luminaries alternate through the four seasons, encountering each other [in due course]: this is the Round Way. [On earth] something stirs and burgeons; burgeoning, it is born; born, it grows; growing, it matures; mature, it declines; declining, it dies; dead, it becomes latent [preceding another birth]. This is the Round Way." (p. 54)
2. Classical Chinese scholar and translator Elizabeth Rochat de la Vallee comments, "In the paired expression jing/shen . . . jing, 'essences,' represents any substance full of life, while shen, 'spirits,' represents the heav-

enly inspiration in each person. The paired expression jing/shen represents the interpenetration of Heaven and Earth at its highest level: the extraction and renewal of the substances which compose every thing, which are the mark of every life, and which can recompose themselves, in each being, according to its particular life pattern, be it on the level of species, race, lineage, or individual attributes. Essences, in this context, belong to the Earth: they are the basis of all transformation and manifestation. Spirits maintain the unity of being, through the various breaths that animate man and the multiplicity of materials he transforms; they give him heavenly inspiration, allowing his heart to guide him towards the best possible natural fruition: his destiny. The couple jing/shen, then, expresses the origin and unfoldment of Heaven and Earth in man. . . . All the key paired expressions . . . show the relational dialectic existing between Heaven and Earth." Paul Unschuld, ed., *Approaches to Traditional Chinese Medical Literature* (Kordrecht, The Netherlands: Kluwer Academic Publishers, 1989), 69–70.

3. Nathan Sivin, *Traditional Medicine in Contemporary China,* 47–53.

4. It is a paradox that although Chinese medical thinking can be considered "unscientific" in Western terms, it is closely allied in outlook with the insights of advanced modern physics. It is as if the venerable Lao-Tse and Einstein were chatting with each other in hushed voices across the millennia. Both advocate the concept that matter and energy are different aspects of one inclusive pattern; that parts can only be understood within the context of the whole; that there is no past or "cause," but merely an as-is-ness or condition of present happening; and that this condition is not separable from the subject for which it is happening—in other words, there is no objective reality that exists "out there," but rather a subjective reality that arises "in here."

Cartesian-Newtonian thinking defined science as discerning the relations between preexisting separate entities isolated by particular boundaries in time and space. But atoms, once regarded as the brick and mortar, the "building blocks," of our universe, now defy measurement and are no longer regarded as discrete entities. The evidence gathered from the new physics theory reveals that matter, which appears passive and static, is actually full of activity and in constant motion, perpetually reorganizing itself. Subatomic particles do not exist as "things," as if they were substantive building blocks: these particles are not isolated entities, but rather "probability patterns" that are said to have "tendencies to exist" and are invisible to us, evident only by their effects. Similarly, *Qi* is not a thing; it is known only by its effect.

In physics, the term *wavicle* was coined because particles act as waves in one situation and particles in another. A vocabulary that distinguishes sharply between the physical and the nonphysical, the substantive and the insubstantial, the artifact and the process, does not apply. There are no more boundaries, no absolute either-or categories; rather, in the words of contemporary physicist David Bohm, there is only one "unbroken wholeness of that-which-is." Bohm says:

> We must turn around. Instead of starting with parts and showing how they work together (the Cartesian order) we must start with the whole. . . . Parts are seen to be in immediate connection . . . their dynamic relationships depend, in an irreducible way, on the state of the whole system (and, indeed, on that of broader systems in which they are contained, extending ultimately and in principle to the entire universe). Thus, one is led to a new notion of "unbroken wholeness" which denies the classical idea of analyzability of the world into separately and independently existent parts. . . .

Because these ideas exist in such sharp contradiction to so many modern beliefs, physicist Niels Bohr says, "Those who are not shocked when they first come across quantum theory cannot possibly have understood it." And physicist Henry Stapp believes that these theories of modern physics are the most profound discoveries of science and will trigger a major revolution, not only in Western science, but in Western thought as well.

Western medicine, founded upon the thought and logic of modern science, often considers itself a science, although this is systematically debated by Pellegrino and Thomasma in *A Philosophical Basis of Medical Practice*. In the sense that the fundamental assumptions of both the new physics and Chinese medicine are distinct from those of modern science, both are "unscientific"—one from the historical vantage point of being prescientific and the other being perhaps postscientific.

CHAPTER 4   CYCLES AND CIRCLES:
A THEORY OF RELATIVITY YIN-YANG

1. Richard Levins and Richard Lewontin, *The Dialectical Biologist* (Cambridge: Harvard University Press, 1985), 3, 136, 179.

CHAPTER 6   FIVE-PHASE THEORY:
EVOLUTIONARY STAGES OF TRANSFORMATION

1. Nathan Sivin suggests that the translation of *Wu Xing* as *Five Elements* was a confused misconception originating with Matteo Ricci, a Jesuit missionary who in 1608 confused the Chinese concept with the Greek elements. Sivin asserts that *Xing* is not a force itself, but that it is a type of *Qi* that interacts in an ordered way to make up complex configurations in space or time. He sums up, "Wu Xing theory provides a language for

analysis of configurations into five functionally distinct parts or aspects. In other words, the Five Phases do what Yin-Yang does, but with finer divisions, analyzing into five aspects instead of two." (*Traditional Medicine in Contemporary China*, 70–76.) Joseph Needham states that *Wu Xing* refers more to five sorts of fundamental processes than to five sorts of fundamental matter, explaining that Chinese thought characteristically avoided substance and clung to relation. (*Science and Civilisation in China*, vol. 2: Cambridge, England: Cambridge University Press, 1978, 243–244.)

2. Philosopher Alan Watts expresses the notion of the holographic paradigm by commenting on the ancient Taoist view: "Pick up a blade of grass and all the worlds come with it. In other words, the whole cosmos is implicit in every member of it, and every point in it may be regarded as its center. . . . This is the bare and basic principle of the organic view. . . . " (*Watercourse Way* [New York: Pantheon, 1975], 33, 35.) Physicist Werner Heisenberg comments on the relationship between the macrocosm and microcosm: "The same organizing forces that have shaped nature in all her forms are also responsible for the structure of our minds." (*Physics and Beyond* [New York: Harper and Row, 1971], 101.)

3. "The *pattern which connects is a meta-pattern*. It is a pattern of patterns. It is that meta-pattern which defines the vast generalization that, indeed, *it is patterns which connect*. . . . The right way to begin to think about the pattern which connects is to think of it as *primarily* . . . a dance of interacting parts and only secondarily pegged down by various sorts of physical limits. . . . " (Gregory Bateson, *Mind and Nature* [New York: Bantam, 1979], 12–14.)

"The conservative laws for energy and matter concern substance rather than form. But mental process, ideas, communication, organization, differentiation, pattern . . . are matters of form rather than substance." (Bateson, *Steps to an Ecology of Mind* [New York: Ballantine, 1972], xxv–xxvi.) Bateson represents the position of the "new paradigm" thinkers—physicists, ecologists, biologists, psychologists, anthropologists, and mythologists—who are crossing conventional boundaries between science and metaphysics in an attempt to articulate a dynamic, nondichotomous view of a living, interconnected universe.

Five-Phase Theory is an example of what medical anthropologist Paul Unschuld calls "patterned thinking"—Chinese medicine links all visible and invisible phenomena by their mutual association with specific lines of correspondence. The emphasis is upon describing the way phenomena fit together, that is, the context, rather than explaining why they occur. (*Medicine in China: A History of Ideas* [Berkeley, Calif: University of California, 1985], 52.) This parallels contemporary paradigmatic thinking in biology, physics, and psychology.

1. By this we mean that the primary terms of *Five-Phase* thinking are descriptive rather than explanatory, and that its primary focus is that which can be known through the human senses. Phenomenology validates the subjective frame of reference by taking the point of view that by seeking to know the nature of our lived consciousness we can comprehend the nature of reality. This is reminiscent of the *Tao Te Ching*: "How do I know the ways of all things at the Beginning, By what is within me" (*Tao Te Ching*, John C. H. Wu trans. [New York: St. John's University Press, 1961]).

2. In *Medicine in China: A History of Ideas,* Paul Unschuld suggests that the correspondence thinking of Chinese medicine is syncretic, not synthetic—it seeks to "build bridges" among divergent views rather than to "distill a homogeneous system of ideas" from all existing views (pp. 57–58). It is common in Western science to sharply divide the disciplines of biology, psychology, and metaphysics from each other. Some contemporary voices argue for the interpenetration of these fields. For example, commenting on modern biologists like Paul Weiss and philosophical anthropologist Gregory Bateson, Fritjof Capra says, "From the systems point of view, life is not a substance or a force, and mind is not an entity interacting with matter. Both life and mind are manifestations of the same set of systemic properties, a set of processes that represent the dynamics of self-organization" (*The Turning Point*, 290). Bioenergetic psychologist Stanley Keleman emphatically argues that consciousness is not separable from our biological experience: "Life makes shapes. These shapes are part of an organizing process that embodies emotions, thoughts, and experiences into a structure. This structure, in turn, orders the events of existence. . . . Feelings are the glue that hold us together, yet they are based upon anatomy. . . . Without anatomy, emotions do not exist. Feelings have a somatic architecture. . . . Existence is a tribute to how life organizes living forms. To be an individual is to follow the urges of one's own form, and to learn its unique rules of organization. . . . Each of us is a process, a whole made up of living events with an urge toward organization. . . . Human form as a whole is made up of living events just as the universe is made up of living sub-systems" (*Emotional Anatomy* [Berkeley, Calif: Center Press, 1985], xi–1). And mythologist Joseph Campbell says, "A mythology is not an ideology. It is not something projected from the brain, but something experienced from the heart, from recognitions of identities behind or within the appearances of nature . . . framing its community to accord with an intuited order of nature and . . . conducting individuals through the ineluctable psychophysiological stages of transformation of a human lifetime" (*The Inner Reaches of Outer Space* [New York: Alfred van der Marck, 1985], 17–20).   397

3. We began with the ancient rudiments of psychological inference that already exist in correspondence thinking: the sensory, mental, and emotional manifestations of *Organ Network* function as well as the dynamic activity associated with the seasons (for example, the *Liver* corresponds with visual clarity, purposeful thinking, and volatile reactions—it also corresponds with the arousing, initiatory, and changeable activity of spring), asking ourselves, What is the organizing principle that links all aspects (season, color, sound, organ, tissue, emotion, climate, faculties) of each of the *Five Phases*? And can we use these five so-called organizing principles as a set of constructs to invent a typology of human character and physique that describes the people we know?

4. In *A Short History of Chinese Philosophy*, Fung Yu-Lan points out a difference in social and cultural values, currently and historically: Western civilization is a seafaring, exploring civilization, and Chinese civilization is a land-based, continuity-preserving civilization. In the former, the qualities of the unique heroic pioneering individual are mythologized, whereas in the latter the qualities of the conforming and adaptive lineage-upholding individual are revered. (Fung Yu-Lan, *A Short History of Chinese Philosophy*. New York: Free Press, 1948.)

5. Constitutional typing classifies people according to an established set of criteria. The concept of constitution incorporates and synthesizes knowledge about the composition, structure, formation, and organization of human mental and physiologic process. Historically many typological systems have been devised to explain the formation and disintegration of human character and structure. The Galenic medicine of ancient Greece classified people according to the four humors: sanguine, choleric, phlegmatic, and melancholic. Eclectic physicians in the late nineteenth century sorted people as constitutionally strong (sthenic) or weak (asthenic). East Indian Ayurvedic medicine catalogs people according to the three doshas: air (vatta), bile (kapha), and mucus (pitta). Each of these systems uses what is perceived to be a set of fundamental principles.

6. We have reinterpreted into our own conceptual language the meaning of psychospiritual faculties classically associated with each *Phase*; thus *Fire* is associated with *Shen* (Transcendent Mind), *Earth* with *Yi* (Intellect or Self-Aware Mind), *Metal* with *Po* (Primitive or Subconscious Mind), *Water* with *Zhi* (Instinctual or Collective Unconscious), and *Wood* with *Hun* (Ego or Executive Mind).

7. Carl Jung states, "I have long been struck by the fact that besides the many individual differences in human psychology there are also typical differences. . . . I must presume unduly upon the goodwill of the reader if I may hope to be rightly understood. It would be relatively simple if every reader knew to which category he belonged. But it is often very difficult to find out whether a person belongs to one type or the other,

especially in regard to oneself. In respect of one's own personality one's judgment is as a rule extraordinarily clouded. This subjective clouding of judgment is particularly common because in every pronounced type there is a special tendency which is biologically purposive since it strives constantly to maintain the psychic equilibrium. The compensation gives rise to secondary characteristics, or secondary types, which present a picture that is extremely difficult to interpret" (*Psychological Types* [Princeton, N.J.: Princeton University Press, 1978], 3).

We know that people share similarities that set them apart from other people, but we also know that these same people compared with one another will reveal important differences that make us wonder whether or not they really were so alike to begin with. This is the dilemma of any typology: to make true generalizations about the various expressions of human nature without ignoring the individual differences that are essential in understanding each person's unique character. No typology will be able to "explain" all of the idiosyncrasies of a particular person: its truths are broad and relative, not specific and absolute. We come back to the statement of general semantics, that "the map is not the territory," merely a device to get us to the neighborhood that we wish to explore. So, within the loose categories of our *Five-Phase* typology—*Wood, Fire, Earth, Metal,* and *Water* types, with *exaggerated* and *collapsed* patterns—we are able to make some useful statements about people that are both explanatory and predictive, such as what is the general nature of their process of development in health and disease, and what kinds of predicaments they are likely to encounter in the future. This is not a method of divination—it is much more like a road map that indicates cities, towns, and intersections along your route of travel or like an almanac that indicates probable seasonal weather conditions and flora and fauna that you may encounter. It is very often wise to consider this kind of information because it enables us to make intelligent choices as we move through our lives rather than "flying by the seat of our pants." These human maps help us form strategies for conscious living rather than simply reacting to events as they happen to us.

8. Nathan Sivin, in *Traditional Medicine in Contemporary China*, quotes Ko Hung (c. A.D. 320): "A human body is the counterpart of a state. The placement of the [organs within the] thorax and abdomen is like that of buildings [in a compound]. The arrangement of the limbs is like that of suburbs and outlying districts. The articulation of the bones and joints is like [the organization of] officials in the civil service. The spirit [for example, the body's governing vitalities, *Shen*] is like the monarch; the xue [*Blood*] is like the ministers; the qi is like the people. Thus we know that one who keeps his own body in order can keep a state in order. Loving care for one's people is what makes it possible to keep the body intact.

When the people are dispersed the state perishes; when the qi [is] exhausted the body dies. What is dead cannot be brought to life; what has perished cannot be preserved. Because all this is so, the perfected man allays catastrophe before it happens, and cures illness before it has developed. He treats it in advance rather than chasing to catch up after it has passed him by. One's subjects are hard to nurture, easy to endanger; one's qi is difficult to keep pure, easily sullied. That is why one cultivates a majestic virtue in order to protect one's lands, and gets rid of desires in order to preserve one's vitalities." Sivin points out that the physician's role is to mediate between the cosmic and somatic, just as the emperor's mission was to mediate between the cosmic and political orders. He says, "The analogy between the body and state implies that the conditions for normality are the same in both" (pp. 57–59).

Glossary of Important Terms and Concepts

Acupuncture Point. Sites along the skin where the channels of *Qi* come closest to the surface of the body. Access to *Qi* occurs through gateways or acupuncture points along the channels that traverse the body to carry the *Qi*. These points provide a communication system, connecting the outside with the interior. Acupuncture points are stimulated to encourage the circulation of *Qi* and *Blood*, to provide analgesia, to affect particular *Organ Network* function, and to influence the equilibrium of the organism as a whole.

Acquired (Postnatal) Essence. The *Essence* transformed from air, food, and fluid by the *Lung* and *Spleen*, the surplus of which is collected and stored by the *Kidney*, supplements and to some degree offsets and postpones the attrition of prenatal *Essence* due to the process of aging.

Adverse Climates. The internal or external pathogenic agents of *Wind, Heat, Cold, Dryness,* and *Dampness.*

Anabolism. The anabolic process of metabolism in which food is converted into tissue. In the context of Chinese medicine, anabolic processes correspond to *Yin* categories of assimilation and storage of *Qi, Moisture,* and *Blood* (known as the material substance of the organism that is the expression of *Jing* or *Essence*).

Anchor. Through its power to consolidate *Qi* (*Essence*), the *Kidney* is able to "grasp" or "hold on to" the *Qi*, thus giving the organism a root, a lower center of gravity, which stabilizes the organism much the way an anchor keeps a ship from drifting. If the *Kidney* loses this capacity, problems such as shortness of breath, dizziness, and hot flashes may arise.

Archetype. A psychological idea articulated by Carl Jung that describes universal human characteristics as symbolized in the figures and characters that appear in myths and dreams. In our discussion, we have constructed archetypal figures who embody the essential physical, psychological, and social characteristics of the *Five Phases.* They are the *Pioneer* (*Wood*), *Wizard* (*Fire*), *Peacemaker* (*Earth*), *Alchemist* (*Metal*), and *Philosopher* (*Water*).

Blood (xue). The most dense fluid substance in the body, which transmits nourishment and provides the material "matrix" for mental and emotional life: "Blood houses the mind." *Blood* is stored by the *Liver*, generated by the *Spleen*, propelled by the *Heart*, and is the mother of *Qi*.

Body Exterior. Includes body hair, skin, subcutaneous tissue, muscles, peripheral blood vessels, and peripheral nerves.

Body Interior. Includes bones, visceral organs, glands, major blood vessels and nerves, and body cavities.

Body Unit. An anatomical measure used to locate acupuncture points. One unit is equal to the width of the second joint of the thumb. Three body units are equal to the breadth of the second, third, fourth, and fifth fingers when held together. Different parts of the body are divided according to specified numbers of body units—for example, the distance from the navel to the pubic bone is five body units; and the distance from the crease of the elbow to the crease of the wrist is twelve body units.

Catabolism. The catabolic process of metabolism in which tissue is broken down to liberate energy. In the context of Chinese medicine, catabolic processes correspond to *Yang* categories of generation and distribution of *Qi, Moisture,* and *Blood* (in other words, the animation of the organism that is the expression of *Shen*).

Channels. Also called meridians, a network of nonanatomical conduit vessels through which the *Qi* circulates. Each of the *Organ Networks* has a corresponding channel: *Liver, Gallbladder, Heart, Small Intestine, Spleen, Stomach, Lung, Large Intestine, Kidney, Bladder, Pericardium,* and *Triple-Burner.* In addition there is the *Conception Vessel,* which travels along the midline in the front of the body, and the *Governor Vessel,* which travels along the back of the middle of the head and down the spine. There are also "extra channels," which are made up of a combination of acupuncture points from different channels.

Character. In our terms, the inborn nature or matrix of the soma and psyche expressed as one of the *Five-Phase* types. Character is distinct from personality insofar as the latter is an aggregate of what is both inherited (genetic) and acquired (experience and development), whereas character refers to the innate tendencies and potentials of the individual.

Chinese Medicine. A methodology of medicine developed in ancient China, also known as Chinese traditional medicine, that refers to a system of thinking and practice rather than a description of current medical convention in China.

Cold. Characterized by aversion to cold, desire for heat, hypoactivity, desquamation, lack of thirst, loose stool, pallor, lethargy, dullness, somnolence, weakness, profuse clear urine, thin odorless discharges.

Collapsed. A subtype of the *Five-Phase* types corresponding to *Yin* categories of attrition and dissipation of *Qi.* When a *Phase* is *collapsed,* the *Organ Network* or individual associated with that *Phase* shows signs of weakness, vulnerability, and passivity.

Consolidate. Condense, tone, astringe: to consolidate is to counter the weakening of body functions or the dissipation of body substances by gathering, densifying, and astringing *Qi, Moisture,* and *Blood.* Herbs and herbal formulas that consolidate aid the body in concentrating and retaining substances and tightening tissue. In the body, consolidation is exemplified by the *Kidney Network,* whose function is to receive, concentrate, and store *Essence.*

Context. The background or environment in which a particular event or phenomenon occurs. In Chinese medicine all considerations are contextual in the sense that no specific symptom, sign, or complaint can be interpreted correctly without reference to the total configuration, that is, all the manifestations of the organism that are accessible to observation or intuition.

Core. The deepest layer of tissue and function of the organism, expressed by the interaction and integration of the *Heart (Shen)* and *Kidney (Jing).*

Correspondence Thinking. A logical system of describing reality in which all phenomena are interrelated by association with a set of categories. In Chinese thought these categories are generated by *Yin-Yang* and *Five-Phase* theories. All events can be described according to the interaction of these primary variables. Entities and processes that can be similarly described are said not only to be related, but, in a profound sense, to influence one another. Paul Unschuld defines Chinese traditional medicine as the "medicine of systematic correspondence." It is based on a nonlinear, synchronistic rather than linear, causal method of analysis. This mode of thinking distinguishes Chinese traditional medicine from modern Western medicine.

Dampness. Characterized by feelings of heaviness, swelling, distension of chest and abdomen, fluid accumulation, nodular masses, watery stool, sore joints, stupor, sticky copious discharges, and phlegm.

Diagnosis. In Chinese traditional medicine there are four modes of diagnosis: seeing, listening and smelling, questioning, and palpating. Primary among these are inspection of the tongue and palpation of the pulse at each wrist, observation of the complexion and facial features, and palpation of acupuncture points.

- To see: complexion, eyes, tongue, nails, hair, gait, stature, affect, quality of excretions, secretions
- To listen and smell: sound of voice and breath; odor of breath, skin, excretions, secretions
- To question: current complaints, health history, family health history, patterns of sleep, appetite, weight, elimination, menses, stress
- To palpate: texture, humidity, temperature, elasticity of skin; strength and tone of muscles; flexibility, range of motion of joints; sensitivity of diagnostic points; radial pulse evaluation

Disperse. Move, circulate, distribute, disseminate: to disperse is to relieve stagnation of *Qi, Moisture,* and *Blood* or the accumulation of *Heat, Cold, Dampness,* or phlegm. In the body dispersion is exemplified by the functions of the *Liver Network* and *Lung Network* in evenly and rhythmically circulating *Qi* and distributing *Blood.*

Dispersing and Descending. The functions of the *Lung Network* whereby the moist *Qi* of the upper body is distributed downward throughout the chest and abdominal regions to be collected and consolidated by the *Kidney Network* in the region of the pelvis.

Earth. The material realm of human existence, belonging to *Yin,* including the soil, seas, and rivers, as well as the visible influences of the seasons and climates. In the human body, that which is below the navel corresponds to *Earth.*

Eight Guiding Principles. Four diagnostic sets of polar categories that define patterns of distress within the organism: *Cold-Hot* (relating to the nature of a disease process); *deficient-excess* (indicating the strength of the organism relative to the virulence of the pathogenic process); *internal-external* (referring to the location of the disease process relative to superficial and deep tissue and functions); *Yin-Yang* (general categories that summarize the interaction of the other six: a *Yin* condition is *Cold, deficient,* and *internal,* whereas a *Yang* condition is *Hot, excess,* and *external.* Mixed *Yin* and *Yang* syndromes are more often the rule, such as *Hot, excess,* and *internal* or *Cold, deficient,* and *external*). Of the eight categories, four (*excess-deficiency, Hot-Cold*) are the most critical in differentiating one pathogenic process from another.

- *Cold*—lack of body heat locally or systemically, subjectively or objectively
- *Heat*—excess body heat locally or systemically, subjectively or objectively
- *Deficient*—lack of basic constituents (*Qi, Moisture, Blood*); organic hypofunction of any organ or physiological system
- *Excess*—surplus, congestion of basic constituents (*Qi, Moisture, Blood*); organic hyperfunction of any organ or physiological system
- *Internal*—affecting the deeper levels of biological activity or occurring in the visceral organs or areas such as body cavities, bones, glands, major blood vessels, and nerves
- *External*—affecting or occurring in the superficial tissues or organs such as the body hair, skin, subcutaneous tissue, muscles, joints, and peripheral blood vessels, and nerves
- *Yin-Yang*—concepts that summarize the fundamental or composite nature of any disease process

Electroacupuncture. The use of battery-powered instruments that generate alternating current to stimulate acupuncture points through metal needles, rubber electrodes, or by direct contact with a metal probe.

Energetic. A term loosely and widely used to identify or describe the intangible processes that underlie and govern the material bodily events that are the tangible expression of the "energy" or "forces" of life. Energetics is often part of the vocabulary of alternative or unorthodox healing systems that do not rely on the conventional empirical scientific model that is the basis of modern Western medical theory and practice.

Essence (Jing). That which is the material basis of an individual's life, which can be transmuted and transformed into a new and separate individual life through procreation. *Essence* is the most refined substance of the body, which forms the basis of all tissue, especially male and female reproductive secretions, including sperm and ova. *Essence* also represents the reserve or stored *Qi* of the body, some of which is derived from parents at conception (inherited or prenatal *Essence*) and some of which is derived continuously from food and air (acquired or postnatal *Essence*). It is the capacity to generate, conserve, and preserve *Essence* that determines a person's freedom from degenerative disease and potential life span. *Essence* can be observed in the luster and texture of the skin, hair, and tongue and in an individual's fertility, creativity, and potency.

Exaggerated. A subtype of the *Five-Phase* types corresponding to *Yang* categories of overconcentration and accumulation of *Qi*. When a *Phase* is *exaggerated*, the *Organ Network* or individual associated with that *Phase* shows signs of dominating and oppressing other *Networks* or *Phases*.

External Illness. Engendered by external climatic conditions; exists in the exterior layer of the body.

Feng Shui. Literally, wind-water; the ancient art of geomancy, involving the design and placement of buildings, farmland, and burial sites according to the movements of *Qi* in the environment, including things such as the shapes of the terrain, cycles of weather, directional flows of winds and streams, patterns of sun and shade.

Five Phases (Wu Xing). Literally, the five movements or processions. The *Five Phases* correspond to the five points of reference of the compass—north, south, east, west, center—and to *Water, Fire, Wood, Metal,* and *Earth* respectively. Because China has been a land-based agrarian society, the earth has been central to its image of the world and nature. The sun rises in the east, reaches its zenith in the south, sets in the west, and barely shines in the north. Each *Phase* acquires its meaning from nature and in turn organizes and describes all processes in nature. The *Five Phases* define five stages of   405 transformation: birth, growth, maturity, decay, and death. Along with *Yin-Yang* theory, *Five-Phase* constructs function as the logical schema of correspondence thinking in Chinese traditional medicine that explains the interaction between the organism and its environment.

There are two ways of depicting these *Five-Phase* relationships: with *Earth* in the center and the other *Phases* as points of the compass; or in a continuum of *Wood, Fire, Earth, Metal, Water* in patterns of generation and restraint. The former describes the macrocosm, and the latter describes functional relationships in the microcosm of the human person.

The *Five Phases* correspond to the five seasons, climates, directions, sounds, colors, emotions, *Organ Networks*, and character types.

Fu Zheng. Literally means "to strengthen what is correct." The term is applied particularly to herbal and nutritional therapies whose primary goal is to improve constitutional integrity and build resistance to disease, promoting health and longevity.

Harmony. The existence of balance, beauty, spontaneity, and creativity in nature; as applied to human health, harmony describes the sense of ease, congruence, and vitality that is experienced when all functions of the soma and psyche are in accord with each other and with the external environment. It is an idealized state of being, and its existence is, on a human scale, transient. From the point of view of medicine, it is a yardstick, a standard by which the relatively healthy or distorted function of the organism is evaluated. The implication is that by adhering to the principle of "living according to Tao," in other words, an appropriate response to the ever-changing dynamic of *Yin-Yang* and the *Five Phases*, one will attain harmony within and without. In a more pedestrian sense, to attain harmony is to achieve a natural ease of living that mitigates the destructive effects of stress, pain, and suffering.

Heat. Characterized by aversion to heat, desire for cold, hyperactivity, inflammation, dehydration, constipation, redness, restlessness, confusion, insomnia, aggressiveness, scanty dark urine, and thick malodorous discharges.

Heaven. The immaterial realm, belonging to *Yang*, including the sun, moon, sky, and atmosphere that surround us, as well as the invisible forces that influence us. In the human body, that which is above the diaphragm corresponds to heaven.

Hedonic. Derived from a Greek word meaning pleasure; in our context, referring to the sense of well-being that arises from a harmonic process, that of being aligned with and acting from one's true nature.

Herbal Properties. The potential of herbal substances to produce particular effects within the body. Four basic herbal properties are tonifying (to augment); consolidating (to gather); dispersing (to distribute); purging (to eliminate).

Holographic Paradigm. A modern concept articulated by contemporary physicists and philosophers that defines nature as an undifferentiated continuum of interrelated events mutually affecting each other. This view of the world as "one unbroken wholeness" is similar to the syncretic, synchronistic theories of "systematic correspondence" in Chinese traditional medicine.

Human. Both the individual person and society that function as the interface or nexus between the forces of Heaven and Earth, *Yin* and *Yang*, the hinge or pivot around which the human universe turns. In the human body, that which is between the diaphragm and navel corresponds to the realm of the "human."

Inherited (Prenatal) Essence. The fundamental substance of life acquired from the parents at conception and during gestation, stored by the *Kidney*, and not replenishable.

Internal Illness. Located within body cavities and affecting internal organ systems and structures.

Ke Sequence. The *Five-Phase* interaction that describes the cycle whereby one *Phase* controls, regulates, inhibits, and oversees another: *Wood* restrains *Earth, Earth* restrains *Water, Water* restrains *Fire, Fire* restrains *Metal*, and *Metal* restrains *Wood.*

Ke Triad. The *Phases* along the *ke* sequence that restrain or are restrained by a given *Phase.* For *Wood: Metal-Wood-Earth*; for *Fire: Water-Fire-Metal*; for *Earth: Wood-Earth-Water*; for *Metal: Fire-Metal-Wood*; and for *Water: Earth-Water-Fire.* This triad is considered to be regulatory and less stable.

Microcurrent. Electrical current generated by medical instruments in the range of millionths of an amp, which is within the same range as the body's own bioelectricity.

Modules. Herbal formulas that have limited properties and effects that are designed to be combined like building blocks to create more complex multipurpose formulas.

Moisture (Jin-ye). Those processes and influences within the body that cannot be classified as *Qi* (insubstantial) or *Blood* (substantial); that is, an intermediate state of *Qi. Moisture* includes cerebrospinal fluid, synovial fluids, interstitial fluids, sweat, mucus, tears, saliva, sexual secretions, sebaceous secretions, urine, and the *Nutritive Essence* that circulates with the *Blood.*

Nutritive Qi. Also called *Food Qi* or *Nutritive (or Food) Essence*; that which is transformed by the *Stomach* and assimilated by the *Spleen* to become the basis of the *Qi, Moisture,* and *Blood* that nourishes the organism. The lighter more refined *Yang Essence* combines with *Air Qi* to become the *Pure Qi* that circulates in the channels. The heavier *Yin* part is transmitted downward to the *Kidney* where it combines with the congenital or prenatal *Essence* to become the pure *Essence* stored by the *Kidney* (the material basis of growth, regeneration, and procreation).

Ontogeny. The pattern of individual development in a living organism.

Organ. Refers not only to an anatomical entity such as the heart or liver, but also to the aggregate of tissues, activities, and channels that constitute the *Network* of which that *Organ* is an integral part. Thus the *Heart* is associated with the *Organ Network* of the *Heart,* which also includes the *Organ* of the *Small Intestine* as well as the channels of the *Heart* and *Small Intestine.*

Organ Networks (Zang Fu). Distinct physiological-psychological spheres of function within the organism. The *Five Organ Networks* correspond to each of the *Five Phases.* These *Networks* organize all physical and mental processes and link together all of the structural components of channels, *Organs,* tissues, fluids, and so on. They are the *Liver (Wood), Heart (Fire), Spleen (Earth), Lung (Metal),* and *Kidney (Water).*

Pathogenic Agent. Any entity of external or internal origin that obstructs or interferes with normal function and that itself can create secondary pathologic changes.

Pattern of Disharmony. The integrated interpretation and identification of an individual's array of symptoms and signs in terms of the categories of *Yin-Yang, Five Phases, Body Constituents, Eight Principles, Adverse Climates,* and pathogenic accumulations; thus, a typical pattern of disharmony of the *Spleen* includes *deficiency* of *Qi,* an accumulation of *Dampness,* and stagnation of *Qi* of the *Stomach.*

Pericardium. One of the six *Yin* channels whose function is subsumed within the *Heart Organ Network.* The *Pericardium,* along with the *Triple-Burner,* is not associated with an anatomical entity. It corresponds with the active function of the *Heart* in perfusing the body with *Blood* (arterial circulation) and with the passive function of harboring the *Spirit* (maintaining awareness).

Phlegm. Mucus, a by-product of dense, congealed *Dampness,* which can cause obstructions, nodules, lumps, or tumors.

Phenomenological or Phenomenology. In philosophy, the attempt to describe both internal and external events that constitute our reality or existence without seeking to understand or identify their ultimate or original causes. Chinese traditional medical thinking tends to be phenomenological rather than causal, in contradistinction to modern Western medical thinking.

Psyche (Shen). A Greek word for "soul," meaning that which is not of the body or matter. In the context of Chinese medicine it refers to all of the mental and psychological processes and immaterial aspects of the organism.

Purge. Eliminate, evict, eradicate, remove: to purge is to rid the body of pathogenic agents or *Adverse Climates* such as *Wind, Heat, Cold, Dryness,* and *Dampness* or phlegm; or to eliminate the undesirable congestion of *Qi, Moisture,* and *Blood.* Herbs that purge oust unwanted conditions by strongly stimulating the eliminative function of the skin, lungs, intestines, and bladder as well as the metabolic and temperature regulating mechanisms of the vegetative nervous system.

Qi (pronounced "Chee"; also spelled *Ch'i*). The creative or formative principle associated with life and all processes that characterize living entities. All animate forms in nature are manifestations of *Qi. Qi* is an invisible substance, as well as an immaterial force that has palpable and observable manifestations.

   Qi has its own movement and also activates the movement of things other than itself. *Qi* begets motion and heat. Within the context of the human person, *Qi* is that which enlivens the body and is differentiated according to specific functional systems. All physical and mental activities are manifestations of *Qi*: sensing, cogitating, feeling, digesting, stirring, propagating.

   One Chinese ideogram for *Qi* is composed of an upper radical representing "rising vapor" and a lower radical denoting "grain." The steam that spirals from a pot of cooking rice symbolizes distilled essence, hence *Qi* can be translated as the vapor of the finest matter. *Qi* refers to resources the human organism consumes, transforms, and transmits.

   The highly refined essence of food (*Food Qi*) and air (*Air Qi*) in the body becomes one entity known as *Pure* or *Righteous Qi.* It is this *Righteous* or *Zheng Qi* that circulates in the channels, regulating and nourishing all body processes and activities. *Defensive Qi (wei)* is the activity of adapting to influences such as weather or mobilizing resistance to pathogenic microorganisms and noxious substances in the environment. *Qi* also implies the totality of *Blood, Moisture,* and *Qi,* the total summation of the life of the organism.

   Qi is regulated by the *Liver,* generated by the *Spleen,* distributed by the *Lungs,* and stored by the *Kidney.*

Sheng Sequence. The *Five-Phase* interaction that describes the cycle whereby one *Phase* produces, gives rise to, or nourishes another: *Wood* engenders *Fire, Fire* engenders *Earth, Earth* engenders *Metal, Metal* engenders *Water,* and *Water* engenders *Wood.*

Sheng Triad. The *Phases* along the *sheng* sequence that are the parent and child of a given *Phase*: for *Wood: Water-Wood-Fire*; for *Fire: Wood-Fire-Earth*; for *Earth: Fire-Earth-Metal*; for *Metal: Earth-Metal-Water*; for *Water: Metal-*

Water-Wood. This triad is considered supportive and usually more stable.

Soma (Jing). A Greek word meaning "corpse" or all that is not spirit. In the context of Chinese medicine it refers to all of the physiological processes and material components of the organism.

Spirit (Shen). In the vocabulary of Chinese medicine, *Spirit* or *Shen* refers to that which both originates and forms the outward expression of the life of the organism, observed in the clarity and luminosity of the eyes and complexion and in the focus, lucidity, and intensity of intellectual and emotional process.

Strange Organs. The brain and uterus are referred to as "strange" in that they are not linked specifically to any *Organ* or channel but are historically identified as important. All channels are said to penetrate and nourish the brain, but insofar as the brain is regarded as the "sea of marrow" and the *Kidney* oversees the marrow, the *Kidney* rules the brain. Primarily the channels of the *Kidney, Liver,* and *Spleen* regulate and nourish the uterus.

Tao. The flowing course of nature or the ways of nature; a cosmological and philosophical term that denotes the universe as an undifferentiated whole— as everything and no-thing. Stephen Mitchell writes in his translation of the *Tao Te Ching:* "The Tao can't be perceived./Smaller than an electron,/it contains uncountable galaxies. . . . " and "The Tao never does anything,/yet through it all things are done."

Tonify. Nourish, supplement, augment, build, support, bolster, invigorate. To tonify is to add to the supply of body constituents—*Qi, Moisture, Blood*—and to promote the proper function of the *Organ Networks.* Herbs that tonify the body assist the *Spleen, Lung,* and *Kidney* in generating *Qi, Moisture, Blood,* and *Essence.*

Triple-Burner. One of the six *Yang* channels whose function is subsumed within the *Lung, Spleen,* and *Kidney Organ Networks.* The *Triple-Burner,* along with the *Pericardium,* is not associated with an anatomical entity. The *Triple-Burner* corresponds with the three main body cavities—pelvis, abdomen, and chest—and the function of transporting fluids and integrating the activities of all the other *Organ Networks.*

Turbid. Refers to the coarse, unrefined elements of food and fluid as they pass through the organism in the process of ingestion, digestion, assimilation, and elimination. The *Small Intestine* and the *Kidney* are primarily responsible for transmitting the impure elements of food and fluid respectively to the *Large Intestine* and *Bladder.* Turbid also refers to the pathogenic alteration of clear or pure substances such as mucus, blood, bile, and urine, which become foul-smelling, cloudy, viscous, and dirty in appearance.

Type. According to *Five-Phase* thinking, there are five primary configurations that express the innate qualities and tendencies (body and mind) of human individuals. Each of these types—*Wood, Fire, Earth, Metal, Water*—can be further differentiated into an *exaggerated* or *collapsed* subtype.

Typology. A system for classifying individuals according to sets of criteria that distinguish one class of people from another. Thus, there are typologies based on categories of race and ethnicity, composition of blood, socioeconomic status, religious beliefs, personality traits, physical structure, and so on. In the context of Chinese medicine, people can be differentiated into five primary types based on sets of criteria that correspond to the categories of the *Five Phases*, including physical shape, mental and emotional habits of perception and response, behavioral tendencies, and physiological patterns of activity.

Vaporize or Precipitate. Refers to the integrative, transformative, and distributive function of the *Triple-Burner* in cooperation with the *Lung, Spleen,* and *Kidney* in regulating the upward and downward movement of *Qi* and *Moisture.* As *Qi* moves downward it "precipitates" from a diffuse vapor to a dense fluid. As *Qi* moves upward the reverse process of "vaporization" occurs. There is moist exhaled breath above and urine below.

Water Decoction. Extracting the useful ingredients from herbs by cooking them in water as medicinal tea. Usually one half to two ounces of raw herbs are cooked in four to six cups of water in a covered vessel for thirty to sixty minutes, at the end of which the liquid is strained out and the solid material discarded.

Wind. Characterized by aversion to drafts, sudden changes, spasms, disequilibrium, tears, migratory pains, dizziness, trembling, itching, headache, stuffy nose, scratchy throat, and numbness.

Yang. Literally, "the sunny side of the mountain"; one of the two fundamental polar forces that organize the universe. *Yang* manifests as form, light, noise, warmth, activity, and birth. It includes the functional activity of the body, and the generation of metabolic heat.

Yang Organs (Fu). Also known as the "hollow organs" that transform matter, liberate its essence, transport substance, and discharge waste. The *Yang Organs* are the *Gallbladder, Small Intestine, Stomach, Large Intestine,* and *Urinary Bladder.* The *Gallbladder* receives and discharges bile; the *Small Intestine* receives and transports digestate; the *Stomach* receives and transforms food and fluids; the *Large Intestine* receives and discharges solid waste; and the *Bladder* receives and discharges liquid waste.

Yang Phenomena. Heat, dryness, activity, growth, expansion, dispersion, full- 411 ness, sudden, acute: when *Yang* decreases, *Yin* dominates; lack of *Yang* generates *Cold* and *Dampness*.

Yin. Literally, "the shady side of the mountain"; one of the two fundamental polar forces that organize the universe. *Yin* manifests as substance, darkness, quietness, coldness, inertia, and death. It includes the material substance of the body, which includes tissue, blood, fluid, and internal secretions.

Yin Organs (Zang). Also known as the "solid organs" that store the *Essences* of the body. The *Yin Organs* are the *Liver, Heart, Spleen, Lung,* and *Kidney*. Palpable *Essence* is manifest in each of these *Organs* respectively as tears, sweat, saliva, mucus, and sexual secretions.

Yin Phenomena. Coldness, wetness, quiescence, deterioration, contraction, congelation, emptiness, slow, chronic: when *Yin* decreases, *Yang* dominates; lack of *Yin* generates *Heat* and *Dryness*.

Yin-Yang. Mutually interdependent polar forces; the principle of duality that fundamentally organizes the universe. *Yin-Yang* symbolizes that interactive process that characterizes life. Wholly relative designations.

HERB NAMES CROSS REFERENCE

Common name	Chinese pin-yin	Botanical
achyranthes rt.	niu xi	Achyranthes bidentata
agastache hb.	huo xiang	Agastache rugosa
agrimony hb.	xian he cao	Agrimonia pilosa
akebia stem	mu tong	Akebia trifoliata
alisma rhz.	ze xie	Alisma plantago
American ginseng rt.	xi yang shen	Panax quinquefolium
anemarrhena rhz.	zhi mu	Anemarrhena asphodeloides
angelica rt.	dang gui	Angelica sinensis
apricot or bitter almond sd.	xing ren	Prunus armeniaca
aquilaria wood	chen xiang	Aquilaria agallocha
areca peel	da fu pi	Areca catechu
artemisia leaf	ai ye	Artemesia vulgaris
asaram hb.	xi xin	Asarum sieboldi
astragalus rt.	huang qi	Astragalus membranaceus
atractylodes rhz.	bai zhu	Atractylodes macrocephala
aurantium fr.	zhi ke	Citrus aurantium
bamboo shavings	zhu ru	Phyllostachys nigra
benincasa pl.	dong gua pi	Benincasa hispida
biota sd.	bai zi ren	Biota orientalis
black date	da zao	Zizyphus jujuba
black mushroom	xiang gu	Lentinus edodes
bugleweed hb.	ze lan	Lycopus lucidus
bupleurum rt.	chai hu	Bupleurum chinense
calamus gum	xue jie	Calamus draco
cardamom sd.	sha ren	Amomum villosum
carthamus fl.	hong hua	Carthamus tinctorius
chrysanthemum fl.	ju hua	Chrysanthemum morifolium
cinnamon bk.	rou gui	Cinnamomum cassia

cinnamon twig	*gui zhi*	*Cinnamomum cassia*
citrus pl.	*chen pi*	*Citrus reticulata*
clove bud	*ding xiang*	*Eugenia caryophyllata*
codonopsis rt.	*dang shen*	*Codonopsis pilosula*
coix sd.	*yi yi ren*	*Coix lachryma-jobi*
coltsfoot fl.	*kuan dong hua*	*Tussilago farfara*
coptis rhz.	*huang lian*	*Coptis chinensis*
corn silk	*yu mi xu*	*Zea mays*
cornus fr.	*shan zhu yu*	*Cornus officinalis*
corydalis rhz.	*yan hu suo*	*Corydalis yanhusuo*
curculigo rhz.	*xian mao*	*Curculigo orchioides*
curcuma rhz.	*jiang huang*	*Curcuma longa*
cuscuta sd.	*tu si zi*	*Cuscuta chinensis*
cyperus rt.	*xiang fu*	*Cyperus rotundus*
dandelion rt.	*pu gong ying*	*Taraxacum mongolicum*
dendrobium hb.	*shi hu*	*Dendrobium nobile*
dianthus hb.	*qu mai*	*Dianthus chinensis*
dioscorea rhz.	*shan yao*	*Dioscorea opposita*
dipsacus rt.	*xu duan*	*Dipsacus asper*
donkey gelatin	*e jiao*	*Equus asinus*
dry ginger rhz.	*gan jiang*	*Zingiber officinalis*
eclipta hb.	*han lian cao*	*Eclipta prostrata*
eleutherococcus hb.	*ci wu jia*	*Eleutherococcus senticosus*
ephedra hb.	*ma huang*	*Ephedra sinica*
eucommia bk.	*du zhong*	*Eucommia ulmoides*
eupatorium hb.	*pei lan*	*Eupatorium fortunei*
euryales sd.	*qian shi*	*Euryale ferox*
evodia fr.	*wu zhu yu*	*Evodia rutaecarpa*
fennel sd.	*hui xiang*	*Foeniculum vulgare*
forsythia fr.	*lian qiao*	*Forsythia supensa*
414 fritillary bulb	*chuan bei mu*	*Fritillaria cirrhosa*

ganoderma fn.	*ling zhi*	*Ganoderma lucidum*
gardenia fr.	*zhi zi*	*Gardenia jasminoides*
gastrodia rhz.	*tian ma*	*Gastrodia elata*
ginger rhz.	*sheng jiang*	*Zingiber officinale*
ginger skin (fresh)	*sheng jiang pi*	*Zingiberis officinale*
ginseng rt.	*ren shen*	*Panax ginseng*
glauber's salt	*mang xiao*	*Sodium sulphate*
glehnia rt.	*bei sha shen*	*Glehnia littoralis*
gypsum mineral	*shi gao*	*Calcium sulphate*
haliotis shell	*shi jue ming*	*Haliotis diversicolor*
hawthorn fr.	*shan zha*	*Crataegus pinnatifida*
honeysuckle fl.	*jin yin hua*	*Lonicera japonica*
ilex rt.	*mao dong qing*	*Ilex pubescens*
isatis rt.	*ban lang gen*	*Isatis tinctoria*
knotgrass hb.	*bian xu*	*Polygonum aviculare*
laminaria hb.	*kun bu*	*Laminaria japonica*
licorice rt.	*gan cao*	*Glycyrrhiza uralensis*
ligusticum rhz.	*chuan xiong*	*Ligusticum wallichii*
ligustrum fr.	*nu zhen zi*	*Ligustrum lucidum*
lily bulb	*bai he*	*Lilium brownii*
lindera rt.	*wu yao*	*Lindera strychnifolia*
litchi sd.	*li zhi he*	*Litchi chinensis*
lobelia hb.	*ban bian lian*	*Lobelia chinensis*
longan fr.	*long yan rou*	*Euphoria longan*
long pepper fr.	*bi ba*	*Piper longum*
loquat leaf	*pi pa ye*	*Eriobotrya japonica*
lotus sd.	*lian zi*	*Nelumbo nucifera*
lotus stamen	*lian xu*	*Nelumbo nucifera*
lycii fr.	*gou qi zi*	*Lycium chinense*
lygodium spores	*hai jin sha*	*Lygodium japonicum*
magnetite	*ci shi*	*Magnetitum*

magnolia bk.	*hou po*	*Magnolia officinalis*
melia fr.	*chuan lian zi*	*Melia toosendan*
millettia stem	*ji xue teng*	*Millettia reticulata*
morus fr.	*sang shen*	*Morus alba*
motherwort hb.	*yi mu cao*	*Leonorus heterophyllus*
moutan peony bk.	*mu dan pi*	*Paeonia suffruticosa*
mulberry lf.	*sang ji sheng*	*Loranthus parasiticus*
mung bean	*lu dou*	*Phaseolus mungo*
mustard seed	*bai jie zi*	*Brassica alba*
myrrh resin	*mo yao*	*Commiphora myrrh*
nutmeg sd.	*rou dou kou*	*Myristica fragrans*
ophiopogon rt.	*mai men dong*	*Ophiopogon japonicus*
peppermint leaf	*bo he*	*Mentha haplocalyx*
peach sd.	*tao ren*	*Prunus persica*
perilla fr.	*zi su zi*	*Perilla frutescens*
pinellia rhz.	*fa ban xia*	*Pinellia ternata*
plantain sd.	*che qian zi*	*Plantago asiatica*
platycodon rt.	*jie geng*	*Platycodon grandiflorum*
polygala rt.	*yuan zhi*	*Polygala tenuifolia*
polygonatum rhz.	*yu zhu*	*Polygonatum odoratum*
polyporus fungus	*zhu ling*	*Polyporus umbellatus*
poria fungus	*fu ling*	*Poria cocos*
prunella spike	*xia ku cao*	*Prunella vulgaris*
pseudoginseng rt. (cooked)	*shu tian qi*	*Panax pseudoginseng*
pseudoginseng rt. (raw)	*tian qi*	*Panax pseudoginseng*
pseudostellaria rt.	*tai zi shen*	*Pseudostellaria heterophylla*
psoralea sd.	*bu gu zhi*	*Psoralia corylifolia*
pueraria rt.	*ge gen*	*Pueraria lobata*
radish sd.	*lai fu zi*	*Raphanus sativus*

rehmannia rt. (cooked)	*shu di huang*	*Rehmannia glutinosa*
rehmannia rt. (raw)	*sheng di huang*	*Rehmannia glutinosa*
red dates	*hong zao*	*Zizyphus jujuba*
red peony rt.	*chi shao yao*	*Paeonia lactiflora*
red pepper	*la jiao*	*Capsicum anuum*
rhubarb rhz.	*da huang*	*Rheum officinale*
rice sd.	*jing mi*	*Oryza sativa*
rose hips	*jin ying zi*	*Rosa laevigata*
rubia rt.	*qian cao gen*	*Rubia cordyfolia*
rubus fr.	*fu pen zi*	*Rubus chingii*
salvia rt.	*dan shen*	*Salvia miltiorrhiza*
sargassum hb.	*hai zao*	*Sargassum fusiform*
saussurea rt.	*mu xiang*	*Saussurea lappa*
schizandra fr.	*wu wei zi*	*Schizandra chinensis*
scutellaria rt.	*huang qin*	*Scutellaria baicalensis*
sileris rt.	*fang feng*	*Siler divaricatum*
sparganium rt.	*san leng*	*Sparganium stoloniferum*
stephania rt.	*fang ji*	*Stephania tetrandra*
sweet almond sd.	*xing ren*	*Amygdalus communis*
tangerine pl.	*ju hong*	*Citrus grandis*
tribulus fr.	*ci ji li*	*Tribulus terrestris*
trichosanthes fr.	*gua lou zi*	*Trichosanthis kirilowii*
trigonella sd.	*hu lu ba*	*Trigonella foenum-graecum*
triticum fr.	*fu xiao mai*	*Triticum aestivum*
turmeric rhz.	*jiang huang*	*Curcuma longae*
uncaria stem	*gou teng*	*Uncaria rynchophylla*
unripe aurantium fr.	*zhi shi*	*Citrus aurantium*
unripe citrus pl.	*qing pi*	*Citrus reticulata*
white peony rt.	*bai shao yao*	*Paeonia lactiflora*
ziziphus sd.	*suan zao ren*	*Ziziphus spinosa*

BIBLIOGRAPHY

Achterberg, Jeanne. *Imagery and Healing.* Boston: Shambhala, 1985.

Augios, Robert, and George Stanciu. *The New Biology.* Boston: Shambhala, 1987.

Bateson, Gregory. *Mind and Nature.* New York: Bantam, 1979.

———. *Steps to an Ecology of Mind.* New York: Ballantine, 1972.

Becker, Robert. *The Body Electric.* New York: William Morrow, 1985.

Bensky, Dan, and Andrew Gamble. *Chinese Herbal Medicine, Materia Medica.* Seattle, Wash.: Eastland, 1986.

Berman, Morris. *The Reenchantment of the World.* Ithaca, N.Y.: Cornell University Press, 1981.

Blofeld, John, ed. *I Ching.* New York: Dutton, 1965.

Bloomfield, Frena. *Chinese Beliefs.* London: Arrow Books, 1983.

Bohm, David. *Wholeness and the Implicate Order.* London: Ark, 1980.

Bowers, John Z., Jay William Hess, and Nathan Sivin. *Science and Medicine in Twentieth-Century China: Research and Education.* Ann Arbor, Mich.: University of Michigan, 1988.

Butt, Gary, and Frena Bloomfield. *Harmony Rules.* London: Arrow Books, 1985.

Campbell, Joseph. *The Inner Reaches of Outer Space.* New York: Alfred Van Der Marck, 1985.

Cannon, Walter. *The Wisdom of the Body.* New York: Norton, 1939.

Capra, Fritjof. *The Turning Point.* New York: Bantam, 1982.

Cheng, Xinnong. *Chinese Acupuncture and Moxibustion.* China: Foreign Language Press, 1987.

Cheung, C. S. *Rationale and Correct Organization of Prescription of Traditional Chinese Medicine.* San Francisco: Traditional Chinese Medical Publisher, 1980.

Cheung, C. S., and U Aik Kaw. *Synopsis of the Pharmacopeia.* San Francisco: American College of Traditional Chinese Medicine, 1984.

Cheung, C. S., Yat Ki Lai, and U Aik Kaw. *Mental Dysfunction As Treated by Traditional Chinese Medicine.* San Francisco: Traditional Chinese Medical Publisher, 1981.

China, The Beautiful Cookbook. Los Angeles: Knapp Press, 1986.

Chinese-English Terminology of Traditional Chinese Medicine. Hunan, China: Hunan Science and Technology Press, 1981.

Chinese Massage. Compiled at Anhui Medical School in China. Washington, D.C.: Hartley and Marks, 1983.

Dharmananda, Subhuti. *Chinese Herbal Therapies for Immune Disorders.* Portland, Ore: Institute for Traditional Medicine, 1988 [ITM: 2442 S.E. Sherman, Portland, Ore. 97214]

———. *Chinese Herbology: A Professional Training Program.* Portland, Ore.: Institute for Traditional Medicine, 1981.

———. *From the People's Pharmacy.* Portland, Ore.: Institute for Traditional Medicine, 1989.

———. *Foundations of Chinese Herb Prescribing.* Portland, Ore.: Institute for Traditional Medicine, 1989.

———. *Pearls from the Golden Cabinet.* Portland, Ore.: Institute for Traditional Medicine, 1986.

———. *Prescriptions on Silk and Paper.* Portland, Ore.: Institute for Traditional Medicine, 1989.

———. *Your Nature, Your Health.* Portland, Ore.: Institute for Traditional Medicine, 1986.

———. *The Golden Mirror of Chinese Medicine.* Portland, Ore.: Institute for Traditional Medicine, 1990.

Dubos, René. *Man Adapting.* New Haven, Conn.: Yale University Press, 1980.

———. *Mirage of Health.* New York: Anchor Books, 1959.

Eisenberg, David. *Encounters With Qi.* New York: Norton, 1985.

Ellis, Andrew, Nigel Wiseman, and Ken Boss. *Grasping the Wind.* Brookline, Mass.: Paradigm Publications, 1989.

Ellis, Andrew, Nigel Wiseman, and Ken Boss. *Fundamentals of Chinese Acupuncture.* Brookline, Mass.: Paradigm Publications, 1988.

Essentials of Chinese Acupuncture. Beijing, China: Foreign Languages Press, 1980.

Flaws, Bob, and Honora Wolfe. *Prince Wen Hui's Cook.* Brookline, Mass.: Paradigm Publications, 1983.

Fratkin, Jake. *Chinese Herbal Patent Formulas.* Portland, Ore.: Institute for Traditional Medicine, 1986.

Garber, Daniel. "Science and Certainty in Descartes." In *Descartes,* edited by Michael Hooker. Baltimore, Md.: Johns Hopkins University Press, 1978.

Garvey, Jack. *The Five Phases of Food.* Newtonville, Mass.: Wellbeing Books, 1985.

Hayward, Jeremy. *Shifting Worlds, Changing Minds.* Boston, Mass.: Shambhala, 1987.

Heisenberg, Werner. *Physics and Philosophy.* New York: Harper & Row, 1962.

Holman, H. R. "The 'Excellence' Deception in Medicine." *Hospital Practice* 11, no. 4 (April 1976): pp. 11, 18, 21.

Hsu, Hong-Yen. *Commonly Used Chinese Herbal Formulas.* Long Beach, Calif.: Oriental Healing Arts Institute, 1980.

Huard, Pierre, and Ming Wong. *Chinese Medicine.* New York: World University Library, 1968.

Hyatt, Richard. *Chinese Herbal Medicine.* New York: Schocken Books, 1978.

Illich, Ivan. *Medical Nemesis.* New York: Bantam, 1976.

Illustrated Dictionary of Chinese Acupuncture. Hong Kong: Sheep's Publishing Ltd. and People's Medical Publishing House, 1986.

Jones, Roger. *Physics As Metaphor.* New York: New American Library, 1982.

Jung, Carl Gustav. *Four Archetypes.* Princeton, N.J.: Princeton University Press, 1959.

———. *Psychological Types.* Princeton, N.J.: Princeton University Press, 1971.

———. *Psychology and the East.* Princeton, N.J.: Princeton University Press, 1978.

Kaptchuk, Ted. *The Web That Has No Weaver.* New York: Congdon & Weed, 1983.

Kaptchuk, Ted, and Michael Croucher. *The Healing Arts.* London: British Broadcasting Corporation, 1986.

Keleman, Stanley. *Embodying Experience.* Berkeley, Calif.: Center Press, 1987.

———. *Emotional Anatomy.* Berkeley, Calif.: Center Press, 1985.

———. *Your Body Speaks Its Mind.* Berkeley, Calif.: Center Press, 1975.

King, Lester. *Medical Thinking.* Princeton, N.J.: Princeton University Press, 1982.

Koo, Linda. *Nourishment of Life.* Hong Kong: Commercial Press Ltd., 1982.

Kretschmer, Ernst. *Physique and Character.* New York: Cooper Square, 1970.

Lad, Vasant, and David Frawley. *The Yoga of Herbs.* Santa Fe, N.M.: Lotus Press, 1986.

Larre, Claude, Elizabeth Rochat de la Vallee, and Jean Schatz. *Survey of Traditional Chinese Medicine.* Paris: L'Institut Ricci, 1979.

Lawson-Wood, Denis and Joyce. *The Five Elements of Chinese Acupuncture and Massage.* England: Health Science Press, 1965.

Lee, Jane, and C. S. Cheung. *Current Acupuncture Therapy.* Hong Kong: Medical Interflow Publishing House, 1978.

Legeza, Laszlo. *Tao Magic.* London: Thames and Hudson, 1975.

LeShan, Lawrence. *Alternate Realities.* New York: Ballantine Books, 1976.

Leslie, Charles. *Asian Medical Systems.* Berkeley, Calif.: University of California Press, 1976.

Levins, Richard, and Richard Lewontin. *The Dialectical Biologist.* Cambridge, Mass.: Harvard University Press, 1985.

Lu, Henry. *Chinese System of Food Cures.* New York: Sterling, 1986.

Maciocia, Giovanni. *Tongue Diagnosis in Chinese Medicine.* Seattle, Wash.: Eastland Press, 1987.

Manaka, Yoshio, and Ian Urquhart. *Layman's Guide to Acupuncture.* New York: Weatherhill, 1972.

Matsumoto, Kikko, and Stephen Birch. *Five Elements and Ten Stems.* Brookline, Mass.: Paradigm Publications, 1983.

Merchant, Carolyn. *The Death of Nature.* New York: Harper & Row, 1980.

Moore, Charles, ed. *The Chinese Mind.* Honolulu: University Press of Hawaii, 1967.

Needham, Joseph. *The Grand Titration.* Toronto: University of Toronto, 1969.

———. *Science and Civilisation in China.* Vol. 2, Cambridge, England: Cambridge University Press, 1962.

———. *The Shorter Science and Civilisation in China.* Abridged version by Colin Ronan. Cambridge, England: Cambridge University Press, 1978.

——. *Science in Traditional China*. Hong Kong: Chinese University Press, 1981.

O'Connor, John, and Dan Bensky, trans. and ed. *Acupuncture: A Comprehensive Text*. Chicago: Eastland Press (Shanghai College of Traditional Medicine), 1981.

Pang, T. Y. *Chinese Herbal*. Eastsound, Wash.: Tai Chi School of Philosophy and Art, 1982.

Pellegrino, Edmund, and David Thomasma, *A Philosophical Basis of Medical Practice*. New York: Oxford University Press, 1981.

Porkert, Manfred. *Essentials of Chinese Diagnostics*. Zurich, Switzerland: Chinese Medicine Publications Ltd., 1983.

——. *The Theoretical Foundations of Chinese Medicine*. Cambridge, Mass.: MIT Press, 1974.

Purce, Jill. *The Mystic Spiral*. New York: Thames and Hudson, 1974.

Reid, Daniel. *Chinese Herbal Medicine*. Boston, Mass.: Shambhala, 1987.

Requena, Yves. *Morphological Hand Diagnosis in Acupuncture*. Marseilles, France: Solal, 1986.

——. *Terrains and Pathology in Acupuncture*. Brookline, Mass.: Paradigm, 1986.

Revolutionary Health Committee of Hunan. *A Barefoot Doctor's Manual*. Seattle, Wash.: Cloudburst, 1977.

Rodis-Lewis, Genevieve. "Limitations of the Mechanical Model in the Cartesian Conception of the Organism." In *Descartes*, edited by Michael Hooker. Baltimore, Md.: Johns Hopkins University Press, 1978.

Ross, Jeremy. *Zang Fu*. London: Churchill Livingston, 1985.

Rossbach, Sarah. *Feng Shui*. New York: Dutton, 1983.

Seem, Mark, and Joan Kaplan. *Bodymind Energetics*. Rochester, Vt.: Thorsons, 1988.

Selye, Hans. *The Stress of Life*. Rev. ed. New York: McGraw-Hill, 1978.

Siegerist, Henry. *Civilization and Disease*. Chicago, Ill.: University of Chicago, 1943.

Sivin, Nathan. *Traditional Medicine in Contemporary China*. Ann Arbor, Mich.: University of Michigan, 1987.

Smith, F. Porter, and G. A. Stuart. *Chinese Medicinal Herbs*. San Francisco, Calif.: Georgetown Press, 1973.

Smith, Fritz. *Inner Bridges*. Atlanta, Ga.: Humanics, 1986.

Sobel, David, ed. *Ways of Health*. New York: Harcourt Brace Jovanovich, 1979.

Sommers, Fred. "Dualism in Descartes: The Logical Ground." In *Descartes*, edited by Michael Hooker. Baltimore, Md.: Johns Hopkins University Press, 1978.

Starhawk. *Dreaming the Dark*. Boston, Mass.: Beacon Press, 1982.

Starr, Paul. *The Social Transformation of American Medicine*. New York: Basic Books, 1982.

Tang, Bick Jane. *The Therapeutic and Preventive Uses of Food*. Self-published: 61 El Camino Alto, 103A, Mill Valley, CA 94941, 1985.

Teeguarden, Ron. *Chinese Tonic Herbs*. New York: Japan Publications, 1984.

Thomas, Lewis. *The Lives of a Cell*. New York: Bantam, 1975.

"The Treatment of Disease and the War Against Cancer." *Scientific American* 253, no. 5 (1985): pp. 51–59.

Unschuld, Paul, ed. *Approaches to Traditional Chinese Medical Literature*. Netherlands: Kluwer Academic Publishers, 1989.

——. *Forgotten Traditions in Ancient Chinese Medicine*. Brookline, Mass.: Paradigm Publications, 1990.

——. *Introductory Readings in Classical Chinese Medicine*. Netherlands: Kluwer Academic Publishers, 1988.

——. *Medical Ethics in Imperial China*. Berkeley, Calif.: University of California, 1979.

——. *Medicine in China: History of Ideas*. Berkeley, Calif.: University of California, 1985.

——. *Medicine in China: A History of Pharmaceuticals*. Berkeley, Calif.: University of California, 1986.

Veith, Ilza. *The Yellow Emperor's Classic of Internal Medicine*. Berkeley, Calif.: University of California Press, 1972.

Wallnofer, Henrich, and Anna Von Rottauscher. *Chinese Folk Medicine*. New York: Crown Books, 1972.

Watts, Alan. *Tao: The Watercourse Way*. New York: Pantheon, 1975.

Wilber, Ken. *The Holographic Paradigm*. Boulder, Colo.: Shambhala, 1982.

——. *No Boundary*. Boston, Mass.: Shambhala, 1985.

Wing, R. L. *The Tao of Power*. New York: Doubleday, 1986.

Wiseman, Nigel. *Glossary of Chinese Medicine*. Brookline, Mass.: Paradigm Publications, 1990.

Wiseman, Nigel, and Andrew Ellis. *Fundamentals of Chinese Medicine*. Brookline, Mass.: Paradigm Publications, 1985.

Woolerton, Henry, and Colleen McLean. *Acupuncture Energy in Health & Disease*. North Hamptonshire, England: Thorsons, 1979.

Yanchi, Liu. *The Essential Book of Traditional Chinese Medicine*. New York: Columbia University Press, 1988.

Yeung, Him-che. *Handbook of Chinese Herbs and Formulas*. Vols. 1 and 2. Los Angeles: Institute of Chinese Medicine, 1985.

Yu-Lan, Fung. *Short History of Chinese Philosophy*. New York: Free Press, 1948.

Yu-Min, Chuang. *The Historical Development of Acupuncture*. Los Angeles: Oriental Healing Arts Institute, 1982.

Zhu, Chun-Lan. *Clinical Handbook of Chinese Prepared Medicines*. Brookline, Mass.: Paradigm Publications, 1989.

Zukav, Gary. *The Dancing Wu Li Masters*. New York: William Morrow, 1979.

Dragon Rises, Red Bird Flies (New York: Station Hill Press, 1990) by Leon Hammer, M.D., was published after *Between Heaven and Earth* was written, so it was not used as a reference, but we recommend it as further reading for those interested in psychology and Chinese medicine. Similarly, *Chinese Herbal Medicine: Formulas and Strategies* (Seattle: Eastland Press, 1990), compiled and translated by Dan Bensky and Randall Barolet, is a resource guide to traditional herbal formulas. Another general source is *The Foundation of Chinese Medicine: A Comprehensive Text for Acupuncturists and Herbalists* by Giovanni Maciocia (London: Churchill Livingstone, 1989).

Many of the books on Chinese medicine are available through the mail-order catalog of Redwing Book Company, 44 Linden Street, Brookline, Massachusetts 02146. Phone: 800-873-3946.

INDEX

acupressure massage, 252–53
acupuncture, xiii, xv–xvi,
  7–8, 10, 14, 235–63
  and bioelectric oscillating
    fields, 242–43
  body area point combina-
    tion in, 253
  contemporary techniques
    and, 252
  diagnosis and, 80, 243
  and distorted patterns of
    Wood, 167–69
  duration and frequency of,
    246–48
  for Fire types, 183–84
  for first aid, 252–54, 257,
    259
  gates in, 236–37
  for high blood pressure, 9,
    250
  how it works, 240–41
  introduction of West to,
    12–13
  locating points in, 255–63
  for Metal types, 211, 213–
    14
  methods of treatment with,
    251–52
  origins of, 240
  point insertion in, 237
  points for self-care in,
    253–55
  powers of, 3
  Qi and, 236–42, 245, 248,
    251
  selection of points in,
    245–46
  sensations from needles in,
    244
  in Shanghai clinic, 248
  specific ailment point com-
    binations in, 253–54
  as treatment method, 44–45
  for Water types, 225
  what it can treat, 248–51
Alchemist, xv, 134–35, 205
alisma, 293
allergies, herbs for, 266, 318,
    320
American ginseng, 346–47

Angelica sinensis (dang gui),
    276, 281–82, 285
Anger, 67–68
angina, herbs for, 281–83
archetypes, xvi, 131–231
  affinities and aversions of,
    144
  challenges, contradictions,
    and knots of, 145
  determination of, 146–57
  equating pathology with,
    136–38
  powers of, 140–41
  solving puzzle of which
    you are, 157
  and understanding sheng
    and ke sequences, 156–
    57
  yearning to be another, 156
  see also specific archetypes
arthritis, xiii, 249
asparagus, 332
asthma, herbs for, 266
Astragalus membranaceus
    (huang qi), 275, 285, 292,
    343–44, 346–47
aurantium, 291–92
Autumn (Li Ch'ing Chao), 204

back pain, 10–11
  acupuncture for, 250
  herbs for, 279
Bateson, Gregory, 6, 87
Becker, Robert, 242–43
Bell, Frank, 251
Bensky, Dan, 274n
Berlioz, Louis, 11
Bernard, Claude, 46–47
bitter foods, 333
Bi Yan Pian, 318–20
Black, Sylvia, 251
black dates, 346–47
black fungus, 343, 350–51
black mushrooms, 13, 343,
    350–51
Bladder, 54, 91
  channel of, 261
  food and, 329
  Heart and, 111
  herbs and, 278

Kidney and, 124–25
Lung and, 119
Qi circulation and, 94–95
Blofeld, John, 29
Blood, 105, 382
  acupuncture and, 236–37,
    240–41, 245, 248
  circulation of, 36, 92–93,
    109–12
  decongestion of, 341, 359
  deficiency of, 38, 116, 165,
    213, 300–301
  diagnosis and, 62–63, 66–
    68, 70, 73–74, 77, 80,
    83
  and distorted patterns of
    Earth, 194–95, 199
  and distorted patterns of
    Fire, 181, 184
  and distorted patterns of
    Metal, 209, 211–14
  and distorted patterns of
    Wood, 166–67, 169–70
  food and, 325, 327–33,
    338, 340
  herbal cuisine and, 342,
    344, 347, 349, 351,
    353, 355, 357–59, 361,
    364–66, 368–71, 373–
    74, 376–77, 379
  herbs and, 266–74, 276,
    278–89, 294–97, 300–
    303, 318
  and interaction of Five
    Phases, 96–98
  interaction of Moisture, Qi,
    and, 34–35
  Kidney and, 124–25
  Liver and, 105, 107–9,
    164–66
  Lung and, 120
  in organization of body,
    33–35
  Organ Networks and, 91–92
  reorganization and replen-
    ishment of, 44
  signs and symptoms of de-
    pletion or congestion
    of, 289
  Spleen and, 112–17